# HOW TO CARE
## *for* AGING
# PARENTS

A COMPLETE GUIDE

# HOW TO CARE
## *for* AGING
# PARENTS

## VIRGINIA MORRIS

*Foreword by Robert N. Butler, M.D.*

WORKMAN PUBLISHING • NEW YORK

Library of Congress Cataloging-in-Publication
Morris, Virginia
How to care for aging parents / by Virginia Morris.
p. cm.
Includes index.
ISBN 1-56305-435-3 (pbk.)

1. Aging parents—Family relationships—Handbooks, manuals, etc.
2. Aging parents—Care—Handbooks, manuals, etc. I. Title.
HQ1063.6.M66 1996                                    94-19321
306.874—dc20                                         CIP

*Workman books are available at discounts when purchased in bulk for premi-
ums and sales promotions as well as for fundraising or educational use. Special
editions can be created to specification. For details, contact the Special Sales
Director at the address below.*

Cover illustration by Mark Braught

Workman Publishing Company, Inc.
708 Broadway
New York, NY  10003-9555

Manufactured in the U.S.
First printing March 1996
20  19  18  17  16  15  14  13  12

# Dedication

*To Dr. John McLean Morris (1914-1993)*

*In your living, you taught me about courage, determination, philanthropy and truth. In your dying, you taught me about love. I will miss you, always.*

# Many Thanks

A t the end of one of his comedy shows, Steve Martin faced his audience to say good-bye. "You've been wonderful and I'd like to thank each and every one of you," he said. He then proceeded to point at individuals in the audience saying, "Thank you. Thank you. Thank you. Thank you. Thank you. Thank you. Thank you. . . ."

I, too, would like to thank each and every person who helped create this book—the doctors, lawyers, researchers, advocates and geriatric social workers who shared their wisdom and time; the public relations people at groups like the Alzheimer's Association, the National Institute on Aging and the American Association of Retired Persons, who fielded my endless stream of questions with patience and thoroughness; and, in particular, the dozens of caregivers who opened their hearts and homes and shared their pain, joy and sorrow with me. These people have all created this book. To each and every one of them, I am grateful. But because it is impossible to offer so many individual thank-you's here, I have limited my acknowledgments to a few essential players.

First, I want to thank those who poured over chapters of my manuscript, checking the facts and adding new ideas: Dr. Margaret Drickamer, a remarkable geriatrician who spent so much time answering my questions that she should be listed as a co-author; Dr. Ronald Miller, who generously opened the doors of his geriatric assessment center and library at Yale to me; Dr. Sherwin B. Nuland, surgeon, friend and author of several outstanding books, including *How We Die*, who provided enormous moral support; Lea Nordlicht Shedd, an elder law attorney whose thoroughness and patience with this project reflects her dedication to her work; Tim Casserly, elder law attorney and financial planner, who tirelessly guided me through the complexities of finance and law; Sara Stadler, estate planner, who selflessly helped with this project even when she was behind in her own work; Mary Pat Tracy, a social worker who provided tremendous insight into the needs and dilemmas of caregivers; and Sarah Berger of the National Citizens' Coalition for Nursing Home Reform, whose entire organization helped me to understand the ins and outs of how nursing homes operate.

Other readers who deserve great thanks are Mary Miner, a geriatric social worker; Ann Kantra, a family therapist; Anna Kavolius, nurse and attorney with Choice in Dying; Colleen Pierre, dietitian; and Beth Burrell, my friend and colleague.

I also want to extend my thanks to Dr. Barbara Parker, Dr. Diane Meier, Gail Wojtyna, Fran Fergusen, Dr. Selby Jacobs, Ken Scholen and Barbara Fussiner.

I am grateful to all sorts of people at Workman Publishing. Robbin Reynolds came up with the idea for this book and had enough faith in me to let me write it. Peter Workman had enough faith in Robbin to make the idea a reality. Ruth Sullivan, who truly helped make this book what it is, edited thoughtfully and meticulously, often over her weekends and into her nights. Sara Blackburn added her own professional and personal touch to the editing process and gave me gentle encouragement along the way. Diane Botnick made sense of the confusion, provided much-needed laughter and coolly handled the steady stream of phone calls, faxes and Federal Expresses. Jenny Mandel and Andrea Rosen have provided an abundance of enthusiasm, as well as dear friendship. Many thanks also to the art designer, Flamur Tonuzi, the proofreader, Janet Hulstrand, and all the Workman typesetters who have devoted tremendous hours and skill to this book.

Last, I want to thank my husband, Bob Plumb, who saw me through—and put up with me through—every step of this project. And I am always indebted to my dear, wonderful mother and my siblings, who are not only my family, but better yet, my friends. They advised me, encouraged me and always believed in me more than I believed in myself.

To each and every one of you, thank you.

# Contents

# Foreword

*by Robert N. Butler, M.D.*

A whisk past midnight, January 1, 1996, the oldest of the Baby Boomers hit 50. This remarkable generation, the largest in American history, accounts for one-third of today's population— the so-called "pig in the python." As such, it has affected the nation socially, economically and politically as no generation before.

The life trajectory of the Boomers is proceeding ahead, yet not necessarily merrily. As they turn 50, their parents are entering their 70s and 80s, and those who have not already experienced the impact of aging on their parents will do so in the next decade. When these older persons need help, and most of them eventually do, it will come almost exclusively from their children, and the caregiver burden on the baby boom generation will rise rapidly.

But there are few role models to follow, since aging itself is a relatively new development. It is only very recently that people could be assured of reaching their mid-70s due to advances in healthcare and technology. Being the first to deal with this phenomenon, the Baby Boomers will confront issues they have either denied or never imagined.

Just as the baby boom generation has all along altered or redefined social issues, in the new task of parentcare it is likely to continue its role as a transformative generation—in this instance, helping to transform old age. In its efforts to do so, it would gain measurably from the knowledge and planfulness offered in this book.

*How to Care for Aging Parents* is well-researched and comprehensive—covering the financial, legal, medical and psychological concerns facing adult children as they care for elderly parents. It is also a practical resource and timely guide to hard-to-find services and subsidies.

Virginia Morris's book can be of enormous assistance to contemporary older persons as well as to Baby Boomers and the generations that follow.

*Robert N. Butler, M.D., founder of the National Institute on Aging, is the Director of the International Longevity Center as well as Professor of Geriatrics and Adult Development at Mount Sinai Medical Center, New York.*

# Introduction

I was finishing this book when a friend asked what my next project would be. "Something a little less depressing, I hope," she said with a sympathetic smile.

Her reaction was one I'd heard before, and I can understand it, to some extent. This is not a cheery subject. On the surface, I suppose my research seems downright dreary—studying incontinence and fading minds, visiting nursing homes, interviewing caregivers whose constant worries and personal sacrifices are heartbreaking. But I discovered two things that have kept me immersed in this project for the past four years and will continue to engage me for years to come.

The first is the need, both the depth of the need of individuals looking for answers and support, and the sheer volume of the need. More than ten million elderly people require assistance getting through the day, and 90 percent of the help they receive—help with shopping, bathing, eating, medical care and getting around—

comes from family members. The numbers, and the need, will only become more profound as baby-boomers begin to care for their aging parents.

More important, I have discovered that there is an aspect to caring for an aged parent, a vital aspect, that is not at all dreary. No matter what story is told, no matter how troubling the details, caring for an aged parent is always about giving. It is about compassion, about family ties that we cannot turn our backs on, about a drive so basic, so powerful, that we cannot ignore it. It is also about closure and saying good-bye. Faced with the reality that life does, indeed, end, that this parent will one day be gone, our most human, most tender, most protective instincts rise to the surface. This response, this need to care, while brought on by heartbreaking circumstances, feels good. It reminds us of what's really important in life and forces us to look beyond the routines of our daily lives. It comes from the heart, and so it can feed the heart.

Caring for an aging parent is trying, there is no doubt about that. It is exhausting, stressful, aggravating and, at times, completely overwhelming. Beyond the day-to-day pressures and practical questions that arise, there are complex emotional issues to deal with—guilt, resentment and grief, the strains of family relationships, the echoes of one's childhood, and the stark, painful visions of one's own old age and death.

However, there are often unexpected rewards. This is, after all, your parent, and no matter how he might infuriate you at times, no matter how he might have erred in his role as parent, no one will ever love you in quite the same way, and, in truth, you will never love anyone else in this way. Helping him now is an opportunity to reciprocate some of that love and attention. It is a chance to say, during quiet moments, things that you might not have said otherwise, to tell your parent how you feel, to settle old conflicts and to care for him in tender ways that you never have before.

Caring for your parent allows you to reaffirm family bonds and, in some cases, to strengthen those bonds.

Of course, these rewards may be hard to see, or even imagine, when you are in the thick of things—hiring home-care workers, sifting through bills, arguing with siblings and conferring with doctors. But at some point, when you look back on your parent's life and this time you had together, you may be glad that you had the chance to give in such an intimate way.

My goal in writing this book is to provide you with reassurance and concrete help—to outline the options, lead you to local services, suggest tips for everyday life. I hope to free you from some of the business of parentcare so you can focus on the emotional aspects of the task and give your parent the kind of love and attention that only you can give. In doing so, perhaps you will not only survive parentcare, but also realize some of its rewards.

* * * *

While reading the information and recommendations offered in these pages, keep in mind that they are addressed to a widely diverse population. Some caregivers live under the same roof with a parent and do this job without break, while others manage home-care services from afar. Some people are just heading into this job with a relatively healthy parent, while others are already well-versed in matters of geriatric care. Most of the advice is aimed at people caring for a lone parent, but some is directed at people who are helping one parent take care of another. The demands of the job, the strengths and strains of your relationship with your parent, and the support you receive from others, all make your job unique. Which advice you follow, how much you give and how you give it is something only you can decide. Do only what feels right for you—no more, no different—and you will be doing it right.

Throughout the book I've included brief quotes to help

convey some points more vividly and to let the people who shared their stories with me speak to you directly. Their words capture the frustrations, pain, courage and humor of their days and will remind you that you are not alone. A few of the quotes are composites of stories and some names have been changed if people asked to remain anonymous.

One of my favorite vignettes illustrates my point about rewards better than I can. It comes from a woman I had known for a long time, but whom I never knew well until the depth of her heart and richness of her soul were exposed to me through her stories about caring for her mother:

*The only time I wasn't the daughter was when I turned into the mother and that was the best feeling ever. It was October. My mother was very sick so I brought her to the hospital, and the doctor ordered some X rays. They had taken Mother's clothes off and she was so weak that I had to hold her up. Her body, which used to be so strong and lean, was thin, her skin was loose and I could feel her bones. I was holding her little body in my arms and there was a great poignancy, a closeness which I was so happy about. She was finally trusting me to care for her. She wasn't fighting me. On that day, I felt what I had always wanted to feel with her. It was like a pouring out of tenderness.*

# HOW TO CARE
## _for_ AGING
# PARENTS

# Chapter One

# GET READY, GET SET

*Talking With Your Parent • Beyond Denial • Gathering Essential Documents • Organizing Your Own Life*

..........................................

N O ONE PLANS TO TAKE CARE OF A PARENT. WE DON'T set aside money or time for the task, or begin reading books such as this one as soon as a parent turns 65. For the most part, a parent's old age, and the needs and dilemmas that typically accompany it, come as a surprise. In fact, even when events begin to unfold, and the reality of the situation becomes apparent, most of us still look the other way, hoping that perhaps things will take care of themselves, that Dad will be all right and our services will not be needed. As a result, we react to each crisis only as it arises.

So here's some advice that's not easy to hear, but truly invaluable to heed: Think ahead and prepare yourself and your parent for what may come. If your father's arthritis is getting worse, talk with him about what might happen if he can no longer manage alone, and start exploring community programs and services that he might need. If your mother has Alzheimer's, learn her wishes concerning her future care, and tour local nursing homes. Get a jump on this. When you use this book, don't read only the chapter that applies to your current situation; read also about issues that you are not yet dealing with—but may very well have to tackle one day.

This point can't be stressed enough. Delaying, postponing or looking the other way is a natural, but risky, approach to take. Your parent will grow older, his health will fail, his needs will intensify. Staying one page ahead, one day ahead, one question ahead, will give you and your parent time to consider the options carefully. It will ensure that your parent receives the best care possible. And, while it may not seem so now, it will provide you with a little peace of mind—a priceless commodity during such times.

# Critical Conversations

Although it can become too late quite suddenly, it is never too soon to talk to your parent about the future—her medical care, housing, finances and personal concerns. Obviously if your mother has been diagnosed with cancer or emphysema, these talks are urgent. But even if she is still relatively healthy and independent, discussing her future is vital. Many preparations, such as buying long-term care insurance or getting on a waiting list for a nursing home, must be done well in advance. And you need to know how she wants things handled if she grows too sick or frail to handle them on her own.

Discussing the future also helps prepare your family emotionally for what may come. If your father is encouraged now to explore the possibility of moving out of his house, it will be easier for him to make the move if it becomes necessary. And these talks give your parent and family members a chance to air their worries and anxieties, to reassure one another, and to learn the truth about any haunting questions. If your mother has been diagnosed with cancer, for example, she may be secretly terrified that she will be in constant pain or be left to die alone in a hospital room. When you create a context within which she can voice such concerns, you can help her learn about pain control and explore various in-home nursing services. And she can be reassured that you will be there for her throughout the time that remains.

## YOUR RELUCTANCE

Admittedly, asking about your father's personal finances, or anticipating a time when he can no longer live alone is not easy. You may have firmly established a relationship over the years in which these personal issues were never discussed. Raising them now may upset that fragile, but relatively comfortable, balance. If he is a domineering or protective force in your life, you risk losing— at least for a moment—the role of the child, a role that may frustrate you, but may also make you feel safe. Furthermore, initiating a conversation about your parent's finances, health care or housing, opens you up to new responsibilities—you brought it up, so now you have to find some answers—and it forces you, and perhaps your parent, to recognize his mortality.

Certain issues may make you particularly uncomfortable. For example, you may be reluctant to ask about assets and wills out of respect for your parent's privacy or out of fear of sounding like a gold-digger. Or you may not want to bring up the subject of death for fear of upsetting your parent. But the truth is that your parent and other family members probably share your concerns as well as your reluctance to discuss them. In fact, your mother may be keeping silent because she is worried about upsetting *you*. Your breaking open the dam and initiating discussions about these taboo subjects is likely to be a welcome relief for all concerned.

Think about your reluctance and the reasons for it. Contemplate your role and the risks of both talking and failing to talk. Remember, as awkward as it may be, talking about the worst case scenarios won't make them come true, and refusing to talk about them won't make them go away. Ignoring the inevitable will only leave you unprepared for a crisis.

## FINDING THE WORDS

If you can't come right out and say what you want to, use an indirect approach. For example, you might express your concern about a friend or family member who is seriously ill or describe your own financial situation and plans to draft a will. Or, use a magazine article or television show as a springboard. *I was reading an article on long-term care insurance. Do you have this kind of insurance, Dad?* If your father had elderly parents, ask how he handled certain matters for them.

If talking face-to-face is too awkward, write a list of questions for your mother. Tell her these are some issues you've been concerned about and ask her to think about them. Then plan a time to sit down with her and discuss them.

## YOUR PARENT'S DENIAL

When your parent is hiding behind denial—*Oh, honey, why do you have to bring up such dreadful things? Let's talk about something more pleasant*—grant her some of that protection. Be patient and try to understand her fears and the reasons why she might not want to face the facts. If the subject isn't pressing, simply ask her to think about the matter and then bring it up another day. Sometimes things have to reach a crisis before such discussions are possible.

When things do reach a critical state and denial becomes an obstacle—when your parent refuses to consider vital legal documents even after months of chemotherapy or refuses to see that her bank account is almost dry—then you need to push, tenderly and compassionately, but very firmly. *Mom, we cannot ignore this any longer. We have got to deal with it.*

If you are still not successful, ask another family member to talk with her. For whatever reasons, she may be more receptive with some-

# BREAKING THE SILENCE

❖ Raise any discussions about your parent's health, finances or other matters at a time when you won't be interrupted, and when you and your parent are calm and rested.

❖ Be open and very clear with the facts—a poor medical prognosis, a major financial hurdle, a less-than-optimal selection of housing options. Don't hide information to protect your father. Lies or half-truths will only hurt him in the long run.

❖ If your mother changes the subject or makes it clear that she doesn't want to talk about something, back off and try again another time.

❖ Keep the discussion focused on your father and his concerns. *You* may worry about who is going to take care of him once the Parkinson's disease gets worse, but *he* may be frightened about becoming helpless, losing people's respect or becoming a burden. You may be surprised to find that your mother has been worried about your well-being should something happen to her. Give her ample room to express her thoughts, for these are important issues that need your undivided attention.

❖ Whenever possible, phrase your concerns as questions, letting your parent draw the conclusions and make the choices. Ask what she thinks should be done rather than telling her what should be done.

❖ Listen carefully, even when you have firm convictions about what's feasible. You may have ideas about where your mother should live or how she should handle her finances, but it's particularly important to listen now. Be open-minded and make a point of really listening to her preferences, and letting her know that you hear and understand.

❖ End each discussion before you or your parent becomes tired or cranky.

❖ Leave the conversation open. One discussion breaks the ice, but these topics need to be discussed repeatedly. Ask your parent to think about whatever subject you have been discussing and conclude the conversation by saying that you'd like to continue the talk in a week or so.

one else. Or urge her to visit a clergyman, a social worker, a lawyer or a doctor to discuss these matters. It's often easier to talk to and accept the advice of someone outside the family circle, especially if the other person is a trusted professional.

If, no matter what you do, your parent continues to deny the facts, you may have to let things be. You cannot force her to act on matters that she simply is not willing to face. But you should have a plan in mind anyway. Think about what will happen if your mother becomes seriously ill or dependent. What help might she need? How much will you be able to give? And where will the rest of the help (services, support, etc.) come from? Who will pay for it? Try to involve siblings as much as possible in planning for future eventualities.

If your father's denial gets in the way of specific actions that absolutely must be taken—he refuses to stop driving even though his vision is very poor, or he won't see a doctor even though his leg is swollen—then you may have to step in and take action, regardless of his wishes. (See page 16 for more on when to intervene.)

## WHAT TO TALK ABOUT

You may know you need to have this discussion with Dad, you may have dealt with your own denial—but where do you begin and what do you ask? Here are a few questions to get you started. (All of these topics are discussed in detail in individual chapters.)

♦ **Your parent's needs and concerns.** What are your parent's biggest worries about the future? What goals in his life does he feel are unmet, what tasks unfinished or conflicts unresolved? What aspects of his life are most important to him at this stage of life? Being near family, hearing the opera, seeing certain friends, practicing his religion?

♦ **Housing.** How important is it to your parent to remain in his

"*After my father died I was very worried about my mom's finances. My dad always took care of everything that had to do with money. Mom never knew about his accounts; I don't think she ever balanced the checkbook.*

*I said to Mom over and over, 'Let's review your financial situation,' and I offered repeatedly to take care of her bills for her. She would say, 'Brenda, don't worry about it. I'm fine.' And then she would change the subject.*

*Then my brother came to visit and within a day he had Mom pulling out folders and showing him bank statements. By the time he left she had handed over almost all of her financial stuff to him.*

*I was stunned. I mean, I was glad to have it settled, but I was also a little annoyed. I'm an accountant. He's a teacher. I guess she feels that money is men's work. I probably should have thought to get him involved right from the start.*"

—BRENDA S.

## THREE CRUCIAL DOCUMENTS

Whatever else you do, be sure your parent has, or has at least considered:

❖ **An updated and valid will** which ensures that his belongings (no matter how extensive or meager) will be allocated according to his wishes. A current will reduces the likelihood of family conflict and an extended and complicated probate process.

❖ **A durable power of attorney** which allows a designated person to make legally binding decisions for your parent, from signing checks to making housing choices, should he become incapacitated. Having power of attorney means the family can avoid the harrowing process of going to court to have a guardian named to oversee his care and finances.

❖ **Advance directives** (a living will and durable power of attorney for health care) which specify your parent's wishes concerning medical care and name someone to make decisions in his stead, should he become incompetent.

(See Chapter Fourteen for a full explanation of these documents.)

own home? Where would he want to live if he could no longer manage at home? What if it isn't possible for him to live with other family members?

◆ **Financial and legal matters.** What are your parent's current financial needs and potential future needs? Is he in a financial position to meet these needs? Is his insurance—including life, health, home and auto insurance—adequate and current? Has he executed all necessary legal papers and are they up-to-date? (See box, above.)

◆ **Health care.** Does your parent have a good doctor whom she trusts? If she is sick, what is her prognosis and how will that affect her housing, finances and care? If you had to make medical decisions for her, what would she want you to know? Does she dread the prospect of a particular disability (dementia, blindness, paralysis)? If so, why? Is she more apprehensive about being in pain or about being groggy from painkillers? Is there a certain point after which she would no longer want aggressive medical care? How does she feel about hospice care?

◆ **Death and funerals.** This may be the toughest subject for you to discuss, but it may be the one foremost on your parent's mind. Try to bring it up, however obliquely, and see if he is willing to talk about it. What, if anything, frightens him about dying? Is he more frightened about death or about what the end of his life will be like? Is there a way that you might be able to alleviate some of his fears? What are his religious beliefs about death? What kind of service does he want? Does he want to be buried or cremated? Has he made any advance arrangements for his burial or funeral?

# Gathering Information

As your mother grows increasingly frail, your family will need certain financial records and other information such as insurance policies, advance directives and the names of her doctors. (See Checklist, on the following page.) Find out whether your parent has all the relevant papers and make sure that you or another family member knows where they are.

If both of your parents are alive, you might simply remind them that these papers are important and suggest that they get them in order and that each has full access to them. If only one of your parents is alive, you might offer some help in finding these documents. If she doesn't want help, impress upon her the importance of gathering these materials, and then follow up later to make sure that she has done it.

If your parent is infirm and you are looking for these papers without his help, you may become shocked or embarrassed as you hunt through his personal papers. If so, get a sibling or friend to help, and

## FALLING ON DEAF EARS

Talking about these issues may not be a problem; getting your parent to heed any advice, however, may be extremely frustrating. You know your mother should sign a will. You are certain that your father should move out of his house. But he refuses to budge. What could possibly be more maddening than a parent who simply won't listen?

You may need to step in regardless of your parent's wishes if the situation is truly dire, but it's more likely that you need to do something far more difficult: Accept your parent's autonomy, and appreciate the limits of your control over his life. You may be convinced that he's making a mistake, but unless he is in real danger, your parent has a right to take risks and make foolish decisions. One day you will have the same rights, despite the better judgment of others.

do it on a schedule that is manageable for you—all at once, like swallowing a pill, or in a series of small doses.

Call your parent's lawyer, accountant or anyone else who has or has had a hand in your parent's financial or legal affairs. Then look

## CHECKLIST

*Documents and information that your parent needs*

❏ Names, addresses and phone numbers of:
—doctors, dentists and other medical providers, such as optometrists, hearing aid suppliers and pharmacists
—lawyers, financial advisors and accountants, insurance agents, real estate agents
—banks and other financial institutions

❏ Your parent's will and codicils (amendments) to the will, as well as his health care proxy, living will and durable power of attorney

❏ The keys to safe-deposit boxes and post office boxes

❏ The location of any hidden valuables

❏ Insurance policies, including life, health, disability, mortgage or loan, homeowner's, accident, auto and credit card

❏ Social security, Medicare and Medicaid numbers and identification cards

❏ Any rental agreements or other business contracts

❏ A complete list of your parent's assets, including
—savings, checking and money market accounts
—stocks, bonds and other securities
—deeds to all real estate
—titles to automobiles, boats, and other vehicles
—business ownership and partnership agreements
—profit-sharing and pension plans
—retirement accounts (IRA, Keogh, SEP, etc.)

❏ A list of debts, including mortgages and other loans, credit card debts, outstanding bills and other liabilities

❏ A list of all routine household bills, such as utilities bills and insurance premiums, that you may have to take care of if your parent becomes ill

❏ Any appraisals of personal property

❏ Copies of federal and state tax returns from the past three to five years

❏ Receipts from property taxes and other large recent payments

❏ Records of any personal loans your parent may have made to family members, business associates or others

in the obvious places—a safe-deposit box, desk and bureau drawers, office files and papers stacked on tables and in corners. If you don't find everything you need, look for leads, such as bills, canceled checks, receipts, address books and letters.

Insurance companies will often provide information about a policy even when the request comes from a family member of the insured. The social security office, former employers and the local office of veterans' affairs may be willing to send you information about pensions and other benefits. Unfortunately, banks are not very helpful in these situations unless you are dealing with a local bank where the manager knows your family. By law, banks can give out account information only to the owner of the account or the owner's legal guardian.

# The Key Is Organization

If you diligently write lists of "Things to Do" on scraps of paper and then routinely misplace them, or if you're constantly remembering things that you shouldn't have forgotten but did:

◆ Keep a tiny spiral notebook in your purse or back pocket at all times. When you think of an essential errand while driving to the grocery store, jot it down at the next traffic light. As a reward for your efforts, you get to cross things off as you accomplish them. Remember, if this book is left at home on your desk, it will be of little use to you.

◆ Have a pocket calendar on your desk or by your kitchen phone (or get one that travels in your purse or briefcase). Record not just the obvious dates and appointments, but every task that must be done on a certain day. If bottles and cans get picked up every other Thursday morning for recycling, make a note to yourself to put them out on Wednesday night. With so much on your mind now, sometimes

*"During my mother's illness, I accumulated so much stuff—brochures from nursing homes, documents from lawyers, forms from Medicare, pamphlets from social service agencies. Every time I got something, I just tossed it into this giant box in my bedroom. Then whenever something came up, like when I wanted to get meals delivered to her while I was away, I would think, 'Oh yeah, I have something on that,' but I could never find it.*

*A friend came over one day and dumped out my box and started sorting through it. She spent the entire day organizing the whole mess. That was the best thing anyone did for me during those two years. Not only could I find things quickly, but it made me feel better. I'd been feeling so out of control, and that gave me a little edge. It made an enormous difference.*

—TERRY B.

remembering your own name can be an effort.

◆ Likewise, each time you call a home-care agency, a lawyer or a social worker, make a note about the call on your calendar, including the name of the person you spoke with and what you talked about, so you can refer to it later if necessary. *(But I spoke to Anne Preston on March 18 and she confirmed that the home health aide would start tomorrow.)*

◆ Whenever you make calls to agencies, doctors, etc., have all the necessary information in front of you and have all of your questions written out. Otherwise you may forget an important question and have to go through all the secretaries and recorded announcements to make contact again. Get into the habit of asking for people's direct lines or extension numbers.

◆ Confirm, confirm. It's better to confirm an appointment the day before than to find out that your father's hearing aid specialist has taken an unscheduled vacation and his temporary assistant forgot to cancel his appointments.

◆ Buy some folders and a sturdy file box or an accordion file, and use it to store all information regarding your parent's care. Label each folder or section in a way that makes sense to you—Medical Information, Nursing Home Brochures, Legal Papers, Community Resources, Letters to Siblings, etc. If you hate to throw things out (you never know when you might need it), keep a file called Information No Longer Needed, or Trash File, just so your other files are current and not overstuffed.

Once you have your files set up, use them. Keep them up-to-date rather than just stacking papers in a "to be filed" pile.

◆ Make a master list of all essential names and phone numbers and store one copy at the beginning of the file box and one copy beside the telephone. (If you're calling certain people or agencies regularly, and if your telephone has a memory feature, you might want to store their numbers into your automatic dialing system.)

◆ If you work better on a computer, set up a computer file that includes all the information and accounts concerning your parent. Be sure to make a back-up disc copy, and keep it in a safe place.

◆ If you're handling your parent's finances or housing, make copies of all medical receipts, insurance claims, nursing home applications and other important documents so that you always have a record of anything that is in the works.

◆ Write a daily schedule. Before scoffing at this idea, try it for a couple of weeks. You may not adhere to it precisely, but it will help structure your day so you are not constantly thinking, "I've got to get to the cleaners. I've got to call the social security office." The task—or the breather you need—will already be assigned to a time slot. Even if you don't use it, writing a schedule for a few weeks will help you to see where your day is going and why you don't have time for all the things you need to do. And it may give you ideas for how you can be more efficient. For example:

| 7 a.m. | *shower, get everyone moving* |
|---|---|
| 8 | *breakfast* |
| 8:45 | *take Mom to the eye doctor for 9 a.m. appointment, read newspaper in the waiting room* |
| 10 | *drop Mom at day care, pick up Bob's pants at tailor* |
| 10:30-11:30 | *exercise class* |
| 12 | *lunch with Ed Farmer* |
| 1:30-5 p.m. | *work on Copeland report—no interruptions!* |
| 5 | *pick up Mom at day care and get last-minute groceries* |
| 6 | *fix dinner* |
| 7 | *dinner is served* |
| 8 | *help Mom get ready for bed* |
| 8:30 | *pay bills* |
| 9 | *call Wendy for a chat* |
| 10 | *watch Picket Fences* |
| 11 | *bed* |

Be reasonable when making your schedule. Give yourself more than the minimum time required to do a chore or to get someplace. If you have an appointment, expect to wait. If a recipe says 30 minutes, give yourself 45. And finally, if you're a morning scrambler, get up 15 minutes earlier than usual to give yourself time to organize the day and start it off calmly.

## ORGANIZING FROM A DISTANCE

When you are caring for your parent from a distance it's even more important to be organized because you have to accomplish tasks during visits or by phone. Whenever you visit, take a mental inventory of your parent's health and living situation and try to foresee trouble before it happens. Does your mother seem wobbly or dizzy? Is the house tidy and clean? Is she well-groomed, or has her personal hygiene deteriorated? Is there ample food in the refrigerator and is it fresh? Are there piles of unopened mail or unpaid bills? If things are askew it may be a sign of serious trouble—depression, confusion, poor appetite because of an illness—or simply a signal to you that she needs some outside help at home.

Establish a support network as soon as possible. Make a list of friends, family or neighbors who live near your parent, people you can call in case of trouble. Also learn about local services such as volunteer visitors, homemakers, adult day care and meal delivery programs.

Organize your visits in advance so you can accomplish as much as possible. If you need to meet with doctors, lawyers, social workers or other professionals, try to set up appointments a month ahead, as their schedules get filled up quickly. Be sure to confirm these appointments closer to the date. Include some time during your visit to talk with nearby relatives or others involved in your parent's care.

Other tips for caring from afar:

◆ When you can't be there, find someone who can. See if a relative, friend or neighbor will stop by occasionally to check on your parent, or contact a visitor service, home-

## A FEW GOOD NUMBERS

Get some basic information about local services, housing options and legal matters early —before your parent, or you, need to use them. With just a few quick calls you can find out much of what you need to know and get leads to other agencies.

❖ **The "area agency on aging,"** which can be found by calling the Eldercare Locator (800-677-1116) or the state unit on aging (listed in Appendix A), has information about services and programs available in your parent's community and may be able to answer specific questions about your parent's care.

❖ **The state long-term care ombudsman's office,** which represents residents of nursing homes and their families, can give you information about local nursing homes and other

available types of housing for the elderly. (The state offices are listed in Appendix A, page 377.)

❖ **The local hospital's discharge planner or social services department** is responsible for placing patients in rehabilitation centers or nursing homes and therefore knows a great deal about services in your parent's community. Many hospital social workers will guide you whether or not your parent is in the hospital.

❖ **The National Association of Professional Geriatric Care Managers** (602-881-8008) provides referrals to local geriatric care managers who can oversee your parent's care when you can't. Care managers' services are not inexpensive, but they are often well worth the price.

care agency or the state long-term-care ombudsman's office, any of which may be able to send someone over periodically.

◆ Buy your parent a medical alert system (see page 138) so if she becomes ill suddenly or falls when she is alone, she will be able to get help immediately.

◆ Leave a duplicate of your parent's house key with a trusted neighbor or friend, or hide one

somewhere outside of her house or apartment in case there is an emergency and someone needs to get in.

◆ Be sure you have a reliable telephone answering machine so your parent or others can reach you in case of an emergency.

◆ Learn about any local elder-watch programs. Some post offices and gas and electric companies train employees to watch for trouble at homes where they know an elderly person lives alone. Sometimes a bank manager will keep an eye out if you are concerned about your parent's finances—is the account suddenly being used up, or has it laid dormant for some time?

◆ From afar, it is especially important to be ready with information and questions when you call doctors or lawyers so you can keep long-distance calls brief. If you are in a different time zone, try to make these calls during off-peak hours.

◆ When things begin to get unwieldy, look into hiring a geriatric care manager or find out if a government agency or charitable group offers free care management. A manager will check on your parent, organize local services for her, handle emergencies and keep you up-to-date. (See page 182.)

# Chapter Two

# YOUR PARENT AND YOU

*Adapting to New Roles • Knowing When to Intervene
•Resolving Old Struggles • Managing Day-to-Day*

P ARENT-CHILD RELATIONSHIPS ARE, BY THEIR VERY NATURE, stressful. Your father makes you feel guilty, expects too much from you or refuses to let you help him. Your mother doesn't understand you, embarrasses you, or perhaps she reminds you a little too much of yourself. Whatever the issue, it stays with you. Long after you think you have outgrown the parent-child power dance, often after decades of work to resolve it, a casual comment or a subtle look can trigger a familiar surge of adrenaline.

Now that your parent needs you, both the bond and the aggravation are magnified. This is the paradox of parentcare. On the one hand, the prospect of losing your parent intensifies your love, and this time together is precious. On the other hand, you are dealing with painful and often contentious issues, and your roles—who is in charge, who is the "parent"—are less clear and sometimes uncomfortable.

You can't change your parent, especially not at his age, but if you can change your reactions to him, it will ease the daily tension. And you can come to terms with the scope and definition of your new role so that you help your parent without hurting his pride or interfering too much in his life. All of this might help you form, not an entirely different relationship with him, but perhaps a more peaceful one.

# Adapting to New Roles

When a parent grows frail, roles shift uncomfortably and both parent and child become a bit disoriented and unsure about how to behave. Who is in charge? When should you intervene? Are you the parent now?

## ARE YOU PARENTING YOUR PARENT?

It is a common remark and a thought that is hard to avoid, especially if you are changing diapers, tying shoelaces or helping your parent walk. But regardless of the circumstances, the answer is a flat-out and very definite NO. You are not parenting your parent.

If your parent is no longer able to care for herself, you may have new responsibilities, ones that may at times resemble those of parenting. But your parent is and always will be your parent, and you will always be her child. Go ahead and use some of the same tricks that help in parenting—diversions to get her onto a new subject or crib sheets for incontinence. But allowing yourself to think that the roles have reversed, that you are now the parent and your father is a helpless child, is a potentially disastrous way to look at this situation—for both of you.

For your parent, it is dehumanizing to be treated or spoken to as a child. No matter how disease and age may have altered your mother's body or mind, no matter how much or how little she can do or think for herself, and no matter how much you are doing for her, she is an adult and deserves to be treated as one. She has a lifetime of experience and a wealth of time-tested opinions. She has earned her autonomy and pride. She may have reverted to childish ways, but that does not make her a child.

### REMEMBER THE GOOD OLD DAYS

If your parent is quite ill, if he has gotten crotchety in his old age, or if he has dementia, find a photo from when he was younger. Put it on your refrigerator or on your desk. It will help you remember better times, when he was stronger. It will help you recall the father who laughed with you and cared for you and taught you things. It will help you remember why you are doing so much for him now.

For you, reversing the roles will only lead to dead ends and frustration. After all, children grow and learn and (usually) do what their parents tell them to do. If you try to parent your parent as you would a child, without perceiving the vast differences in the two situations, you will make things much harder for yourself. You will beat yourself up wondering why you are having such trouble with the task, and you will be angry at your parent for not behaving more like a child. *Why doesn't he listen and do what I say?*

If you can behave as an adult and treat your parent as an adult, both of you will fare better.

## FOSTERING INDEPENDENCE

Not only should you avoid parenting your parent, but go a step further: Make a point of strengthening his independence. Rather than cleaning his room, making his lunch and doing his errands, find a way for him to do these things for himself. (See Chapter Eight for ways to make daily tasks more manageable.) Rather than taking over his finances and legal affairs, keep him at the helm as much as possible. Your role now is not to control your parent's life, but to help him maintain control of it.

Activity and independence are good for your parent's body, mind and spirit. Physically, it is good for him to move, lift, bend, walk and carry. He may not want to wash the dishes or walk to the mailbox because his arthritis makes it difficult, and you may want to help by doing these things for him. But the truth is that inactivity is deadly for the human body. Movement, any movement at all and as much of it as possible, is valuable medicine.

"Use it or lose it" applies to the mind as well as the body. Mental exercise, such as keeping track of one's own finances or composing letters, can keep the mind well-oiled and running smoothly and it can ward off or slow down the onset of dementia.

**"***Now that my mother's dementia is worse, she's given up and wants me to take over. I have to help her dress and get her to day care and feed her. It's to the point now that if someone asks her a question, she'll answer but look to me to make sure it's right.***

*Sometimes I get so frustrated and tired that I yell at her. I tell her what to do and then get mad when she doesn't do it right. And then I feel awful and I think, 'What in the world is happening here?'*

*I have to keep reminding myself over and over that she's my mother and I love her dearly and I respect her. But it's hard.* **"**　—LINDA K.**

More than anything else, independence boosts the soul. Your parent may welcome your help, but when people are constantly catered to, when they no longer make their own decisions, when they are treated as needy and helpless, they grow only more needy and helpless. As they give up increasing amounts of control, they also give up their self-esteem, spirit and drive. They wither.

Your parent has already lost a good deal. Help him hang on to whatever abilities and independence he still has. Help him to help himself, whenever possible.

## WHEN TO INTERVENE

The need to respect your parent's independence can collide with the need to protect his safety and welfare. So when do you intervene and when do you bow out? And how do you step in without taking over? What do you do, for instance, if your father insists on staying in an unsafe home, or refuses to call the doctor after a fall? What if your mother is losing her vision but refuses to stop driving?

If your parent has a mentally competent mate, remember that it is her job to decide when and how to intervene. Don't usurp her role. She will make decisions, as well as she still can, about her mate's care. And it is your role to support her, nurture her and help her to do what she thinks is best. Offer your help and encouragement, but remember that you're in the back seat.

If you are caring for a lone parent or handling the care of two parents, you must step in when your parent's (or someone else's) safety

## WHOSE LIFE IS THIS, ANYWAY?

Early on, when a parent is newly ill or suddenly widowed, adult children often jump in with both feet to help. With all the best intentions, they discuss Dad's living situation, his social life, his health, his finances and his future—often among themselves, with little or no input from Dad. After a number of conversations and a little research, they call Dad with their consensus: "Now that Mom is gone, we think you should move. We've found a wonderful housing complex on the west coast of Florida. It would be just perfect for you. There's golf and a swimming pool and, if your arthritis gets worse or you get sick, it has visiting health aides and a nursing home unit. It will be so much easier than living in that old house. . . ."

The problem is that Dad loves his old house, all his friends live nearby, and he has no intention of moving. The conversation immediately becomes touchy. He feels betrayed and justifiably angry over the fact that decisions are being made for him, as if he were a problem that needed a solution. His children are hurt that he is not happy about this plan they have worked so hard to develop, and annoyed that he refuses to do what is clearly best.

Unless your parent is mentally incompetent, he is still an adult and still in control of his own life. He doesn't need anyone making decisions for him—and certainly not without him. And he doesn't need the unsolicited advice of well-meaning family members. If you are concerned about an aspect of your parent's life, express your concerns, but don't direct him. It is his life, after all.

**❝** *Very late one night as I was returning to the city, I saw an elderly actor I knew getting off the train. He was very frail, and I was astonished to see that he was not only traveling alone, but that no one was there to meet him at the station. I took him home in a taxi, and he seemed very grateful.*

*I was furious at his kids, affluent people whom I also knew slightly, for letting him travel on his own at that hour. I hated to think what might have happened to him, out alone in the city so late at night.*

*A few years later, when my own father became old and frail, he insisted on traveling on his own. He wouldn't put up with our telling him that it wasn't safe, and we finally realized that we couldn't cover his activities in a way that made us feel secure. I understood for the first time the actor's kids and felt foolish that I'd been so self-righteous and critical. What can you do? You have to contain your anxiety. You have no choice.* **❞**          —SARA B.

or health is seriously threatened. You may have to take your sick father to the doctor's office against his wishes. You should be sure he pays his bills, to protect him from utility cutoffs and eviction. You have to have the gas to the stove disconnected if your mother, in her confused state, is at risk of burning the house down. You must stop her from driving if she is a hazard to herself and others on the road.

You also have to step in when your parent becomes incompetent and can no longer understand her options or make a rational decision. (See page 286 for information on obtaining guardianship.) You may have to make decisions about her health care, housing and finances if she can no longer make those decisions for herself.

But beyond these issues of dire risk and mental incompetence, your right to control your parent is superceded by her right to make her own decisions. All of us make decisions about personal health and safety every day—when we get into a car or have a cigarette, for example—and some of these choices are unwise. Your parent, even at her advanced age, retains the right to take risks—even ones you may consider foolhardy.

So what do you do? Urge your parent quite firmly to move if you think her living alone is dangerous. Get others—a doctor, social worker, clergyman or another family member—to talk to her as well. But the final decision is hers. At some point you have to accept what is and make the best of it—move her bedroom downstairs, sign her up for meals on wheels and find or hire companions to stay with her.

Keep in mind that your parent is basing her decisions on different criteria than yours. Your main concern is her health and safety, but at this point in her life she may place greater value on comfort or independence. She may be willing to take certain risks in order to stay in her own home, take care of herself or go out with her friends when she pleases. She

**"***My mother had a stroke about a year ago that left her very unsteady. She needed a cane to get around, and climbing stairs was almost impossible for her. What was difficult for me was that she started going back to her old routines almost immediately. She lives in the city and loves the theater, the opera, going out with her friends. About two weeks after her stroke, I realized that she had resumed her old social life. I was worried sick. It was winter and the sidewalks were slippery and I was afraid she was going to fall or have another stroke.*

*But she got around pretty well, with the help of friends. And I began to realize that for her to stay in her apartment, to sit alone and watch television, would be a fate worse than death. My mother is going to get out and do things as long as she is alive. That's her nature. I worry, but I respect her immensely for it. I hope I have her gusto when I'm her age.* **"**                    —FRAN M.

may be more interested in living fully than in living longer. Understanding her point of view will help you let go of the battle.

Sometimes a support group can help you gain perspective about when and how you should intervene. If you face a troubling situation and don't know how much to intervene, geriatric social workers and case managers are well versed in these matters. You can find a geri-atric social worker or case manager through a hospital's social work or geriatric department, or sometimes through a local home-care agency. Or call the National Association of Professional Geriatric Care Managers (520-881-8008).

# Resolving Old Struggles

While it's tempting to ignore deep-rooted problems between you and your parent—*He's not going to change, so what's the point of talking about it?*—this may be a good time to explore and address them. In fact, it may be your last opportunity to make peace.

The work won't be easy—in fact it's likely to be painful. It may require that you dig back into your childhood, dredge up and inspect buried emotions and let go of some firmly-held hopes. In the process, you may upset the status quo and, in doing so, rattle yourself and perhaps others in the family.

This takes a lot of courage and determination. But if you can do it, sorting through some of the struggles in this relationship will help you survive and perhaps even grow during this stressful time. After all, this is a primal bond; it is the basis of all the other bonds in your life. Understanding it may help clarify some of the other intimate relationships in your life.

Of course, if your father is seriously ill or confused, it may be too late to explore his thoughts, talk with him about painful issues, make

*"No matter how difficult she is or how much we disagree, I can't shut her out. Never. It would be like shutting something in myself out. She needs me now tremendously. The most I'll miss is about three days, and then I have to see her or call her.*

*There must be something so deep in this relationship between mothers and daughters, more than we can ever realize. We're so connected, even when we're so different."*

—BETTY H.

amends or involve him in any real-way in this effort. Even if he is relatively healthy, he may not be willing or able to engage in a dialogue with you, or to hear your concerns. Let him be. You can still deal with these issues on your own.

Where do you start? How do you alter a relationship that is so much a part of who you are, and is so rooted in the past? First, step back and look at the big picture.

◆ **Pinpoint the problem.** What is it that troubles you about your parent and the way you relate to him? What is it that you want and are not getting, or what exasperates you and why does it affect you so much? Think very carefully about this. Try to be precise. Does your parent's personality bother you because it is grating, because it has stood in the way of your being close or because you see the same trait in yourself? Do you withdraw from your mother's helplessness because it places too much of a burden on you or because it has caused you to

become painfully self-sufficient? Do you cringe because of the way your father behaves or because you still feel wounded by something he did in the past?

Or is the root of your anguish simply your parent's power over you? Few of us adequately break away from our parents, but continue to fight for autonomy well into our own old age. Perhaps the real trouble lies not in your parent's actions, but in your own need to sever childhood ties.

◆ **Tackle some issues.** If there is a specific issue—a recurring argument or an unresolved conflict—talk about it if your parent is still able. You may get somewhere, but even if you don't, you will find some peace of mind in knowing that you tried, that you broke the Code of Silence and did what you could to settle the matter.

If the subject is taboo or deeply painful, you may want to do this with a therapist who specializes in family relationships. But do it now—today—while your parent can still take part in the discussion. Here are a few tips that might help:

• Bring up the topic at a time when you are calm. Instead of jumping into a heated discussion just when your mother has said the one thing that really exasperates or hurts you, wait until the emotional climate is more temperate.

• Try to stay composed. If you are confrontational or accusatory, you will only put your parent on the defensive, and blaming him will prevent you from moving forward. Instead, try to turn things around and describe the problem as *yours*. (Try this even if you know that the problem is your parent's fault—it isn't easy to do but it can be very effective.) As a general rule, use statements that begin with "I" rather than those that begin with "You." Instead of telling your mother that she manipulates you and makes you feel guilty, tell her that *you* have a problem with guilt. Talk about how easily and how often you feel guilty and how bad it makes you feel. Ask her if she or others in the family tend to feel a lot of guilt, and how they handle it. If your father constantly criticizes you for being overweight, instead of berating him for his insensitivity, talk to him about your need for his approval and the insecurities you feel about your appearance.

• Avoid old arguments. Steer the conversation away from familiar eddies with a history of going nowhere. As soon as you sense things slipping into old patterns, ask a new question. If certain old comments elicit strong reactions in you, take a moment before responding—count to ten—to give yourself time to decide whether you want to follow this particular route or change course.

♦ **Let go of unreasonable hopes.** There will be some matters, especially those having to do with your parent's personality, that you can't change. Personality traits are hard to change at any age, but they tend to become only more fixed later in life, and for some reason this is particularly true of less desirable traits. Someone who is gentle, giving and selfless may become more saintly as the years pass, but more often someone who is a little trying will become very difficult indeed.

## WHAT HAVE YOU GOT TO LOSE?

If there is an issue that you've been wanting to raise with your parent but you haven't done it, think about what may be stopping you. What's the worst thing that could happen? What do you fear? Are you afraid of breaking some unwritten family rule? *We don't talk about Dad's drinking.* Are you afraid that your parent will be hurt, get angry or be disappointed in you? Are you worried about getting into the kind of painful argument that always ends in tears? Are you afraid of hearing what your parent has to say, or of losing your role as the child?

Weigh the potential cost and gain of raising the subject or leaving it alone. Then decide which way you want to go. If you leave it alone, do so because you have considered the matter and made a conscious decision, not because you put it off or avoided it. Then, try to accept the consequences of your decision and move on.

A parent who has never asked you about your life or your feelings is not apt to want to get to know you now; a parent who has been frugal with compliments is not likely to shower, or even sprinkle, you with praise; a parent who has never been loving or intimate probably won't be able to open his heart now.

Of course, somewhere in your logical mind, you know all this, but accepting it in your heart can be devastating. Recognizing that your parent won't change means accepting that this will never be the kind of relationship that you wanted. All of us want, deeply and profoundly, to have a loving, intimate bond with a parent, one that is based on mutual respect and trust. Accepting that such a tie will never exist, at least not in the way you believe it should, is almost like accepting the death of your parent—the parent you had hoped for and the parent you can never have.

Recognizing all this may leave you feeling intensely alone, and perhaps betrayed. But accepting, and then mourning, this loss allows you to move on. Once you let go of your hopes, you can stop struggling to make this relationship into something it isn't. And once you stop looking to your parent for approval and validation, you are free to get these things from yourself.

You may also find that your relationship with your parent develops new strengths. You may notice qualities in your parent that you never saw before. Your parent may be able to appreciate certain qualities in you for the first time. You may find that you actually enjoy

> **"** *For years I thought I would finally have a really wonderful relationship with my mother. I envied people who had such relationships and I was sure that I could have one too. But I've gotten a little more perspective on that. I'm doing the best I can by my mother, but I realize that we can never be close. We are just too different from one another.*
>
> *Now I don't expect her to understand me. I used to open up to her, tell her something that I felt deeply or was upset by, and she would say, 'But you're doing fine, aren't you?' And that would be the end of it. She would end the conversation. She doesn't want to hear about any of the darker sides of my life. It makes her anxious, and she needs me to be happy and effervescent. But I don't expect intimate conversations anymore. And things are much better between us. The less need I bring to this, the better it is for the relationship.* **"**          —FRAN M.

what *is*, rather than constantly feeling cheated by what isn't.

One final note on this business of letting go. Remember that even though your parent may not be able or willing to change, you still can. You can work on your personality and relationships, you can learn to be more open, honest, loving or tolerant. In other words, you are not your parent. You are your own person.

◆ **Learn about him.** Sometimes we expect our parents to understand

YOUR PARENT AND YOU

## WHAT DOES HE WANT FROM ME?

You have just spent the day zipping around your parent's house, doing his laundry, changing the bed and fixing his dinner. Two days later he says that you never visit him. What's a daughter to do?

It may be that your parent doesn't want more of your time, just more of you. That is, your company and affection may be more important to him than clean socks and hot meals. So while you are busy as a bee, he is feeling ignored. Later on he wonders why he never sees you because the truth is, he hasn't.

The dilemma is that these tasks have to be done and, truth be told, it may be easier to be in the kitchen cooking than in the living room talking with him. Find a compromise —a little time in the laundry room, a few minutes by his side. Or have some conversation while you fold the laundry. Ask your parent what household chores he most wants done, and then cut out some of the others. By addressing his most fundamental needs for companionship and affection, you will be giving him far more help, and you may head off some of the I-never-see-you laments.

If he still complains that you don't visit enough, avoid arguing—*I was here just two days ago! What do you want from me?*—and simply reassure him that you love him, that you will come to see him again as soon as you can. His comments may be more a reflection of his own loneliness and insecurity than a criticism of you.

and respect us for who we are, but we fail to give them the same courtesy. Get to know your parent—really know him—as a person. Ask your father about his life—his upbringing, the loves he had, his travels, successes, failures and role models. Get him to tell you stories he's never told you or to add new details to the old stories. Next time he makes some vague comment that you've heard many times before, rather than brushing it away, encourage him to explain it. *Why do you think I don't care about you? What could I do to make you feel more loved?*

While you are at it, get him to talk about his current situation. Whether he says so or not, your parent has probably suffered great losses recently. He may have lost friends, a spouse, a job, his financial security. He may have lost his mobility, his health and some or all of his independence. Perhaps he is grieving about all this, or perhaps he is afraid of what he believes his future now holds—dependency, abandonment, helplessness, isolation and death.

Hearing about your parent's past, getting to know what makes him who he is, understanding something about how he feels now—all of this should help you to see your parent as human, vulnerable and limited, a person who did the best he could by you and who is still doing the best he can. It won't change what has happened, but it might help you to let go of some anger and be more forgiving. It might give you a little more patience and tolerance. And if your parent is able and willing to open up as a result of your gentle probing, these talks may relieve some of his pain and fear.

*After my father died I found his old letters and journals, and as I read them I realized that there was this whole other side of him that I never knew, a sensitive and caring and emotional side that he never, even once, revealed to me. It makes me sad because I keep thinking, if only I had known this part of him we might have had a very different relationship.*                —ALICIA B.

◆ **Stop blaming.** Whatever your mother did in the past is done. She probably intended to be a good parent, just as you want to be a good parent to your children. If you need an apology, or if you think it would make you feel better if you told her what you are feeling, then discuss the subject with her, but do it carefully. Remember that the past is over.

# Managing Day-to-Day

Moving from the big picture to the small picture, if your parent has a trait or habit that makes your chest tighten and your shoulders tense, there are steps you can take, day-to-day, to ease the stress and lower your blood pressure.

◆ **Pass by the hooks.** Find ways to ignore those little comments or looks that make you so hopping mad. Pretend you are a fish swimming along a mountain stream on a beautiful day and that you spot a big, fat worm. It lures you, but you know that there's a big, sharp hook behind it. You have two choices: Bite at the hook and get hurt, or swim on by and enjoy your day.

Next time your parent says something that makes your blood pressure rise, say to yourself, "Aha, that is a hook and as much as I am drawn to it, I have no intention of biting." Count how many hooks you pass by and then try to do better the next time. It will be your own inner victory. With each hook you pass, unfazed and unaffected, you really do win.

◆ **Pause before responding.** When your parent does or says something that's abrasive, count to ten before responding. Take in a deep breath from your stomach and then exhale slowly as you count. That brief pause will help you to stay calm and give you a moment to consider your response.

*"My mother is very dependent, always has been, but she never says thank you or shows any appreciation or cares that she is putting you out. I said to her, 'Mom, don't you realize what you are putting us through? Don't you realize the anxiety and worry that you cause?' And she said, 'That's your problem.'*

*I had to laugh at that. I mean, she's your mother. What are you going to do?"* —RHODA B.

♦ **Recognize your habits.** How do you typically react to problems in this relationship? Become angry and combative? Withdraw, or tense up? Throw yourself into your work? Take it out on other people? Eat a pint of ice cream?

Once you're aware of your reaction, you will be better able to alter it. If you start yelling at the children or shutting out your friends, ask yourself "What is this about?" Perhaps you'll notice that it's not about the kids being demanding, but about your visit with your mother that afternoon.

♦ **Forget victory.** Instead of trying to win a fight with your parent, make it your goal simply to end the discussion peacefully. That will be a true victory. Rather than saying, once again, "Why do you always bring up that same story from my childhood? Why can't you just let it go?" say, in your calmest voice, "You know, whenever you tell that story we end up in an argument that goes nowhere. I really don't want to fight

with you. I want to have a nice time with you. I wonder if there's some way we can either resolve or avoid this discussion. What do you think?"

♦ **Head for new ground.** If you find yourself falling into the same uncomfortable or annoying ruts with your parent, change the pattern. Play cards, go for a walk, talk about something new or plan your visits for a different place and time. If you always visit in the evening when your parent is tired or has had a drink, stop by in the morning instead. If you always visit at her house, bring her over to your house. The change may do you both good.

♦ **Reward yourself.** Ignoring the hooks, staying calm, avoiding old fights and generally being more tolerant requires enormous patience and personal strength. These are no small feats. Reward yourself for a job well done. Buy yourself a little present, treat yourself to a bubble bath, take a drive in the country, immerse yourself in some activity that has nothing to do with your parent and her illness.

♦ **Introduce your parent to you, the adult.** If you constantly fall into the old role of your childhood, pull your parent into your adulthood. If she is mobile, take her with you to your office or bring her to a local meeting where you are involved. If she is less mobile, introduce her to your friends, show her your latest business report or bring her some of your artwork. Let her see you as an adult, be firm in your resolve to

**«** *The difficult thing for me is the nonstop talking. I've heard the same conversation over and over, the same exact stories. My mother is a compulsive talker and those are long hours.*

*What I do now when I'm visiting is to ration myself. After I've been with her for a while, listening to her talk, I'll either go out and take a long, long walk by myself, which is great, or I'll try to get her out of the house. This is a new thing and it works quite well. I now get her out every day.*

*It was so important to break that pattern of sitting in the living room, with her in her chair and me on the couch, opposite each other. It opened things up a little.* **»**

—BETTY H.

act as an adult, and she may start to think of you as one and treat you accordingly.

♦ **Adjust your expectations.** Not just your grand expectations about this relationship, but your hopes about each visit, about holiday gatherings, about family to-

getherness. Lower your expectations to as close to zero as possible.

If you envision your family as a Norman Rockwell painting, you are doomed to disappointment. Likewise, if you approach your parent's door poised for a fight, it will probably happen. Family arguments can be ignited simply because you are primed for them. When it happens, you explode. *I knew that's what you would say. You always . . . .*

When you visit, keep your mind open and let things go as they will. Enjoy what's good and try not to make too much of the bad.

♦ **Make note of the good times.** When you have a wonderful visit or a moment of closeness, share a warm hug, or receive a rare word of praise or thanks, don't sell it short. Make a note on your calendar or write a brief description of it, and keep it close at hand. It will help get you through the tougher times.

While you are at it, write a little note to your parent about that special moment or warm feeling you shared. Mail it or leave it by her bed. When a relationship is tense, this is an opportunity to connect in a positive way.

# Chapter Three

# CARING FOR THE CAREGIVER

*Setting Limits • Dealing with Guilt, Anger and Grief • Achieving a Healthy Mindset*

.........................................

W HY WOULD A BOOK ABOUT CARING FOR A PARENT feature a chapter on caring for yourself? Because it's probably the one thing you'll fail to do and it may be the most important thing you can do—both for yourself *and* your parent.

Don't flip past this chapter too quickly, thinking, *My mother needs me. I don't have time for myself right now.* Your parent's care can easily consume an ever-expanding part of your life. It may begin with a few calls here, some visits there, questions for doctors and lawyers. Then, more visits. More worrying. More phone calls. Before you know it—and sometimes without your even realizing it—you are too busy for friends, distant from your spouse, distracted at work and constantly trying to shake a cold.

You need to use all the help that is available, decide how much you are able to give, and then accept that there are limits to what you or anyone else can do in this situation. Gain some perspective, pace yourself and curb your instinct to want to "fix" everything.

You need to take care of yourself, find ways to get away from it all, even to enjoy yourself, in the midst of this ongoing crisis.

# Setting Limits

If there were such a thing as Care-givers Anonymous, the first step in the program would be to get rid of that little voice inside you that says, *I can do it all, I am responsible for everything, and whatever I do, it's never enough.*

Of course you want to make your parent well, make her happy, make her safe. In fact, if it were possible for you to be with her every minute of the day, perhaps you would be. But the truth is that you can't personally do everything that needs to be done for her, and trying to do so will only exhaust and frustrate you without really helping your parent over the long haul.

So how do you use your energies most effectively? If your mother has a sudden and severe illness, of course you'll want to be there. But when her needs are more chronic, when you find yourself taking on

**"***For a long time I visited my mother twice a week, but I was always running and always tired. I started to dread each visit and I was angry at her because I felt it was all her fault. She was ruining my life.***

***Then a friend said to me, 'This isn't her fault. It's your fault.' And, you know, she was right.* "**
                    —FRAN M.

more and more responsibility over a matter of months or years, you must step back, take a realistic look at the situation and draw some boundaries for yourself. Determine what you can reasonably do for your parent and, more important, what you have to stop trying to do. As hard as this is, you may be surprised to discover that setting some limits will relieve your guilt and ease some tension. And you will have more patience and energy for those things that only you can give.

♦ **Examine your motivation.** Why are you helping your parent? It sounds like an odd question, but it's a healthy one to mull over. Do you view your parent's care as a burden that was dumped upon you? Do you feel that you have a duty to care for her? *She's my mother, after all!* Or are you helping because, given your parent's situation, this is what you choose to do?

If you are helping your parent hoping to get the praise, respect or love you never had before, you're headed for disappointment. This relationship isn't going to change now. If you are trying to repay your parent for all she did during your childhood, you can't. It's not possible. In fact, it's not a debt anyone ever intended for you to repay.

Take a moment to consider your motivation, think over your options and make a conscious choice about your involvement in your parent's care. Then, accept this as your choice, not as something your parent or an unfair world has imposed upon you. The work you do for your parent will still be difficult, but it will feel more like an interruption and less like an imposition. It will be about love, not about debt.

♦ **Accept and enlist help.** One way to limit what you do is to let others help. And you need to get them involved as soon as possible. If your father needs some assistance around the house, encourage siblings and other relatives to pitch in. If a friend or neighbor offers to lend a hand, say yes. Other people not only can help, but they often want to help. Let them.

Siblings, in particular, should be called on right away. They might have different ideas about your father's care or ways of doing things you might not agree with, but they too have a right to care for him, and besides, he needs them now. You need them, too. If you begin this as a family effort when the tasks are smaller, you will have each other further down the road when the needs and responsibilities tend to be more monumental. (See Chapter Twelve on dealing with siblings.)

If you don't have siblings or your siblings can't or won't help for some reason, draw on neighbors, aunts, uncles and cousins, local volunteers, and your parent's healthier friends. When more help is needed, consider meal delivery, housekeeping, adult day care and other local services. (Some of these services are free or inexpensive; a few are covered by insurance and Medicaid.)

*"I used to spend hours trying to convince my parents to move out of their big house and to organize their finances. But they didn't do anything. They would ask me questions and listen and act like they were going to do something about it. But they never did.*

*And then I realized, they are not going to change. They are not going to move until something forces them to. And there is nothing I can do about it. It was terribly difficult to back off. You want so much to help and you know things are only going to get worse. It took me three years to give up and let go, and I still struggle with it sometimes. I just have to go along and see what happens next."* —DIANE P.

It's important to get hooked up with such supports early because it gives your parent time to get used to them when he is relatively well, and it makes him less dependent upon a sole caregiver—you.

Let other people give *you* a hand as well—pick up your dog at the vet, bring over a casserole, water your plants, or stay with your parent on occasion so you can get some rest.

♦ **Let go of futile efforts.** Don't waste precious energy trying to get your parent to change her ways if it's clear that she won't. Tell your mother what you think, get others to help in the effort, but if she still refuses to heed your advice, you have no choice but to give up. For example, if you are spending a lot of time researching group homes for the elderly, and she has absolutely no intention of moving, stop the hunt and move on to more productive tasks (like safeguarding the house that she's in).

You may feel that you have failed. You haven't. You may leave your mother in a risky situation. She may fall or run out of money. But you have done all you can and you cannot do anything more. You can't blame yourself if your parent's refusal to accept help leads to an illness or injury. (See page 16 for more on when to intervene.)

Letting go of hopeless crusades is an enormous accomplishment. It enables you and your parent to live within the current situation until events provide a new perspective.

♦ **Reign yourself in.** Be candid with yourself in determining what help is essential. Day-to-day your parent's care may seem more pressing than other matters in your life—*everything* you do for your parent at this point may seem essential—but think about it. Visiting your mother every day may be valuable for both of you, but wouldn't she be okay with fewer visits? Try to distinguish between your impulse to relieve your own anxiety about your parent's welfare and the true demands of the situation.

As you decide what's truly necessary, consider what you may be ignoring or giving up because of the burden of your parent's care. Are you willing to jeopardize your own health? Neglect your children? Damage your career? You may decide to skip a trip to Florida because your father is in the hospital, but when he is in the midst of a prolonged illness, should you cancel a special dinner out with your husband or miss a deadline at work?

Now create a pared-down schedule for yourself that meets your parent's most pressing needs—the things that only you can do for her—while still respecting your own needs. Even if you live with your parent, set some parameters—what hours you will be with her each day, which tasks you will do for her. Schedule time away from her just for yourself.

Be conservative in your plan; it always feels better to increase your commitment than to decrease it. Don't promise to make three visits a week or three visits a month if that puts you over the edge; keep it at two. Then, when you talk with your parent, focus on what you will do for her, not on what you won't.

One quick word of warning: Don't use no-mate-no-kids as an

*"When I retired, I didn't tell my mother. I didn't want her to think I was more available, that I had more time for her. I had been taking care of her for several years and when I retired I realized there was a lot that I wanted to do for myself, a lot that I had neglected because of her.*

*I told her that I was working from home more, in case she called and found me there, but I didn't tell her that I had retired. And I have never regretted it."* —BARBARA F.

excuse for doing more than you can reasonably manage or tolerate. Your time is no more expendable, no less important because you are single. You have a career, relationships, and other commitments that need your attention. Don't underrate yourself or your needs, or let a family member make judgments about when you "should" be available.

◆ **Learn to say "no."** Caregivers are often as bad at saying "no" to requests for help as they are at saying "yes" to offers of help. Learn to say no to your parent, certainly, but also learn to say no to yourself. It may be your own psyche and your own needs that drive you to do more than you can handle, while your parent may be fine with less help, with assistance from a community service and with fewer visits.

Women, in particular, often have trouble saying no; they feel they must be the "good girl" or "strong daughter." This martyr syndrome is neither helpful nor "good."

Convince yourself that saying no to certain things is not only okay, but necessary. Practice. Try it out on the dog. Say "no" to the mirror. But get the word out. Confronted with a parent's escalating needs, you may learn, perhaps for the first time in your life, how to act on your own behalf.

◆ **Stick to your guns.** Sure, you can decide to cut back on some visits, even put a plan in writing, but how do you stick to it? Say you decide that your marriage or some other primary relationship needs more attention, but just as you and your mate settle in for a quiet evening together, the first in weeks, you find yourself wondering if your father is all right and feeling guilty for not being with him. You're short with your mate when he asks what's troubling you, or you call your father and feel even worse when he asks why you don't come see him.

Be firm in your resolve. If you decide that you are not going to concern yourself with your father's financial affairs anymore, don't spend an evening researching home equity loans. If you've told your mother you cannot be interrupted during work and she continues to call, remind her quickly and gently that this is not the time to talk and that you'll call her when you get home.

And don't be unduly influenced by how someone else is handling a comparable situation. Just because a colleague sees her mother every weekend and once during the week doesn't mean that you should further strain your schedule. Just because your cousin cared for her mother at home for twelve years and is critical that you aren't doing the same, don't feel apologetic. Only you can create the right balance for yourself. Find it and keep to it.

**❝** *The last time I went to my support group, this woman was talking about her father, who has dementia. She was taking care of him twenty-four hours a day, and she was so warm and had such a nice sense of humor about it all that I thought, 'This woman is a saint.' It made me feel terrible.* **❞**   —LINDA K.

# Emotional Minefields

Taking care of yourself, simply surviving parentcare, requires that you deal with some potent emotions. Believe it or not, reactions you are experiencing now, even the ones that seem disturbingly out of character for you, illogical or childish, are normal and quite common. And most of them can be tempered once you recognize what it is you are feeling and why.

## GUILT AND HELPLESSNESS

These are the constant companions of caregivers, with women more often plagued by guilt and men more often frustrated by feelings of helplessness. Women seem to have inherited a burden of guilt from their mothers, and their grandmothers before them. *I'm not doing enough, I'm not doing it right, I should have done something else.* Men, on the other hand, tend to want to fix problems, and become exasperated when they can't be fixed. In general, they also aren't as experienced as women in the hands-on care and empathy that is required when a parent is frail or sick, so they feel all the more helpless. And whatever your gender, distance can compound feelings of guilt and helplessness.

Getting a grip on these emotions is essential, and you'll have to do so again and again, for they have a habit of reappearing. Consider for a moment whatever it is that you

think you should be doing for your parent and are not. How reasonable are your expectations? Can you realistically do these tasks? Would performing them help your parent significantly?

Now look at the situation from the opposite perspective. Instead of berating yourself for not doing something, focus on what you *are* doing for your parent. Make a list of these things and be sure to include absolutely everything that

*"I wish I was there with my father. Absolutely. I saw him a lot over the summer and that really made me happy. I loved being there for him. But I guess that's easy for me to say from a distance. While I feel a bit at a loss, the grind of being there on a daily basis is very hard on my brother. Because I'm far away, I appreciate each visit, each minute. I am always afraid when I leave that it might be the last time."* —JANE C.

you provide—emotional support, regular phone calls, visits, letters, talks with doctors, help with financial matters, assurance that your parent will be cared for in the future and that his wishes will be respected. Recognize and be proud of what you are giving and give it generously.

## ANGER AND RESENTMENT

Try to alleviate any anger or resentment as soon as you recognize that you are feeling it.

## THOSE UNTHINKABLE THOUGHTS

Many people caring for an aged parent wish, at some point along the way, that this parent would die. It may be a fleeting thought or a constant presence. Either way, it's very disturbing.

If you are wishing your mother would die because she is terminally ill and in pain, then you shouldn't have any guilt about such thoughts. They are normal and, in most cases, even merciful.

The trouble comes when you are wishing your father would die because he has become a burden to you, or because caring for him is using up all the family money, or because you are simply tired of worrying and wondering. In other words, you want him to die less for his sake than for yours. This is a common and natural reaction, but it is jolting when the thought first comes into your mind, and it can produce a great deal of guilt and shame. *I can't believe I'm thinking such things. I must be a really horrible person.*

Watching and caring for an ill parent over time is draining—emotionally, physically and financially. Since there is really no other possible outcome, it is natural to want the struggle to end, for everybody's sake. You are not a bad person for feeling this way. You are only human.

Reframe your resentment. That is, rather than wishing that the person or the situation you're resenting would change, think about what you can do to change things. If you resent your parent because you are doing too much and missing out on your own life, then back off. Do less. If you resent your spouse for not sympathizing or helping, try to understand his perspective and then talk to him about what *you* might do to remedy any conflict.

Anger is more difficult to deal with because it is so hot and blinding. Be careful. Anger can lead to rash acts and regrettable words. When you feel angry, try not to take any action right away. Distance yourself from the situation and wait until you simmer down. Once you're calmer, address the reason for your feelings. You don't want your anger to explode, but you also don't want to suppress it or it will implode.

Ask yourself what made you so stomping mad. What would ease the fury? Can the enraging situation be changed? If not, how can you respond to it differently so you don't become quite so angry the next time?

If you have trouble thinking clearly about this, try writing it down. Writing can help blow off

## AROUND AND AROUND WE GO

Don't fall into the anger-guilt-anger cycle. *My mother annoys me. I get angry with her. I feel guilty for getting angry. I resent her for making me feel bad, so I find her even more annoying. Then I get angry....* Recognize the cycle, determine what gets you on this merry-go-round, and then next time, try to stop it before it starts. If you do get angry, forgive yourself immediately. Don't feel guilty. Snapping at your parent and other emotional outbursts are typical reactions to this kind of stress.

a little steam without burning anyone in the process. It can also, with time, help to clarify some issues—and sometimes, as a result, lead to solutions.

Keep a diary for several months, or just let loose on any handy piece of paper whenever you find yourself on emotional overload. If you are uncomfortable addressing a diary, write a letter to the person who caused the anger, a friend, or some made-up therapist, describing the problems and your feelings (but don't send it). While you write, don't think about sentence structure or grammar or legibility, just scribble down the thoughts as they come to you—they will come fast once you let it happen. If it's easier, talk into a tape recorder that you keep by the bed or take along in the car.

If anger or the situation that is precipitating it get beyond your control, talk to a therapist. Therapy can be enormously helpful in sorting out overwhelming feelings of anger.

### SORROW AND GRIEF

All of us grieve in our own way, at our own pace. The sadness can be constant, or it may crash over you in waves at odd times. Go with it and allow yourself time to grieve. There is nothing weak or selfish about grieving. And holding in the feelings may make you tense or withdrawn from your parent, when it's the opposite you want. Take some time away from work. Spend time alone if you feel the need, or share your pain with others. Then, while

**"***My mother has always been my best friend, and after my father died we only became closer. The idea of losing her is too painful for me to bear. She has always been there for me, always understood me. When she is gone, no one will do that for me. I can't imagine my world without her.*

*Sometimes after I hang up the phone when she sounds down or weak, I feel helpless and sad. I cry so hard that I can't breathe. I guess I'm lucky to have a mother that I love this much, but sometimes I think that if I didn't, it wouldn't hurt so much.* **"**    —CAROL P.

you still have time, let your mother know that you are sad, that you love her, that you will miss her. Don't miss this opportunity to tell her how you feel. (See Chapter Eighteen for more on grief.)

## SUPPORT GROUPS

More than anything else, support or self-help groups help you to see that your situation is not unique, that others face many of the same difficult issues and turbulent feelings. This in itself can be an enormous relief. Because group members are usually strangers, it's a safe arena in which to air intimate problems, vent anger or talk about feelings you might be ashamed of. And because you all

*" Sometimes in the evening I reach a point when I think, 'I'd just rather not go out tonight.' But I always come home from the support group feeling better. Because everyone in the group is dealing with someone with dementia, it helps me see that what my mom is doing is perfectly normal for this disease. I also see that what I'm feeling isn't cruel or selfish or crazy. Even if I never see these people again when this is over, I'll never forget them. "* –BARBARA F.

face similar situations, you understand each other in a way that others, even best friends, cannot.

Support groups are particularly

## DEEP IN DEPRESSION

Depression is a physical illness that needs immediate medical attention. If you have symptoms of depression—feelings of extreme sadness, relentless waves of self-criticism, apathy and hopelessness, changes in eating or sleeping habits, trouble concentrating, thoughts about death—consult a doctor immediately. Depression can usually be treated quite effectively with counseling and/or medication. (See page 106 for more on depression.)

For immediate help call the local crisis intervention, suicide or depression hotline, or 911. For information about depression and a referral to a local specialist, contact:

**The National Foundation
for Depressive Illness
(800-248-4381)**

**The National Mental
Health Association
(800-969-6642)**

**The National Institute of
Mental Health's Depression
Awareness, Recognition and
Treatment (DART) Program
(800-421-4211)**

wonderful for people who feel isolated either because they have no other friends in the same situation or because they aren't interested in opening up to friends or siblings about the subject. They are also a godsend for people who simply feel overwhelmed by the situation at hand and want to see how others handle it (or fail to handle it).

The nature of support groups varies widely in terms of purpose and membership, and you may need to try two or three before finding one that meets your needs. Some groups are designed for people caring for a sick parent, while others zero in on specific issues—family relationships, Alzheimer's, stroke, cancer, death. Some are set up so people can share practical information and resources for help, while others function purely as emotional outlets. Some have leaders, others are group-led. Although support groups are usually for the caregiver, some encourage the parent to attend as well.

To find a support group, call your area agency on aging (see Appendix A), Children of Aging Parents (215-945-6900) or the National Self-Help Clearinghouse (212-354-8525). Most nursing homes, adult day-care centers and mental health clinics should also be able to refer you to nearby support groups. If you are interested in a specific topic, look in the phone book for the appropriate association, many of which either run support groups themselves or can refer you to one (for example, the Alzheimer's Association, the American Cancer Society, Emotions Anonymous).

# 12 Steps to a Healthy Mindset

Setting limits and coping with guilt take a lot of discipline and practice. Here are some more modest and perhaps enjoyable ways to ease stress and take care of yourself. Think of it as your own 12-Step Caregiver Program.

## TAKE FIVE

If you are caring for your parent on a regular basis, especially if you are living with him, remove yourself completely from the situation once in a while. You need to refuel and you can't do it without some distance. Do it before you are too distraught to plan or enjoy such a break.

Make arrangements for any necessary fill-in help (a schedule of family, friends, volunteers, home-care workers), or get your parent into one of the many respite programs available at a hospital or nursing home. (See page 188.)

Then, while you are away, be completely away. Do something just for yourself. Think about something else. Talk about anything else. Clear your head.

## A FRIEND INDEED

When you are caring for an aging parent, quite often the first thing that goes is your social life. Invitations are turned down and friendships are put on hold because you simply do not have the time or the energy for them. If you are living with your parent, social isolation can become a serious problem.

But friends are more important now than ever. They can provide a sympathetic ear, make you laugh, get you thinking about other things and remind you that you are not alone. Studies show that caregivers who have social supports, and use them, experience less depression and illness and generally are less overwhelmed by their responsibilities than those who don't. So rather than cutting yourself off, reach out to your friends. Find a way. Make it a priority. Go out for lunch with them, go for a walk or at least call them on the phone. Just as you would be there for them, your friends want to be there for you.

## SHIFT GEARS

Whenever you are feeling Type A, think Type B. Researchers have actually timed people who run through red lights and blast their horns at pedestrians, and they have found that these racers don't save themselves any time at all. In fact, hurrying often slows things down because in the rush you are more apt to spill food on your shirt or misplace your car keys.

Slow down. If you are driving somewhere and it takes twenty minutes to get there, don't try to make it in nineteen. Leave extra time and then relax and use that time to listen to your favorite music or a book-on-tape, or to think about an issue that needs some solitary meditation.

Or simply relish the silence. Stay in the slow lane, wait until the light turns green and leave the honking to the geese.

## THE WORRY HOUR

Caring for a parent means worrying—lots and lots of worrying, most of it useless, but nonetheless unavoidable. Rather than stewing during a meeting at work or lying awake at three o'clock in the morning, set aside a specific time, 15 minutes or half an hour each day, just for worrying. It sounds ridiculous, but it works. When you can't stop fretting, jot down whatever it is you are thinking about and know that you will contemplate it during your "worry hour." Then, go back to sleep.

## LOVE TO LAUGH

Laughter is a forgotten healer. It makes the world sane (or at least it makes the insanity more fun) and

**"***My mother had a mastectomy and sometimes she forgets to put her prosthesis in. She'll come downstairs with her shirt all askew and sagging and, after standing there for a minute or two, she'll say, 'Something is not right.'*

*And I look at her and I have to laugh. 'Mom,' I say, 'you forgot your boob.' And we'll both laugh. She thinks it's funny, too. It could happen to anyone. If we didn't laugh, we would cry. It's that sort of thing.***"**
—CAROL G.

# HEALTHY BODY, HEALTHY MIND

The mind-body connection works in two directions. You can boost your physical health with a positive outlook, but you can also improve your outlook by tending to your physical health. Now, when your energy and optimism may be taking a bit of a beating, it is more important than ever that you eat well, exercise and get plenty of rest. Yes, you've heard it all before, but now give it a real try. Make a concerted effort for two or three months to take care of your body, and see if you don't notice a dramatic difference in your mood and attitude.

## Good Eating

Good eating habits take up very little extra time, if you follow a few general guidelines. (See Appendix D, page 407, for details on nutrition.)

❖ Don't eat on the run, wolfing down a sandwich in the car or eating stew out of a pot while you talk on the phone. Make meals a time for enjoyment, dinner in particular. Slow down, and even if you are eating alone, set the table, light some candles and put the stew in a dish. Savor the meal.

❖ Plan the week's meals in advance and make a detailed shopping list so you don't have to run to the store for forgotten items or rely on take-out food every night.

❖ Keep your cupboard shelves and freezer packed with good, healthful food (pasta, canned tomatoes, tuna, frozen vegetables, etc.) so there is always something for dinner.

❖ When you cook, make plenty. Freeze extra portions for another day, or turn leftovers into new meals. A large, roasted chicken can be used for sandwiches, a chicken omelette, cream of chicken on rice, and then soup.

❖ When buying prepared foods, look for ones with the least amount of fat and sodium.

❖ Make better choices, even when you're in a hurry. Rather than racing out the door in the morning with a cup of coffee and a muffin (most muffins are full of fat), have a hunk of dark, grainy bread and a glass of orange juice. Rather than getting a quick burger at the lunch wagon, opt for a salad or bring your own healthful meal to work.

## A Little Sweat

There is nothing like a workout to shed pent-up emotions, clear a muddled head and revive a tired body.

❖ Make it doable. Weight training and rigorous workouts are great for you, but if you hate that sort of thing, find something else. It's better to walk two miles a few times a week and stick to it than to run four miles daily and give up after three weeks. Whatever exercise regime you choose, try to find one that lasts at least 20 minutes and includes some variation.

❖ Make it social. If you find an exercise partner, you will be less apt to excuse yourself from the routine, and you get the added benefit of socializing while you sweat.

❖ Make it useful. If you don't think you have time for exercise, combine errands and physical activity. Rake the yard, walk to work, or clean out the basement. Read the newspaper while you ride on a stationery bike. Talk to a co-worker about a new project while you walk along a track. Or chat with your parent while you stretch.

❖ Make it fun. Exercise doesn't have to be boring. Play tennis, go swimming, skate on a frozen pond, or dance to your favorite Motown songs.

### Regular Check-ups

Are you urging your parent to see a doctor but neglecting your own health? Stop postponing that physical or your appointment with the dentist. Don't put off your mammogram or your eye exam any longer. Your parent may provide a handy excuse for you to cancel medical check-ups, but don't.

### Zzzzz

In studies of laboratory rats, scientists have found that severe sleep deprivation is always fatal. In humans, it certainly feels deadly, causing irritability, poor concentration, lack of coordination and forgetfulness. Make rest a priority—go to bed early and take time out for naps when necessary—because it enhances far more than your physical appearance; it bolsters your immune system and keeps your mind clear, alert and calm.

### Some Pitfalls

For people under stress, one cup of coffee each morning can gradually turn into three. A glass of wine with dinner can become a scotch before dinner and half a bottle of wine during the meal. Be aware of how much caffeine and alcohol you are consuming because without realizing it you can start imbibing more and more. Avoid using drugs of any kind, including sedatives, antidepressants and antianxiety pills, unless you are taking them under the supervision of a doctor. And be careful not to use food to calm your frazzled nerves. When you reach the bottom of the Pepperidge Farm bag, you won't feel any better; in fact you'll probably feel a little sick.

## MAINTAINING A SOCIAL LIFE

If you and your parent live together, you can still have a social life. You just have to be a little flexible.

❖ Leave your parent at home and get a sitter or companion to stay with her, rather than skipping a night out or dragging her into a social situation that will be tiring for her. Even though it may seem like an extravagance *(I don't really have to go out tonight)*, make yourself do it. It's a worthwhile investment in your mental health.

❖ If you want your parent to be involved in a social event, have the guests come to your house rather than going out. Home is a more familiar and comfortable setting for your parent. It also means she can leave the room when she needs to rest, without breaking up the party.

❖ Have a pot-luck supper, with each guest bringing a course, so you're not cooking everything yourself. (If it's a casual gathering, you can ask guests to help prepare and clean up, too.) If you don't feel comfortable having a pot-luck party, at least ask guests to bring wine or dessert to ease some of the workload and expense.

❖ If you decide to cook dinner for guests yourself, make something that's easy to prepare in advance like lasagna or stew, put something on the grill, buy prepared food or order out. And while they are not great for the environment, paper and plastic make for much easier clean-up.

(See page 320 for tips on socializing when your parent has dementia.)

it also makes the body healthier. Scientists have found that a good dose of humor strengthens the immune system, improves circulation, relieves stress and bolsters the spirit.

Of course howling with laughter when someone you love is ill can feel like some sort of sacrilege. You may think that you have to be serious and solemn to reflect the severity of the situation and to show respect for your parent. But you don't. You really don't. It's okay to

laugh, no matter how sick or incompetent your parent may be. In fact, the worse things get, the more aggressively you should seek out things to laugh about.

Find something funny about the situation and your parent probably will, too. (Dentures are funny. Certain sourpuss hospital personnel are funny. The Jell-O served in nursing homes is funny, especially if you jiggle it.) See a slapstick movie, visit a goofy friend, scan the comics, play

a joke on someone, read a Dave Bar-
ry or Molly Ivins book, clown
around with your sisters. Whenever you are exhausted and depressed,
find some way to laugh—a long,
side-splitting, teary, wet-your-pants
kind of laugh. It's good medicine.

## GET SOME PERSPECTIVE

Take time to read the morning
paper or listen to the news. Stay
abreast of what's happening in the
world, in your community and with
your friends. It will help put your
problems into perspective and get
your mind off your situation.

Likewise, if your parent's illness
and needs are a major topic of conversation in your house, or the only
topic, plan a meal during which you
agree they will not be discussed. Talk
about the school play, world events,
or just gossip. Do whatever it takes
to get away from the subject from
time to time.

## TAKE ACTION

Anyone caring for a parent is
bound to have disagreements with
professionals, disputes with institutions and arguments with relatives.
Don't just complain to your friends
about a chronically late home-
care worker, a rude orderly or a
poorly-run meal service. Talk to the
person involved, and if he's not re-
sponsive, speak to a supervisor. Take
action. Without being belligerent,
move up the ranks until you get an
acceptable response. Be pleasant but
persistent.

Also, get informed. Ask questions when dealing with profes-

sionals. Learn about your parent's
ailments, ways to appeal Medicare
decisions and patients' rights within a nursing home. Be an educated
advocate for yourself and your parent, and don't be afraid to speak up
when necessary. It's better than letting problems fester and it often
leads to solutions.

## AVOID THE COULDA-
## SHOULDA-WOULDAS

Also known as the If-onlys or
the More-better-different syndrome,
it's a dangerous mindset: *I should
have . . . If only . . .* ad infinitum.

Wishing for things that can't
be, regretting what is, or day-
dreaming about how things used
to be is futile and potentially de-
structive if it keeps you from more
productive tasks. It's human nature
to think this way, but try not to focus on what might have been, and
look instead at what is and what
can be.

## PURSUE OTHER INTERESTS

Hobbies, sports and other such
pursuits are not frivolous pastimes.
Clearing your mind of your worries
—even for brief interludes—will
allow you to regain balance and
energy. So don't forgo your pottery,
gardening, tennis or oil painting, or
feel guilty about enjoying them.
Make it a point to find time for
them. Take pleasure in them.

## SPIRITUAL SUPPORT

Whether you are religious or
not, spiritual issues often arise when

**"**_During my father's illness I got very depressed and closed in. I realized that I needed some outlet, some way of dealing with the constant anxiety. So I started drawing._

_I hadn't done any sketches since I was a little girl, but I bought a pad and some pens and began sketching. For some reason, I can express my rage and fear in drawings better than I can with words. I sketch each night. It's my sanity. I've actually gotten pretty good at it._**"**
—ELEANOR R.

a parent is sick, for the situation provokes troubling questions: _Why would a loving God do this? How do I ease my anguish or grief? How do I face my own mortality?_ Caring for an aging parent can also try one's patience and kindness. A little guidance may help strengthen your will and focus your life. Nearly 75 percent of caregivers say they use prayer as a way of coping.

If going to religious services doesn't interest you, or if you simply want a more personal discussion, most clergy are happy to meet with people individually. Just call. (You can send a little donation if you want to repay the favor.) Sometimes friends can provide spiritual support, even if they just sit quietly with you and listen.

## MEDITATION, MASSAGE AND RELAXANTS

You don't know how much stress you are carrying around until you sit in a relaxation class and let go of it. The techniques you learn there can be used anywhere, anytime, to ease the pressure. Classes in tai chi, meditation and yoga, as well as in general relaxation, all relieve stress. To find out about them, call local gyms, spas, and recreation centers or check the bulletin board at a local health-food store.

If you can afford it, give yourself a real treat by having a massage. You can get the name of a good masseuse or masseur from a doctor or physical therapist or sports medicine center, or by calling the American Massage Therapy Association (312-761-2682).

## INDULGENT NECESSITIES

It may sound like an oxymoron, but some indulgence is a necessity. Everyone needs some pampering occasionally, for both physical and mental health. So treat yourself to a long, hot bath, a shopping spree, an exquisite dinner, room service in a hotel, a facial, an afternoon in the sun, a morning lounging in bed, a new hair style—whatever brings you that special, mischievous pleasure that comes only from indulging yourself.

# Chapter Four

# Doctor Do's and Don'ts

*Rx for the Elderly • A Geriatric Assessment • Finding
a Good Doctor • An Informed Patient*

ALTHOUGH YOU MAY BE DOING THE LION'S SHARE OF THE work, seeing your parent through her senior years is a team effort. And a key member of that team—one who is going to become more important over time—is your parent's personal physician.

Whether your mother is having a routine check-up or a series of tests and treatments for an advanced stage of cancer, she needs a primary physician at the helm who is experienced in treating elderly patients. One doctor should keep track of all of her ailments and medications, refer her to specialists when necessary, and then coordinate her care so that treatments for one problem don't aggravate another—an all-too-common phenomenon in the medical care of elderly patients.

She also needs to be a good advocate for herself, or, if you are managing her care, you need to be an informed advocate for her. That means familiarizing yourself with her treatment options and participating in decisions about them. It means being willing to ask questions, to seek second opinions and, when your parent's medical care is not satisfactory, to find a new doctor. Once your parent has a trusted physician and you become comfortable in your role as her advocate, your work and your worries will be much lighter.

# Rx for the Elderly

Old bodies are not the same as younger ones, so they require slightly different medical care. The operating systems are weaker, which means that an otherwise treatable illness may be life-threatening, a common disease may cause uncommon symptoms, and a recommended dose of medication may produce dangerous side effects. A drug that a young person can use without difficulty can cause confusion, incontinence or blurry vision in an older patient. Symptoms may vary as well. Withdrawal and apathy in an older patient may not signal depression, but stroke or heart disease.

Aside from the fragility of an older body, the sheer number of ailments and the diverse medications they require often complicate the medical care of an elderly person. A doctor caring for an older patient can't simply fix a broken ankle. He or she needs to recognize that the patient has fallen because her vision is waning or because the combination of her arthritis medication and her heart pills is making her dizzy.

For all these reasons, geriatric medicine, more than general medicine, must be holistic. A doctor has to look beyond one or two ailments and examine the entire body within the context of the patient's past and current life. A geriatric doctor needs to be aware of your parent's housing arrangements, exercise regime, diet, daily habits, social supports and perhaps even her financial situation, because each of these plays a role in her general health and well-being.

## A GERIATRIC EXAM

An annual physical of an elderly patient typically includes:

**The body.** A physical exam for an elderly person includes most of the same tests that would be part of any check-up—blood pressure, temperature, weight, and blood and urine tests, as well as any necessary screenings and special tests that are required because of a particular illness, risk or symptom. In addition, the doctor will look for ailments that are common in the elderly (arthritis, weight loss, thyroid problems, heart disease, etc.). And he or she should review your parent's medical history and medications, as older people often take a number of drugs which are not appropriate, either alone or in combination.

Unlike other routine physicals, a geriatric exam focuses on physical ability and function. A doctor will check your parent's legs for rashes or tenderness, but he or she will also be concerned about gait and dexterity. With a few quick and simple tests the doctor can find out if your parent can reach, bend, walk, turn, sit down and get up without difficulty; hear a soft whisper; pick up a spoon; or read his own pill bottles.

**The brain.** The exam will include a quick test of your parent's cognitive abilities and mental state. Elderly people who are in the ear-

## A SEAT IN THE BLEACHERS— OR BEHIND HOME PLATE?

What if your father doesn't want your input or help? What if he doesn't tell you about his medical care or doesn't listen to your advice? As maddening as it may be for you, as long as he is competent he has the right to manage these issues for himself—up to a point.

If you are concerned about your parent's choice of doctors, express your concerns and offer your assistance. Mention that there have been advances in geriatric medicine and point out the benefits of having a doctor who knows about these advances. Likewise, if you are concerned about a medical problem, urge him to talk to the doctor about it.

If he blocks your efforts and the issue isn't dire, you may have to back down. But when you think the problem is serious—your mother fainted while walking to the car, she has become uncharacteristically contentious and disoriented, or she has occasional but acute chest pains—you have to be more aggressive. Urge, nudge, push and, finally, demand. If, for example, your mother refuses to mention a serious symptom to her doctor, ask her to "do it for me." If she keeps her heels dug in, call the doctor yourself and talk about the problem, or take your mother to the doctor yourself.

It may agitate her or make you feel like the villain, but when your parent's health is in serious jeopardy, there's no time to worry about her privacy or delicate feelings.

liest stages of dementia can usually compensate for mental lapses with family members, but it's not so easy to cover things up in an exam. And it's helpful to get a diagnosis early.

To check your parent's cognitive abilities the doctor might, for example, ask her to think of three items and then recall them a minute later. If there is any question about her mental abilities, the doctor will conduct a more comprehensive exam. (The exam and follow-up tests are described on page 304.)

The doctor should also ask about any past psychiatric care and your parent's current mental state, including moods, fears and anxiety. If there is any suggestion of depression, an anxiety disorder or other mental illness, the doctor might refer your parent to a geriatric psychiatrist for further evaluation.

**The person.** The doctor or a staff nurse or social worker should ask about your parent's eating, sleeping, exercising and toileting habits. They should also inquire, at least briefly, about her housing situation and social supports. Such information can alert a doctor to medical

## THINK PREVENTION

Prevention is the most important and most ignored aspect of health and medicine today. For the elderly, who cannot bounce back from an illness or an injury as easily as their younger counterparts, prevention is critical.

But prevention may not have been part of your parent's upbringing. He may come from the school of if-it-ain't-broke-don't-fix-it, which means that you may have to do some gentle but forceful persuading.

Make sure your parent's living situation is as safe as possible, see that he is eating healthfully, urge him to get a little exercise (see page 155), encourage him to remain mentally active, and keep after him to have regular physicals, eye exams and dental check-ups. He should also have a one-time pneumococcal vaccine to fight pneumonia and should get an influenza shot each fall, as elderly people are highly susceptible to the flu. (Flu shots are often offered for free at senior centers and nursing homes.)

ailments such as depression, insomnia or incontinence, and also point up practical problems and potential risks. If your mother can't get to the toilet, would a commode placed by her bed be helpful? If she is losing weight, does she need to be put in touch with a meal-delivery service? If she lives alone, is she at risk of falling or other accidents?

If your parent needs social services, the doctor's office may be able to refer her to some. If not, you may have to consult a geriatric social worker or care manager.

## A GERIATRIC ASSESSMENT

Because the medical care of the elderly can be so complex, many hospitals and clinics have established geriatric assessment centers (also called geriatric evaluation units). In these centers, a geriatrician heads a team of specialists (neurologists, psychiatrists, rheumatologists, etc.), nurses, social workers, physical and occupational therapists, case workers and dietitians, who address all facets of your parent's health and life. Studies suggest that for very frail or incompetent patients, such comprehensive care can mean fewer accidents, less illness, longer lives and greater independence.

While some of these centers provide primary medical care, replacing the family doctor, most act as consultants in cases where the patient has dementia, multiple ailments, difficult-to-diagnose symptoms, or a lot of problems managing at home. Patients are typically referred to a geriatric center by their personal doctors, but you or your parent can make an appointment directly if you have nagging concerns that aren't being answered by his doctor, or if you believe that he needs more comprehensive care than his doctor can offer.

A geriatric assessment lasts anywhere from three hours to several days and includes a detailed physical, neurological and mental exam, as well as evaluations by social workers and nurses who will talk with your parent, and perhaps with the family, about your parent's daily life and future. The team will provide counseling as well as practical help, hooking your family up with local services and housing options.

Geriatric centers are usually found in big medical centers or hospitals in large cities, although some are now opening elsewhere. To find

## IN THE EXAMINING ROOM

If you stay with your parent during any segment of the exam, stay in the background as much as possible. Be careful not to answer questions addressed to him because quite often, the doctor is not simply looking for an answer but is observing how your parent responds. You also need to give your parent and the doctor a chance to develop some rapport. If possible, wait until the discussion period to add any information that may have been omitted.

one, ask your parent's doctor or call hospitals in the area. The American Geriatrics Society (212-308-1414) has a partial list of geriatric centers around the country.

# A Good Doctor

Just as children see pediatricians, who specialize in caring for the young, your parent needs a doctor who is familiar with the ailments that are common in old age and savvy about the symptoms, treatment regimes and side effects that are unique to elderly patients.

While it is preferable to have a doctor who specializes in geriatrics, it is by no means essential. Family practitioners and internists are perfectly capable of caring for your parent, especially if they have had a good deal of experience with elderly patients.

If your parent has a primary doctor whom he trusts, he may not need to look any further. But if he needs to find a specialist to treat a specific ailment, or if he is hunting for a primary doctor, a number of issues are worth considering.

◆ **A matter of instincts.** The healing process starts in the mind. If your parent becomes very sick, she will fare better in the hands of someone who is competent and who also instills confidence in her. For this reason, choosing a doctor is partly a matter of personality. A good primary doctor should be one whom your parent trusts and feels comfortable with. If your parent doesn't like a doctor, but can't quite explain why, help her to find someone else.

Open, two-way communication is essential. The doctor should be honest about your parent's health and prognosis and should explain, in simple terms, the necessity for and the results of all tests. In addition, your parent or you should be informed of all treatment options. The doctor should be willing to admit when he or she is uncertain about something or when answers simply don't exist. Likewise, your parent should feel free to ask questions, even those that may seem silly, and to talk openly about any delicate matters or embarrassing symptoms.

Gut instinct is less important when you are looking for a specialist who will treat a specific medical problem. Then, credentials and experience should receive more weight.

◆ **A credential check.** Take a look at the prospective doctor's background—medical school, residency training, board certifications and any other qualifications. You can learn about these either by asking the office secretary or by looking in the *Directory of Medical Specialists,* which can be found in most public libraries (the directory may not be complete, so it's best to ask the office secretary or receptionist).

◆ **Beyond credentials: experience.** A Harvard degree does not always a good doctor make. Just as important as credentials is the doctor's experience in treating elderly patients or treating the problem that plagues your parent, whether it's Parkinson's disease or diabetes. If

*"My father had several doctors. When he had his stroke and we brought him home to take care of him, I didn't know who to turn to. His oncologist had been called in while he was in the emergency room, but our family doctor was the one who read his X rays. It was such a horrible time and I was juggling phone calls and information from three or four doctors and trying to sort through this tray of medications that Dad was taking. Finally I called our family doctor and explained the situation and asked if he would oversee his care. Then I called the other doctors and explained the situation to them. I was worried about alienating them, but they were relieved. One of them said, 'This was just as confusing and frustrating for us as it was for you.'"* —ALICIA B.

your parent's doctor is not a geriatrician, find out what percentage of his or her practice is devoted to elderly patients.

◆ **Financial considerations.** You or your parent also need to find out whether a particular doctor "accepts assignment," which means that he or she accepts Medicare's predetermined fees as full payment for services. If not, and if the doctor charges a higher fee, your parent will have to pay the difference out of her own pocket unless she has Medigap insurance. (See Chapter Thirteen for details on Medicare and Medigap.) Before making an ap-

## WHAT TO BRING TO THE DOCTOR'S OFFICE

Before going to the doctor's office for a non-urgent visit, you or your parent should gather all pertinent health insurance cards—Medicare, Medicaid, Medigap, or other identifying health insurance documents—and make a list of all relevant medical information as well as any questions you have. (It's often difficult to remember these matters once an exam begins.) The doctor will need to know about:

❖ Past illnesses or injuries, tests, hospitalizations, surgery

❖ Any current symptoms—dizziness, fatigue, confusion, swelling, bleeding, nausea, weight loss or gain, bowel or bladder problems, personality changes. When did they begin and how? Were they sudden or gradual? The doctor will find it very helpful if you or your parent ranks these concerns in order of their importance rather than mentioning them vaguely or with equal emphasis.

❖ Medications taken in the past and those being used currently, including prescription and over-the-counter drugs as well as diet supplements (also diet aids, nicotine gum, vitamins, laxatives, decongestants, sedatives, eye or nose drops, medicated creams, patches, etc.). You might have to search your parent's medicine cabinets and drawers to compile a complete list.

❖ Allergies or sensitivities to medications or other substances

❖ Daily eating, sleeping, toileting and exercise habits

❖ Eyeglasses, hearing aids, dentures or other such devices

❖ Any obstacles faced in daily life—problems with bathing, getting dressed, balancing the checkbook, climbing stairs, communicating clearly

❖ Family history of physical or mental illness—including parents, siblings, grandparents, children and blood-related aunts and uncles—which can provide clues to hereditary risk

❖ Information about tobacco, alcohol or other substance use

❖ Prior exposure to heavy metals or chemicals (usually in a workplace)

❖ Names and phone numbers of previous doctors who might have your parent's medical records.

## BEWARE OF AGEISM

Ageism—prejudice against old people—is rampant, even among doctors, social workers and other professionals who routinely deal with the elderly. Many people expect those who are aged to be frail, confused, depressed and riddled with disease, so they don't do anything to help change the situation. They fail to treat many of an old person's ailments, or to address his loneliness or his worries. *What does he expect at his age?* Sometimes professionals even further the deterioration by corralling elderly people into situations in which they have few challenges and no control.

But many of the ailments, as well as the loneliness and boredom, that are common in old age can be treated.

Beware of ageism in yourself, in others and even in your parent, who may feel that he is just a worthless old man. Encourage him to get adequate medical care, to go out and do the things he loves, to make friends and pursue hobbies. Your parent should enjoy life to its fullest despite his age—and because of it.

pointment, ask the office secretary about the doctor's policy or look in the *Medicare Participating Physician/Supplier Directory,* found in libraries, social security offices, area agencies on aging and senior citizens' organizations.

◆ **Affiliations, associates and emergency back-up.** Check whether a doctor has admitting privileges at a respected hospital. And, if possible, find a doctor with a broad range of contacts who will be able to recommend qualified specialists, if needed. If the doctor is in a group practice, find out whether your parent will see this particular doctor only, or whether he may be assigned to whoever is available that day. Is the doctor available on an emergency basis? Some stick to an eight-to-four schedule. Does he or she have an associate who covers during vacations?

◆ **A shared philosophy.** Get your parent to discuss with the doctor her feelings about medical care, specifically treatment at the end of life. She needs a doctor who respects—and will uphold—her wishes, whether that means forgoing aggressive medical treatment or fighting to the end.

## HOW TO FIND A GOOD DOCTOR

You or your parent can find a good geriatric doctor by talking to friends, relatives or colleagues. Or you can get a recommendation from a trusted gynecologist, pediatrician

*"Mum has one general doctor, who is what I would call a social doctor. He's kind and he's sweet-looking, but he is not a help. He has missed so many things it's amazing. When she was in the hospital after her hip operation, he was going to let her go home without night nurses even though she couldn't get out of bed. Then last fall he failed to realize that she had severe congestion in her lungs. He'd prescribed diuretics for her, but never checked to see whether or not she was taking them. He's not thorough at all. He just reassures her and says, 'You're doing splendidly.'*

*She says, 'I know he isn't a good doctor but I can't leave him. He's been Dad's doctor and my doctor for too long.' I can't push her to do anything once she's made up her mind. It just means that we have to keep closer tabs on her health and keep pressing him when we think something is wrong. Once I called to see when he would be on vacation and then made an appointment for her during that time just so another doctor in the practice would examine her.*"

—BETTY H.

or another medical professional. If you happen to be visiting a geriatric unit in a hospital, ask the nurses about good local geriatricians. Or call the head of internal medicine or geriatrics at a well-reputed local hospital or medical school and ask for guidance. If you live far away from your parent, a geriatrician in your own vicinity may be able to make a recommendation, as doctors often get to know each other at medical conventions.

Local medical societies and hospitals can give you the names of doctors from their lists of members and employees. (Tell them that you are looking for a board-certified geriatrician or a doctor who treats a lot of elderly patients.) Most public libraries, social security offices, area agencies on aging, hospitals and senior citizens' groups have directories of doctors, such as the *Directory of Medical Specialists* and the *American Medical Association Directory*.

Once you have a list of potential doctors, call and ask the receptionist or nurse some questions, and take note not only of the answers, but of the person's degree of courtesy and helpfulness. It's worth asking for a brief interview with the doctor. (Some doctors will agree to give one and some won't.) Generally speaking, if the doctor can't schedule a routine physical within the next four to six weeks, he is overbooked and your parent should find someone else.

## ALTERNATIVE MEDICINE

Alternative, or unorthodox, medicine—acupuncture, herbs, imagery, homeopathy, osteopathy—has gained enormous popularity in recent years, partly because many people have become disenchanted with traditional medicine, and partly because a growing number of people claim to have had success with alternative techniques.

There is virtually no solid scientific data available on the value

## CHANGING DOCTORS MIDSTREAM

Small disagreements or doctor-patient tussles can often be remedied by talking about them (or writing a letter, if that's easier), but when the problem is insurmountable, urge your mother to find another doctor. Thank the first one for his or her time, but explain that your parent has found someone with whom she feels more comfortable.

People are often reluctant to switch doctors, no matter how dissatisfied they are, because they are embarrassed or afraid of hurting the doctor's feelings. But most doctors understand that different patients have different needs.

If a doctor implies that you are ungrateful for his or her past devotion, or that the care your parent receives elsewhere will be of a lower standard, don't let it affect your decision. Your parent deserves the best care available.

of alternative medicine, however. Some of these therapies may have true medicinal properties, some may heal through a "placebo effect"—healing occurs purely because the patient believes in the process—and some may help heal the body by soothing and calming the mind, which in turn bolsters immunity, circulation and other bodily systems.

Whatever the reasons, some of these practices seem helpful and most are not harmful as long as they are approached with care and are used to augment modern medicine, not replace it.

Your father should check with his doctor before adopting any alternative medical regimens, not to get the doctor's approval of the therapy, but to make sure that it won't interfere with his ongoing medical care. Certain herbal medicines, for example, can be potent drugs and may be hazardous if used with your parent's current medications.

**❝** *I wouldn't say that my mother is into alternative medicine—she doesn't try anything terribly radical. But when she was diagnosed with cancer I bought her a couple of books on diet and nutrition. She started taking a lot of vitamins and drinking what I call her "power drinks," which are loaded with healthy stuff. She also started reading books about emotional states and healing— Bernie Siegel stuff. I think it really helped. She is stronger both physically and mentally. I can see the change in her. It makes her feel like she still has some control, like she can take charge and really fight this thing herself.* **❞**
—DIANA M.

## A WORD OF CAUTION
## ABOUT QUICK CURES

Beware of any claims of quick fixes and medical breakthroughs. Certainly, ads claiming to restore hearing, revitalize skin, reverse baldness and repair arthritis (this last one uses extracts from New Zealand green-lipped mussels, no less) may be tough to pass by. But pass them by you must.

Medical discoveries take place over time and, once made, still must be proved, disproved, tested and re-tested. If you or your parent hear about something that piques your interest, ask the doctor about it. But don't pin your hopes on a cure that sounds too good to be true. It probably is.

# An Informed Advocate

A good doctor is only part of the medical care team; the patient must play an active role as well.

Normally, your parent and his doctor will have their own relationship, which you will have little, if any, part in. But as your parent grows sicker, you may become his advocate if not his spokesperson. The medical world can be confounding and intimidating to an outsider, but try to be bold.

◆ **Ask questions.** If you are overseeing your parent's medical care, feel free to ask questions. If your parent is handling her own care, remind her to ask questions and to note the answers. Don't be embarrassed that you don't know exactly what the liver is, where it is or what it does. Don't pretend that you know what hydrocephalus, an antigen or a fistula is, nodding your head agreeably as the doctor races on. Ask.

Write down any questions that occur to you prior to an appointment and then give them to the doctor so he or she can allot time for them and address the most critical problems first.

If you have questions that can't wait until the next visit—*Is she supposed to take the new medication with dinner or before going to bed?*—call. Don't be intimidated or worry about whether the question is important enough. The doctor may not be able to talk to you, but an assistant should be able to answer your questions, and if necessary the doctor will get back to you later.

◆ **Take notes.** Every time you talk with a doctor or nurse, have a pad handy and take notes. It's easy to forget specifics when you are upset or uneasy about a diagnosis or a procedure. If your parent is still in charge, encourage her to take notes, or ask the doctor to write down any diagnosis or specific instructions. This will be helpful for your parent, who may not remember the details, and it allows her to relay any important information to you or others helping in her care. *He said I had some kind of bowel disorder, oh, what did he call it? Irreversible? Irrational? I don't remember. Something to do with the bowel.*

◆ **Do your homework.** When the doctor hasn't explained the facts clearly or your parent gives you only partial information, do a little research on your own. You don't have to look up every study ever done on coumadin, but find out what blood-clotting is about, what the drugs do to prevent it, what they shouldn't be mixed with and what side effects are possible.

Be sure that your resources are reliable; be leery of sensational articles from popular magazines or advice from friends. Ask the doctor if there are any brochures or other literature about your parent's condition that you might read. Or go to the library and consult a medical encyclopedia or drug handbook for consumers if there's something you still don't understand.

◆ **Be a keen observer.** If you are involved in your father's medical care and you see him fairly regularly, keep a mental note of his moods, habits and complaints. A minor fall, a dull pain, or changes in weight, sleep habits or moods can all indicate a serious medical problem and should be brought to the doctor's attention. Your parent may not alert the doctor to the problem—he may not be aware of the change, he may not want to talk about it or he may not remember to talk about it. So the doctor may have no way of knowing what is going on without your intervention.

◆ **Keep records.** Maintain an updated list of all your parent's medications, including the dose, the date that she began and ended any medication, and any adverse side effects from medications; any allergies; the names, addresses and phone numbers of all doctors seen; special dietary needs; and the dates, places and reasons for any hospitalizations or surgery.

◆ **Use one spokesperson.** If your parent can't oversee her own medical care, one person should be chosen to be the family spokesperson. He or she should be in contact with the doctor's office and then relay information to the others. Of course, it's important that your family spokesperson is sensitive to the concerns of siblings and willing to bring their questions to the doctor's attention. (See Chapter Twelve for more on dealing with siblings.)

◆ **Get a second opinion.** Even if your parent's doctor is the greatest, it's important to get another opinion on any serious matter, particularly when surgery is recommended. Another doctor will either offer new options or be able to reassure you that this is the best way to proceed.

Because a doctor may be reluctant to disagree with a colleague, seek out the second doctor on your own if possible. You are more apt to get an unbiased opinion that way and you are more likely to get a different viewpoint, as doctors tend to recommend people who share their medical philosophy.

◆ **Use caution when comparing.** Don't give too much weight to the tales of other people who had a similar illness. A stroke is not a stroke is not a stroke, particularly when it happens in an elderly body. So don't second-guess the doctor just because Aunt Ashley was cured when she had these same symptoms.

## QUICK ACCESS TO MEDICAL DATA

The Internet is loaded with medical information (as well as caregiver support). Some good starting points are the American Medical Association (www.ama-assn.org), the National Library of Medicine (www.nlm.nih.gov), and the National Cancer Institute (www.nci.nih.gov).

If you don't have Internet access or don't want to do the work yourself, a number of companies will do a search for you for a price ($25 to more than $200, depending on the job). These companies include Health Resource Inc. (501-329-5272), Planetree Health Resource Center (415-923-3680) and Medical Data Exchange (503-471-1627).

The National Rehabilitation Information Center (800-346-2742) will send you a variety of free brochures or supply you with a list of research citations from its computer base ($10 for 100 citations, $5 for each additional 100 citations).

Also, almost every identifiable disease is represented by a corresponding organization that can provide information about the disease and referrals to local resources. For the names of such organizations, call the National Health Information Center (800-336-4797); for information about less common ailments, call the National Organization for Rare Disorders (800-999-6673).

◆ **Be a team player.** While you should be a staunch and persistent advocate for your parent, you also need to work with the doctor and other health professionals. Be open about your concerns and questions, but also try to be patient and understanding. Doctors work under enormous pressures and there are limitations to what they can do.

◆ **Understand the process.** Be aware that no one test or treatment is likely to provide "the cure" or "the answer;" it is just part of an ongoing process. Your desire for clarity and complete relief for your parent may push a doctor to act in ways that are not in your parent's best interests. A doctor might, for example, prescribe a potent drug simply to appease anxious family members who want something done. A linear "cure" mentality is apt to lead to disappointment, and it also might distract you from your parent's more important day-to-day care and comfort.

# Chapter Five

# The Body Imperfect
## Part I

*Vision • Hearing • Sleep Disturbances • Overmedication • Temperature Regulation • Skin Problems • Dental Care*

YOUR OVERRIDING CONCERN RIGHT NOW MAY BE STROKE, cancer, dementia or heart disease, and understandably so. But don't lose sight of your parent's more mundane complaints, such as blurry eyesight, incontinence and restless nights. The doctors will attend to your parent's severe illness, but are apt to ignore these other ailments. And they can add tremendously to your parent's discomfort, dependency and despondency. In fact, for your father they may be more troublesome day-to-day than any life-threatening disease. His poor hearing may distance him from people he loves, his itchy skin may keep him awake at night, his crippled knees may prevent him from doing the things he most enjoys.

Be careful not to pass off these complaints as unavoidable aspects of old age. *That's what happens at 86. What does he expect?* Certainly, many ailments are more common in old age, but that doesn't mean they are less worthy of attention. Your father isn't suffering because he is old; he is suffering because he is sick. And the fact of the matter is that something can be done about almost all of his symptoms. Some are preventable, most are treatable and a few are curable. And life with virtually any disability can be made more manageable.

The information supplied here is not meant to replace the advice of a doctor, but if you're aware of what to expect, if you know the common afflictions of old age and recognize their symptoms, you can be on the lookout for problems that need medical attention. You can also make changes around your parent's house and in his daily life to keep him comfortable and independent for as long as possible.

Understanding what your parent is up against—why he doesn't remember what you said (he didn't hear it), or why he is so grumpy (he is in pain)—should also give you more patience and compassion as you try to help him now.

## ON THE LOOKOUT FOR SYMPTOMS

| | |
|---|---|
| ❏ Vision loss | Squinting, pulling back to read small print, failing to notice stop signs, trouble following sporting events or driving at night |
| ❏ Hearing loss | Saying "what?" a lot, constantly turning the volume up, or staring vacantly while others talk |
| ❏ Insomnia | Complaints of fatigue, long periods spent in bed, frequent naps, wandering at night |
| ❏ Overmedication | A cabinet filled with current prescriptions from multiple physicians; confusion, drowsiness or agitation |
| ❏ Alcohol abuse | Flushed face, confusion, instability and irritability |
| ❏ Hyperthermia | Sweating, dizziness, nausea or, in severe cases, hot and dry skin, rapid pulse and confusion |
| ❏ Hypothermia | Lethargy, confusion, paleness, shallow breathing (even in normal temperatures) |
| ❏ Skin problems | Unusual-looking moles; itchy, cracked, red or irritated skin |
| ❏ Mouth ailments | Pain, dry mouth, difficulty chewing |

# Vision

When your mother squints and then stretches out her arm in order to make out the numbers in the phone book it is probably because she has presbyopia, a type of farsightedness that sets in around age 40, when the lens of the eye becomes more rigid. In most cases, presbyopia is easily remedied with a pair of reading glasses or bifocals. Magnifying glasses from the local drugstore are fine if the condition isn't complicated by other factors.

But there are a number of more subtle changes in vision that typically occur in old age, changes that your parent may not be aware of but that will impede her functioning. For example, older eyes can't see well in dim light, are more easily blinded by glare and can't refocus quickly, from near to far, or from light to dark. They also don't discriminate easily between colors and contrasts, such as the edge of a step, and they have trouble following moving objects, such as cars on the highway. Even if your parent insists that her vision hasn't changed, assume that it has and try to compensate wherever you can around the house. (See box, page 60.)

## EYE DISEASES

In addition to the normal vision changes that happen with age, there are four eye diseases that frequently afflict older people:

◆ **Cataracts.** Ninety-five percent of people over age sixty-five

*When my mother's vision began to fade, she became quite depressed. She always loved to read, but that became more and more difficult until finally she couldn't do it at all. She started listening to the radio and watching television up close. But she missed her reading terribly.*

*It was a nurse at the home who set her up with books-on-tape. She has a good tape player, and each month she receives a stack of tapes in the mail. She listens for hours, and the funny thing is that she has expanded her reading repertoire. She used to just read mysteries. Now it's political books, biographies, racy romances, classical books, everything. She listened to a book last month about World War II planes, and she was telling us all about them. She's like a kid again, learning all this stuff.* —MEL T.

have cataracts, although in most cases the symptoms are mild. With age, the transparent lens of the eye becomes cloudy or filmy, hindering vision, especially if the cataract is in the center of the lens. Even mild cataracts can make the eyes extremely sensitive to glare and bright light, which makes driving at night dangerous.

Having cataracts is a little like viewing the world through a pair of fogged-up goggles, but the change happens so gradually that your parent may not realize anything is wrong. He may simply have trouble doing things, and then become frustrated and embarrassed. This is why it's so important that your parent have regular eye exams.

Cataract surgery for severe impairment has become a relatively simple and painless procedure. And studies show that 95 percent of patients experience dramatic improvement. The surgery is accomplished in about an hour, usually in a hospital clinic or doctor's office, and your parent can return home the same day.

The eye takes about a month to heal fully and several more weeks to adjust. In the meantime, your parent can resume his regular daily activities, including driving, reading and working, although he may have to wear large dark glasses to protect his eyes from harsh light.

◆ **Glaucoma.** People usually don't experience any symptoms of glaucoma until irreversible damage is done—another reason to get your parent to the eye doctor regularly! Untreated, glaucoma can lead to partial or total blindness.

The disease occurs when fluid inside the eyeball fails to drain adequately, and builds up until it squeezes the optic nerve in the back of the eye. As this nerve is damaged, one loses peripheral vision. In some cases, the fluid can be drained through surgery, but sight lost from glaucoma usually cannot be recovered. Glaucoma tends to run in families and is more common among African-Americans and people with diabetes or previous eye injuries.

When the trouble is spotted early, medications can stop or slow the damage. If your parent is given eye drops or other medications for glaucoma, it is critical that she continue to use them even if she doesn't notice any symptoms.

 **FOR MORE HELP**

**National Association for the Visually Handicapped 212-889-3141 (415-221-3201 on the West Coast)** Referrals to low-vision specialists and clinics; information on eyes, vision, diseases, and low-vision aids; a catalogue of low-vision aids; and a library of large-print books and tapes.

**National Federation of the Blind 410-659-9314** Support, advice and information for people who are legally blind.

**The Glaucoma Research Foundation 800-452-8266**

**Association for Macular Diseases 212-605-3719** Information, emotional support and referrals.

For a more complete list of the organizations that serve people with vision loss or blindness, see Appendix B, page 401.

## MAKING THE WORLD MORE VISIBLE

❖ Brighten the house, especially in stairways and places where your parent reads. Older people need nearly three times as much light as younger people. A 75-watt bulb placed one or two feet away is usually fine for reading, but try different intensities to see what's most comfortable for your parent. (A reading light should be positioned behind the shoulder on the same side as your parent's better eye.)

❖ Decrease glare by covering shiny surfaces and avoiding waxy floors. Aim lights at a wall or ceiling to create indirect light. Add blinds or curtains to windows that tend to be filled with bright sunlight.

❖ Distribute light evenly because old eyes have trouble refocusing when going from light to dark.

❖ Get your parent some sunglasses with 100 percent UV (ultraviolet) protection to cut down on glare and to protect her eyes from future damage.

❖ Put night lights in the bedroom, hallways and bathroom as your parent's night vision may be poor.

❖ Use reflector tape or colored tape on the edges of stairs to make the steps easier to see.

❖ Make sure light switches are accessible at the entrance to all rooms.

◆ **Macular degeneration.** This disease occurs when the macula, which is responsible for seeing the fine details in the center of the field of vision, breaks down, or degenerates. It slowly creates a blind or fuzzy spot in the center of one's vision, where straight lines become curved and printed words become disjointed. It usually affects both eyes (sometimes one at a time) and worsens steadily until the blurry area covers several words—the very words the person is trying to read.

Your parent should get medical help early. Once the damage is done, he should consult a low-vision specialist. With the low-vision aids that are available today and some motivation, your parent should be able to read and continue to engage in other activities he enjoys.

◆ **Diabetic retinopathy.** Blood vessels in the retina of the eye leak, blurring vision and sometimes causing blindness if left untreated. The longer someone has diabetes, the greater chance he has of developing this disease. The best prevention is proper care of the diabetes and annual eye exams. Laser treat-

Install lights that are triggered by dusk.

❖ Your parent might want to buy a larger television or perhaps a black-and-white one, which is sometimes easier to view.

❖ Buy lubricating eyedrops, sometimes called artificial tears (not saline solution or eyedrops for redness), available in most pharmacies. Dryness, a common problem, makes eyes itch, sting and burn. (If dry eyes persist, your parent should see an ophthalmologist, as chronic dryness can lead to more serious problems.)

❖ Check your parent's medications and then follow up with a call to the prescribing doctors' offices if you are concerned. Certain medications can disturb vision or make eyes dry.

❖ Review your parent's driving habits and urge him to avoid highways and night-driving.

❖ Wear bright colors when you visit if your parent's vision has grown quite poor.

❖ Write notes in big, clear letters with a black-ink, felt-tipped pen.

❖ If your parent's vision is very faint, encourage her to touch things—hold your hand, feel your face, or explore a new object with her hands.

ment or surgery can often improve vision and slow the decline, but only modestly.

## LOW-VISION AIDS

There is a vast assortment of low-vision products now available that can help make the world more visible—from magnifying glasses and large-print calculators to computers that talk. These products can be found in the catalogues listed in Appendix E, page 416 and in some medical supply stores. Or an eye doctor or other low-vision special-ist should be able to guide your parent to appropriate aids.

Many companies have special services for people who are totally or partially blind. For example, some telephone companies offer dialing aids, free operator assistance and a list of special products to people with vision or hearing disabilities. Other companies may be willing to send catalogues, bills or newsletters in large-print format.

Large-print books, magazines and newspapers that are printed in

18-point type like this,

## MEDICAL ALERT

Your parent should see an eye doctor immediately if:

❖ her vision becomes blurred, distorted or she complains of "seeing double"

❖ her eyes are sore, swollen, or leaking unusual amounts of discharge

❖ she sees flashes of light or halos

❖ she has wandering or crossed eyes

❖ she loses her peripheral vision or her vision in one eye

❖ she becomes acutely sensitive to light and glare.

Even in the absence of symptoms, the American Academy of Ophthalmology recommends that people over 65 have their eyes examined every two years, or more often if a person has an eye disease, a family history of eye disease, or another risk factor, such as diabetes.

for example, are a godsend. *The Complete Directory of Large-Print Books and Serials* can be found in the reference section of most local libraries. Any books not on the library's shelves can be borrowed through an interlibrary loan. You can also make articles or documents more readable for your parent by duplicating them on a photocopy machine that enlarges the original.

The National Library Service for the Blind and Physically Handicapped (800-424-8567), which is part of the Library of Congress, lends books and magazines on cassette tape or floppy disc, as well as the equipment needed to play them—all for free. Postage is also free when returning equipment, tapes or discs. Anyone with poor eyesight or a physical handicap that prevents them from holding a book or turning a page is eligible for these services, through your local library. The National Association for the Visually Handicapped (212-889-3141), also has an extensive lending library of large-print books.

# Hearing

Hearing loss among the elderly is a silent epidemic, so to speak. Estimates suggest that *more than a third* of people over 60 have significant hearing loss! But how many older people visit hearing specialists or wear a hearing aid? Very few. Which means that thousands of older people are walking around with little or no idea of what others are saying.

Loss of hearing can have a dramatic impact on people, more so than loss of vision. As Helen Keller put it, blindness cuts people off from the environment; deafness cuts them off from other people. Over time, poor hearing can make your parent withdrawn, irritable and depressed.

But hearing loss often goes untreated because it develops so gradually that the loss is almost imperceptible. A person doesn't suddenly realize that he can't hear and call the doctor. Instead, he turns up the television a little louder, asks to have things repeated and occasionally misunderstands a comment. And eventually, conversation becomes a chore, not a pleasure.

Furthermore, many people don't lose volume as much as they lose clarity, so again, they aren't aware that they are losing their hearing. A person with sensorineural hearing loss (also known as presbycusis or nerve deafness), which is almost universal among the elderly, may hear you, but he may not understand you. High-pitched sounds, in particular, can become fuzzy, and consonants, such as "s," "f" and "z" may be indistinguishable from one another. Your father may ask you to repeat yourself and when you do so in a louder voice, he says, "Don't shout! I'm not deaf, you know!"

If your parent is saying "What?" a lot, urge him to have his hearing checked by his doctor, or see if his doctor can recommend an otologist or otolaryngologist (doctors who specialize in disorders of the ear). Sometimes the problem can be treated—for example, if an infection, earwax or another obstruction is found. And when it can't be treated, it can usu-

ally be allayed by making changes in the way people communicate (see box, page 64) and by the use of various types of aids.

Because this can be a sensitive subject, approach it gingerly. Ask your father if *he* thinks there is a problem, rather than telling him that there is one. And avoid criticism or accusations. *You never hear what I'm saying. You are as deaf as a doornail.* Instead, try to take some of the blame yourself. *I'm probably not speaking clearly and I need to work on that. Let's approach this together.*

## HEARING AIDS

The move to hearing aids, with all the stigma that is attached to them, may be a tough one. Your father may resist this with his heels dug in.

If you can convince him to get his hearing checked, then the onus of discussing hearing aids is on the doctor. If you are doing the convincing, be sympathetic to your father's distaste for this idea. Explain that a hearing aid will be less embarrassing than fumbling through conversations and missing what people say. Suggest that he try it out at home first, which will save him any embarrassment. If he finds that it helps him he may be willing to wear it in public. If you hit a wall, try the old standby, "Dad, do it for *me*, just try it for *me*. If you hate it I promise never to mention it again."

If your parent agrees to try a hearing aid, his doctor should recommend someone to fit it for

## MAKING THE WORLD MORE AUDIBLE

❖ Sit or stand within three feet of your parent when talking to him (don't yell to him from the kitchen).

❖ Make eye contact. Get your parent's attention—say his name, if necessary—and be sure he is looking at you before you begin speaking. (And make sure he is wearing his glasses.)

❖ Sit in the spotlight. There should be ample lighting, and it should be aimed at you, the speaker.

❖ Turn off the television, the running water or other background noise.

❖ Speak clearly. Don't try to talk to your parent while you are eating, chewing gum or smoking. Enunciate clearly, but don't exaggerate your lip movement, as that can make it difficult to read lips (which we all do a little, even without formal training).

❖ Don't shout, because it will only make your words more difficult to understand. Increase your volume slightly, without raising your pitch.

❖ Use simple and direct sentences. Rephrase the sentence when you are asked to repeat it. Different words may be easier for your parent to grasp.

❖ Use body language (touching, pointing, nodding) and lots of facial expression.

❖ Introduce the subject matter before starting a conversation. "Dad, about Thanksgiving. . . ." If you switch topics midway through a conversation, make that clear: "Okay, now let's talk about your friend Ralph. . . ."

❖ If your parent has tinnitus—ringing or buzzing in the ear—she can buy a tinnitus mask, which fits on the ear and emits "white noise" to drown out the humming inside her ears. Or she can create her own white noise with a loudly ticking clock, or the static of a radio or television. Biofeedback, in which a person learns to control certain bodily functions by becoming familiar with them, can also help. And antidepressants can ease some of the depression and anxiety that often accompanies tinnitus.

him—a certified audiologist, who has a graduate degree in hearing impairment; a licensed hearing aid dealer, who has less training, but usually plenty of experience; an oto-laryngologist (ear, nose and throat physician) or an otologist (ear specialist). Be sure your parent sees someone who is experienced and reputable, because he will be extremely frustrated if a hearing aid is not properly fitted or suited to him.

The specialist should do a complete exam, including hearing tests and evaluations, and then try out various kinds of hearing aids. Models range from tiny ones that fit snugly inside the ear to very powerful packs that are carried in a pocket and connected by a wire to an ear piece. While the smaller models are less visible, they are also less powerful, and they have tiny control knobs that can be challenging for stiff fingers.

A good specialist will not only fit your parent with a hearing aid, but also train him to use it correctly. Whether or not he agrees to wear a hearing aid, your parent might also consult a speech therapist who can help with other ways of improving communication, such as speech reading, or lip reading, which can be taught to people of all ages.

When buying a hearing aid, your parent should shop around because prices vary. If a supplier offers the testing free, the price of the equipment is usually higher. Be sure to shop for good service—proper warranties, repairs and maintenance—in addition to good quality. The aid should come with at least a 30-day trial period, during which one can return the device with a full refund (many suppliers will charge a minimal service fee).

Getting the right hearing aid is only half of the battle. Now your parent needs to grow accustomed to wearing a piece of plastic in or

> **"**My mother had terrible trouble with her hearing aids. They were always beeping or ringing. It was very sad, because she became so cut off from everyone and everything.
>
> One night I took her to see a show in New York, figuring that even if she couldn't hear everything, she would enjoy the colors and lights and dancing. They had these plug-in amplifying headphones, and it was a miracle. For the first time in years she could hear everything. She lit up. From then on, she went to the theater every chance she could.**"**
>
> —WILL B.

around his ear, and figure out the dials. Most difficult of all, he has to adjust to a cacophony of new sounds. A hearing aid not only makes the world louder; it also makes it sound hectic and distorted. Hearing aids are not like human ears; they can't tune in one noise and tune out others.

Because it is so hard to adjust to a hearing aid—and even harder late in life—and because a lot of hearing aids aren't fitted properly in the first place, nearly a quarter of the people who buy them end up not using them.

If your father gets the right device, however, and some training, and then can be convinced to wear it for, say, three to six months, it is likely that he will adopt it for good. Give him a lot of encouragement and support during this period, and try to be understanding. He might want to start slow-

## FOR MORE HELP

**American Speech-Language-Hearing Association Helpline**
**800-638-8255**
Referrals to audiologists and speech pathologists.

**Self Help for Hard-of-Hearing People**
**301-657-2248**
**301-657-2249**
Referrals to support groups, and information on the technical and emotional aspects of hearing loss.

**The American Tinnitus Association**
**503-248-9985**
Information about tinnitus and referrals for care.

**National Information Center on Deafness at Gallaudet University**
**202-651-5051**
Information on any aspect of deafness and hearing loss. Gallaudet, the national university for people with hearing impairment, also has a legal service for deaf people, and offers a course for the elderly through International Elderhostel on hearing technology, coping with hearing loss and dealing with stress in the family.

For a more complete list of helpful organizations for people with hearing loss, see Appendix B, page 391.

ly, wearing it only occasionally and with the volume on low while he gets used to the noise. Even when both ears are affected, many users find that one hearing aid works better than two.

When whistling or ringing is a problem, which it commonly is, it means that the microphone is picking up noise, or feedback, from the amplifier inside the ear, and the ear mold may need to be refitted. (The supplier may not be able to get rid of the feedback entirely, but your parent should not have to tolerate a substantial amount of it.) If he changes hearing aids, he will need time to adjust to a new sound, as each hearing aid is different.

## OTHER GADGETS

Other useful devices that aid hearing include amplification devices for the telephone, headphones for the television or radio, vibrating alarm clocks, and doorbells and telephones that flash instead of ring. Inexpensive microphones and headsets that amplify conversations of small groups of people are also very useful.

Consult an audiologist about the possibilities, or call one of the associations that deal with hearing problems. Many of the catalogues listed on page 416 sell gadgets to aid people with hearing problems.

# Sleep

Sleep, wonderful sleep. It's an elusive state for many older people. More than a third of people over 65 have trouble getting to sleep and staying there. It's not that old age changes a person's need for sleep—Dad isn't napping necessarily because he needs more sleep than he used to—but after age 40 people typically spend less time in the deepest stages of sleep. Their sleep is lighter and they wake up more easily during the night. In fact, people may not know they are waking up; sometimes they drift in and out of sleep without any recollection of it, and then don't understand why they are so tired the next day.

In addition to age, stress, hormonal changes, inactivity and poor diet are all to blame for disrupting normal sleeping patterns. So are drugs, especially diuretics, drugs used to treat Parkinson's disease, certain antidepressants, antihypertensives, steroids, decongestants, painkillers and asthma medications, as well as caffeine and alcohol. Illness and pain certainly hinder sleep, and depression keeps people awake or wakes them at early hours. Dementia, which upsets a person's 24-hour clock, can drive wake-sleep patterns even further out of kilter.

If your parent complains of insomnia, be sure his assessment is correct. Sometimes elderly people have misconceptions about sleep, believing they need more than they do. If your parent is bored, he might rather be asleep than awake, and consequently spend a lot of time in bed. The best indication of whether he is getting enough sleep is how refreshed and rested he feels when he wakes up.

If he is truly suffering from insomnia, whatever the underlying cause, it can plunge him into a downward tailspin. Worrying about sleep is the surest way to stay awake. Alcohol, sleeping pills and going to bed too early—all intended to make resting more restful—just make matters worse.

Sleeping pills require special caution because they can have such dire effects on an elderly person. Yet the elderly use them disproportionately, consuming more than 25 percent of the sleeping pills sold in this country. Sleeping pills (including non-prescription ones) should be used only as a last resort, for no more than several days at a time, and always under a doctor's guidance. They can cause confusion and anxiety in elderly people, especially when taken for long periods of time or in conjunction with other drugs. (It is possible for an older person who is using sleeping pills to become so disoriented that he is misdiagnosed as having dementia.)

## SLEEP DISORDERS

The elderly are prone to a number of sleep disorders, among them:

♦ **Restless leg syndrome and periodic leg movements.** In this condition a person's legs become fidgety, almost eager to run or move, just as he is trying to fall asleep.

With periodic leg movements, the limbs jerk suddenly after a person has fallen asleep, disturbing rest but not waking the person fully. The movements last for only a few seconds, but they can recur often, every 30 seconds or so. (Periodic leg movements may disturb a spouse's sleep as well, so both your parents may be tired during the day. If so, they should move into separate beds.)

Both of these syndromes can be treated with short-acting sleeping pills, or with the drugs used to treat Parkinson's disease.

◆ **Sleep apnea.** The airways become blocked and breathing stops for ten seconds or more, often repeatedly through the night. The sleeper is jarred awake as he gasps for a breath, but the awakenings are so brief that he usually isn't aware of them.

Sleep apnea, which is most common in overweight men, may be caused by an obstruction in the airways—the muscles in the throat relax and block the airway—by faulty breathing muscles in the chest or by a problem in the brain's ability to regulate breathing during sleep.

The most common symptoms are loud snoring and daytime fatigue. The only way to get it diagnosed with certainty, however, is to visit a sleep laboratory or clinic. Sleep specialists have a number of ways of treating apnea, including weight loss, the use of an air pressure gadget that pushes the airways open at night, medications and, in the case of an obstruction, surgery.

### TIPS FOR A GOOD NIGHT'S SLEEP

There is no standard recipe for success, so get your parent to explore several approaches and see what works for her.

◆ Stick to a routine of going to bed and getting up at the same time each day, which will help regulate the body's clock.

◆ Stay awake. Oddly enough, your parent will do better spending less time, not more, in bed. She might start on a schedule of going to bed at, say, 11 P.M. and setting the alarm for 6 A.M., and then slowly increase her sleep time, as necessary. She will be sleepier and, therefore, should sleep better.

◆ Limit napping to no more than an hour each day—too much sleep during the day will mean less at night. Naps taken around the middle of the day—at about 2 or 3 P.M.—are the most refreshing. If your parent is nodding off in the late afternoon or early evening, this snoozing will interfere with a good night's rest. (Try to find out if she is dozing off in front of the television without realizing it.)

◆ Reserve the bedroom for

 **FOR MORE HELP**

**The National Sleep Foundation**
**202-785-2300**

For information about sleep disorders or for the name of an accredited sleep clinic in your area.

sleeping and sex. Your parent shouldn't be getting in bed at 8 P.M. to read or watch television for an hour before turning the light out. She should wait until she is ready to sleep before she goes to bed.

◆ Make the bedroom safe and familiar. If your parent is in a new bedroom, fill it with familiar objects, photos and mementos.

◆ Check all medications. Ask the doctor to review your parent's drugs to see if any might be affecting her sleep patterns. If so, see if the medication can be taken earlier in the day, if the prescription can be changed or the dose reduced.

◆ Dinner should be light, low-fat and not excessively spicy, and it should be served several hours before bedtime. It's fine for your parent to have a snack before bed if she is apt to be awakened by hunger.

◆ Tobacco, alcohol and caffeine are stimulants that interfere with normal sleeping patterns. Even though a drink helps people relax, it also keeps them from falling into the deepest phases of sleep, and causes them to wake in the middle of the night as the effects of the alcohol wear off.

◆ Exercise, the elixir for so many problems, is a good antidote for insomnia too. A brisk walk in the fresh air during the afternoon (but not right before bed) is sure to help with sleep problems.

◆ A warm glass of milk just before climbing under the covers helps some people sleep. For others an aspirin or acetaminophen does the trick. It's not clear whether there's any biological basis for this; it may simply be a matter of getting into a routine or believing in a placebo. But if it works, use it. (The doctor should okay any regular use of aspirin, acetaminophen, ibuprofen or other drugs.)

◆ A pre-bed ritual, such as bathing, reading or listening to music, may help your parent relax and tell her body to prepare for sleep. (She should not discuss stressful topics, play competitive card games or watch upsetting late-night television just before bed.)

◆ You might teach your parent some mind-relaxing techniques or buy her a relaxation tape. For example, ask her to close her eyes and imagine herself lying on the beach. In a slow calm voice, tell her to smell the salty air, listen to the gentle rhythm of the waves, and feel the warmth of the sand against her body. Have her take deep, slow breaths as she feels the sun warming her skin and relaxing each muscle and joint . . . first her toes, then her ankles, legs, lower back, stomach, chest, shoulders, and eventually the muscles of her face. If she doesn't like the beach, create another favorite spot for her. You can do this over the phone if need be, but with time, she should be able to do it for herself.

## YOUR SLEEP

If your mother lives with you or others, her lack of sleep can affect everyone in the household. She may be grumpy, distractable, depressed and increasingly susceptible to illness as her immune system tires out. She may keep others awake at night if she is pacing, tossing about or watching television, and then expect them to be quiet during the day while she naps.

If your mother lives with you and is keeping you awake at night, buy yourself some earplugs and be sure your parent's room is set up so she can get whatever she needs—put a glass of water on the night table and a commode by the bed—and doesn't have to leave her room. If she can't get to the toilet without your help, you may have to insist (being sensitive to her protests) that she wear adult diapers at night.

If she is still keeping you awake, you may have to put your needs above hers in this instance. As a caregiver, you are pushed to your limit during the day and need your sleep at night. Talk to the doctor about the possibility of prescribing sleeping pills for her. While careful monitoring is required, it's sometimes necessary to give an elderly person sleeping pills so the rest of the family can sleep. If this is not medically advisable, you might consider hiring someone to cover for you during the evenings or you may have to start looking into other housing options for your parent.

# Medications

The thought of your father as a drug addict may seem absurd, but take another look in his medi-

"*My Mom, who's always been one of the most chipper, upbeat people I know, became very depressed last fall. She was lethargic and mopey and didn't want to go out with her friends. On one visit I brought up the subject of her granddaughter's upcoming wedding, knowing she'd been looking forward to it for a long time. She sort of shrugged and said she'd go, 'If I'm still around.' That was so uncharacteristic of her that I urged her to see a doctor.*

*He took her off the blood pressure pills that she'd been taking since she was 65—that's about 18 years. He said that age had changed her body chemistry so he changed the medication and greatly reduced the dosage. And sure enough, as soon as her medication was adjusted her spirits returned to normal. Not only did she get to the wedding but, as usual, she was the life of the party!*"
—LORETTA R.

cine cabinet. A prescription for chest pain, a little something to calm him down, a pill to aid digestion, medication to keep his blood pressure stable. It's not uncommon for an older person to make weekly visits to the pharmacist. (Studies show that nursing home residents take, on average, eight medications at any given time.)

Inappropriate drug use among the elderly has been referred to as "the nation's other drug problem." The elderly make up 13 percent of the population, but they buy 30 per-

# MEDICATIONS: QUESTIONS TO ASK

*When a new medication is prescribed, get full information from the doctor and write it all down. Ask the pharmacist to clarify anything you don't understand.*

❖ What is this drug intended to do? Is it treating the cause of the problem or only the symptoms? If it's the latter, is there any way to treat the cause?

❖ Is there another way to treat the problem, such as a change in diet, exercise or lifestyle?

❖ When and how should my parent take this drug?

❖ Is it safe for her to use it with the other medications she now uses?

❖ Should she avoid any particular foods or activities while taking it?

❖ Is this the proper dose for someone my mother's age, or could she start on a lower dose? (Because the elderly tend to be sensitive to drugs, they should be started "low and slow," and gradually increase the dose until there are benefits.)

❖ How long does it take for this drug to have an effect, and how will we know if it's working?

❖ How long should my parent use this medication? Should she continue to take it even after she feels better? (Your parent or you should check regularly with the doctor—perhaps every few weeks, depending on the potency of the drug and the side effects—to find out if the drug is still needed or if the dose can be lowered.)

❖ What are the possible side effects? What should I do if my parent has a bad reaction? (There are usually trade-offs to be made in treating elderly patients—for example, your parent may need to take a drug that worsens her confusion in order to get rid of the far more troubling hallucinations she is suffering. Weigh all the pros and cons with the doctor.)

❖What if my parent forgets to take this medication?

❖ Is it habit-forming? Will it be difficult for her to stop taking it?

❖ Can you prescribe a generic version that is just as good, but less expensive.

## GOOD MEDICINE

❖ Always get a doctor's okay before making any change in a medication routine. Your parent should not take more of a drug to increase the effect or stop taking a drug because she feels better or is experiencing some side effect.

❖ Make sure any doctor who sees your parent knows about all her allergies and medications, including any non-prescription drugs she might be taking.

❖ Your parent may be taking medications, especially over-the-counter medications such as antihistamines or sleeping pills, out of habit, unaware that it is time to quit. If the pills are addictive, she may need help from the doctor. Check with him or her and find out which ones should be stopped or at least taken in lower doses.

❖ Keep pills intended for emergencies in a place where they can easily be found.

❖ Never let your parent take a friend's pills, even if he has the same symptoms as the friend.

❖ If your parent has skipped a day or two of medication, call the doctor or pharmacist to find out what to do, rather than blindly returning to the original routine.

❖ Don't crush or break a pill without first securing the approval of the pharmacist. You might destroy a coating designed to protect the stomach, or you might upset the long action of a time-released medication.

❖ Don't leave pills out where a child can get at them. More than one-third of all incidents of children poisoned by prescription drugs involve a grandparent's pills.

❖ Throw out drugs that are old—as a general rule, after one year. (Over-the-counter drugs now have expiration dates on them. Prescription drugs don't, but the pharmacist will mark the bottle for you if you ask.)

cent of the prescription drugs sold each year. Many of these medications are warranted, as an older person's vulnerability to disease is greater. But many, many are not.

Doctors are partly to blame. They sometimes prescribe drugs to alleviate symptoms, rather than treating the underlying disease. They are also apt to keep renewing the same prescription when the patient has outgrown the need. Out of ignorance or the stress of treating large numbers of patients with limited time, some also prescribe drugs in dangerous combinations and fre-

## SAVING MONEY ON MEDICATIONS

Whenever your parent will be using a drug over a period of time, shop around because pharmacy prices vary widely, as do prices for drugs purchased through mail-order companies (which aren't always cheaper than pharmacies). Furthermore, one supplier may have the lowest price on your mother's asthma medication but another may have less expensive estrogen pills, which means she should comparison shop any time she gets a new prescription.

Call the area agency on aging to learn about what discount medications are available for seniors. Some states offer such discounts for low-income residents, and the Patient Assistance Program (800-762-4636) of the pharmaceutical industry will send you a directory listing various company programs that distribute free prescription drugs to people living on low incomes.

If your parent is in a nursing home, check the costs for her medications (scan her bills if the facility is not forthcoming with the information). Many nursing homes charge wildly inflated rates—sometimes two or three times what a drug would cost elsewhere. If that's the case, demand the right to buy your parent's medications yourself.

quently order drugs that are totally inappropriate for the elderly. (A 1994 study showed that a quarter of elderly people are taking drugs that are unsuitable for older patients, including Valium, Librium, Dalmane, Seconal, Nembutal, Elavil, Indocin, Darvon and Darvocet, Diabinese and Persantine.)

Some blame must also be placed on the lack of studies involving the elderly. Older bodies do not tolerate drugs in the same ways young bodies do. Changes in hormones, body fat and water content, metabolism, blood flow, stomach acids and kidney function all affect the way their bodies absorb, use and discard drugs. In the absence of solid, scientific data, many doctors continue to give older people the same medications in the same doses that they prescribe for younger patients.

Lastly, the elderly themselves are at fault because they often fail to tell the doctor all of their symptoms, their medical history and what medications they are using. Or they see too many doctors and don't tell each one what the others have prescribed. And even when prescriptions are appropriate, many elderly people fail to use them correctly, discontinuing the medication regime before it has run its proper course or forgetting to take the medication at all.

If you are involved in your parent's medical care, ask questions when a new drug is prescribed. Keep careful records of the drugs she takes—the names of the drugs, the reason for them, the dates they are started and stopped, side effects and any instructions.

If your parent has a new symptom, look back in these records to see when she began taking any new medications, then alert the doctor. Side effects common among the elderly include restlessness, poor balance and falls, sedation, loss of memory, confusion, depression, constipation, incontinence, tremors and skin problems such as rashes and unusual sensitivity to the sun (causing burns, blisters or swelling).

If you are concerned about your parent's medications, get a good consumer drug guide (such as *The PDR Family Guide to Prescription Drugs*) so you can look up which medications clash with one another, what side effects each may produce and what foods or activities are to be avoided in conjunction with each. Busy doctors and pharmacists cannot be relied on to keep you fully informed about drug hazards.

## KEEPING TABS ON COMPLIANCE

Most of us have trouble remembering to take medication, especially if the pills have no immediate effect or if the symptoms they're treating are already gone. For the elderly, who are apt to be using multiple drugs simultaneously and who tend towards forgetfulness any-

way, noncompliance is a serious problem. Studies show that more than half of older people fail to take their medications as prescribed.

If you are in the role of watchdog or caretaker, there are a few things you can do to improve your parent's habits. First, impress upon her the importance of following the prescribed routine in order to treat the illness completely and avoid complications.

Next, buy her a pill box, not a pretty little one, but a serious pill box with multiple compartments for different drugs and separate labels indicating the time of day each is to be taken. Large pill boxes which hold daily doses for the entire week are useful if you are filling the boxes for your parent during a weekly visit. You can find an assortment of pill boxes in medical supply stores and large pharmacies.

If the pill-box method doesn't work, put the pills in a place where your parent will see them and be reminded to take them. For example, pills to be taken at bedtime might be placed on the toothbrush stand, and those to be taken in the morning, on the breakfast table. Then be sure to label each bottle in clear, dark letters, "Take one with breakfast" or "Take two before bed."

When more than one person is dispensing your parent's medications, make a chart like the one on the facing page, with boxes to check off when a pill is taken. If your parent is in charge and has trouble reading the pill bottle labels, color-code the chart, matching the color of the bottle or pill with a similar color on

## MEDICATION SCHEDULE
*Fill in name of drug and dosage to be taken.*

| | MONDAY | TUESDAY | WEDNESDAY | THURSDAY | FRIDAY | SATURDAY | SUNDAY |
|---|---|---|---|---|---|---|---|
| MORNING | | | | | | | |
| AFTERNOON | | | | | | | |
| EVENING | | | | | | | |
| BEDTIME | | | | | | | |

the chart (*blue pills at 2, white pills at 6, pink liquid at 10,* etc.)

If your father forgets because of dementia or another illness, it is best if someone actually sees him take his medication. If you can't be with him, call him (or have someone else call him) at pill time and have him take his medicine while you wait on the phone.

# Alcohol

Alcohol is a drug, and as with other drugs, it has a more pronounced effect in older bodies, which absorb, use and dispose of alcohol differently than do younger bodies. The amount your parent used to drink without any trouble may simply be too much for him now. (Studies show that when a 60-year-old and a 20-year-old drink the same amount of alcohol, the older person's blood-alcohol level is 20 percent higher than the younger person's. A 90-year-old has a blood-alcohol level that is 50 percent higher.)

Although a drink with dinner is not cause for concern in most cases, be aware that alcohol mixes poorly with most medications and it can exacerbate problems with confusion, incontinence, insomnia or depression. It also hinders coordination and slows a person's reactions, increasing the chances of falls. And alcohol consumption makes one more susceptible to infections, colds and other illness.

Unfortunately, boredom, insomnia, pain and stress can make alcohol a welcome analgesic for elderly people. If you are worried about your parent's alcohol use, talk with her about your concerns or ask a doctor to talk with her. Let her

**❝**My mother used to love to have a couple of old-fashioneds every night. Then we decided that her drinking might be contributing to the dizziness and the falls, so Elizabeth, Mom's companion, got her down to one small glass of sherry. I was amazed, but Elizabeth can get Mom to do almost anything—things that I could never convince her to do.

One evening when I was visiting, Mom said, 'Oh I think I'll have a _real_ drink tonight.' And I said, 'No, Mom, please don't do that.' I was a little nervous about what her reaction would be, but she didn't say a word, and she didn't have the drink. I was truly shocked. And very relieved.**❞**   —GRETA N.

know that even though she is older now, cutting back or quitting can help. And failing to abstain, or being drawn into a cycle of drinking more and more, can lead to serious problems, including malnutrition, serious accidents and permanent damage to the kidneys, brain, heart, stomach, liver, mouth and throat.

### Watch for Withdrawal

If your parent routinely drinks alcohol and is placed in a situation in which alcohol is not available, such as a nursing home or hospital, he may go through withdrawal. The symptoms include shakiness, sweating, agitation and, sometimes, hallucinations and seizures. Alert the personnel about his previous drinking habits, because they may not un-

 **FOR MORE HELP**

For information about alcoholism or referrals to treatment centers and self-help groups, contact:

**National Council on Alcoholism and Drug Dependence Hopeline 800-622-2255**

**National Clearinghouse for Alcohol and Drug Information 800-729-6686**

**Alcoholics Anonymous 212-870-3400**

**Al-Anon Family Groups, Inc. 800-356-9996**

derstand the cause of his problems. Be sure the information is entered in his record so you're not depending on the person you've told to pass it along to other staff. Withdrawal is a medical emergency that requires immediate treatment.

# Temperature Regulation

Older people can become severely chilled simply sleeping in a cool room, or dangerously overheated in temperatures that the rest of us find quite comfortable. Much

## UP IN SMOKE

Everyone knows the potential ravages of cigarette smoking, but what's the point of stopping so late in life? According to a recent report from the U.S. Surgeon General, the benefits of quitting, even at an advanced age, start immediately. Within hours of that last cigarette the body begins to repair and restore itself—oxygen levels increase, nerve endings regenerate, blood pressure falls. Within months your parent should be more energetic, have a better appetite, sleep better and generally feel better.

At least one study suggests that a 65-year-old person who stops smoking can add four or more years to his life.

Your parent can't reverse any severe ailments caused by smoking, such as emphysema or lung cancer, but if he quits at least he won't be making the condition worse, and he will bolster his immune system and improve his general health.

To find out how to quit, call the American Cancer Society at 800-227-2345. To learn about classes, call the local chapter of the ACS.

of the problem is biological. Older bodies have less protective fat and aren't as adept at constricting and dilating blood vessels, or shivering and sweating. Also, in certain situations the brain fails to get the message that it's too cold or too hot. As a result, your parent might stay out in the hot sun for a dangerously long time, or fail to use a blanket on a cool night.

Some of the problem is also practical. A person with a physical disability or a painful ailment may not want to pull himself up out of a chair to get a sweater or to move into another room. If your parent is living on a fixed income, and even if he is not, he may try to save money by keeping the thermostat dangerously low.

So when the the snow is falling or the mercury rising, remind your parent to protect himself. When you are nearby, be aware of his comfort. As a summer day heats up, give him plenty of cool drinks and keep physical activity to a minimum. In winter, his house should be kept no cooler than 65 degrees, even at night. Be sure there are plenty of blankets, slippers, sweaters, long underwear and hats on hand. Your parent might wear a light hat to bed, as body heat escapes through the head, especially when a person's hair has thinned.

Hyperthermia (when the body's temperature gets too high) and hypothermia (when it gets too low) are both medical emergencies. They are particularly worrisome in people who have dementia, stroke or other neurological disorders, thyroid

## RECOGNIZING TEMPERATURE CRISES

*Warning: Hyperthermia and hypothermia are both medical emergencies and require immediate medical attention*

| SIGNS AND SYMPTOMS | WHAT TO DO |
|---|---|
| **Hyperthermia**<br>Heat exhaustion:<br>  Clammy, pale skin<br>  Heavy sweating<br>  Dizziness<br>  Weakness<br>  Nausea<br>  Headache<br>  Cramps<br>  Rapid, shallow breathing | Get your parent to a cool room or shaded area. Make him lie down, with his feet raised about 12 inches. Remove or loosen clothing and sponge his forehead and body with cool (not cold) water. Give him water, preferably with a little salt in it, or a drink like Gatorade. Do not bring his temperature down too quickly. Call the doctor. |
| Heat stroke:<br>  Hot, dry, red skin<br>  No sweat<br>  Rapid pulse<br>  Body temperature above<br>    104° F<br>  Unconsciousness or<br>    confusion | Call an ambulance immediately. While waiting, keep your parent in a sitting position. Sponge him off and wrap him in a cool (not cold), wet sheet. Give him plenty of water. Do not bring his temperature down too quickly (because it can cause a heart attack) or over-cool him. |
| **Hypothermia**<br>  Listlessness<br>  Weakness<br>  Drowsiness<br>  Paleness<br>  Confusion<br>  Slow and shallow<br>    breathing<br>  Slurred speech<br>  Body temperature below<br>    95° F<br>  Unconsciousness | Turn off the air conditioner, turn up the heat or move your parent to a warmer room. Do not warm him too quickly. Get him into blankets, sweaters and a hat, or into a slightly warm bath. Offer warm (not hot) fluids. Do not let him go to sleep. Call the doctor. |

disorders, Parkinson's disease, diabetes or cardiovascular disease, or are taking medications that make the body's temperature fluctuate. So be on the alert.

# Dehydration

Normally when a body is low on fluids, the kidneys go into an emergency mode and hold on to water, and the brain screams out, "I'm thirsty." But older kidneys are less efficient at conserving fluids and the thirst messages don't travel as efficiently, especially if a person suffers from dementia. Even when the message does come through, mobility problems may hinder a trip to the tap.

As a result of all this, an older person can become dehydrated easily, and grow confused, tired, light-headed and faint as his body dries out, yet still be unaware that he needs water. Over time, ignoring the body's need for fluids can cause bowel problems, kidney trouble, urinary tract infections and even delirium.

Get your father to keep a glass of water (or some other non-caffeinated fluid) nearby, and to make a point of sipping from it as often as possible. Eight glasses of fluid a day is the usual recommendation, but he doesn't have to measure the ounces; he should simply drink as much fluid as he can. Unless the doctor wants your father to cut down on fluids for medical reasons, he cannot drink too much water. Make sure that he isn't limiting his drinking because of incontinence. Con-

suming less water won't help; it will only cause new problems.

# Skin Care

Skin announces the onset of old age with cracks, wrinkles and spots long before any of us are ready for it, but usually the sags and blemishes are simply ego deflaters or cosmetic nuisances. When we become quite old, however, skin can present serious medical problems.

The three most common skin problems facing the elderly, aside from skin cancer (see box on page 82), are itchiness, fungal infections and bedsores. Older skin is thinner and less oily, so it tends to be drier and more susceptible to bruises, infections and rashes. When injured, it doesn't heal as quickly as it once did, and minor irritations can become serious wounds. All of this means that your parent's skin needs a little extra TLC.

**Itchy, dry skin** is the most common skin complaint among the elderly, especially in the winter when the air is less humid. It may not seem particularly important in the overall scheme of things, but severely itchy skin (known as pruritus) can be extremely annoying and, over time, it can make your parent irritable and weary from lack of sleep. Here are some ways your parent can ease the dryness and the itch:

♦ Take fewer showers or baths (two or three a week is fine) and keep them short and not too hot. Water and heat draw moisture away from the skin.

## MEDICAL ALERT

If itching comes on suddenly and severely, it may be the result of a disease, such as kidney or liver disease, gallstones or thyroid disorders. Severe itching on hands, wrists, underarms, abdomen and groin may be the sign of mites (scabies), which are found more often in people staying in a hospital or nursing home, and are usually treated with lindane cream. Either situation should be checked by a doctor.

◆ Use a minimal amount of soap, which removes the skin's natural oils. Avoid deodorant and perfumed soaps which contain chemical irritants. Instead, use a glycerin soap with cleansing cream, such as Dove, Basis or Tone, and rinse well.

◆ Avoid scrubbing harshly. Use a soft cloth or natural sponge instead of a brush or rough washcloth.

◆ Moisturize. After a bath or shower, your parent should pat his skin dry gently, leaving it moist, and then immediately apply an oil, lotion or other moisturizer to lock in moisture. Find a moisturizer made with lots of petrolatum—it should be high on the list of ingredients—and avoid moisturizers that contain alcohol, which dries the skin. (Your father may not be in the habit of using lotion, but buy an unscented one and give him a nudge.)

If your parent bathes, add oil (bath oil, mineral oil—almost any oil will do), colloidal oatmeal or cornstarch to the tub water. Do so with caution, however, because the oil can cause your parent to slip, producing a far more serious problem than dry skin.

◆ Apply pure petroleum jelly to very dry areas after a bath or shower. Your parent might wear pajamas, socks or something else to protect good clothing or sheets from the grease.

◆ Keep sheets and clothing clean. All new clothing should be washed before wearing. Avoid bleaches, fabric softeners and heavily-perfumed detergents, which can irritate skin. Rinse clothes well.

◆ Get your parent to wear cotton, which is less irritating than wool or synthetic clothing.

◆ A humidifier can put a little moisture into dry, winter air. But change the water daily and keep the unit clean, as it can breed bacteria and other germs.

◆ Be sure your parent drinks lots of fluids (to moisturize from the inside out).

◆ Steer him away from alcohol, spicy foods and caffeine.

◆ If itching becomes severe, try calamine lotion, cold compresses or cortisone creams. Urge your parent to control his scratching (short fingernails and/or gloves will help), which may only aggravate the itch.

◆ If your parent's itching or dryness is severe and doesn't let up, or if itching becomes a nervous habit and is causing sores and bleeding, be sure he sees his doctor or his dermatologist.

**Fungal infections** can crop up if your parent's immune system is weak or his circulation poor, if he has diabetes, or if he takes antibiotics or corticosteroid drugs.

Fungus grows in warm, moist pockets of the body, like armpits, genitals, the scalp, the mouth and the spaces around nails and between toes. It causes itchy, cracked skin which can become infected. If your parent has a fungal infection, she should consult her doctor about it. In the meantime, to prevent or help get rid of fungal infections:

◆ Keep skin clean and dry. Use a hair dryer on a cool setting to dry hard-to-reach places.

◆ Wear loose, cotton clothing, including underwear and socks (synthetics don't let air circulate as well). Avoid pantyhose.

◆ Change shoes and socks once or twice a day and, if possible, wear sandals or shoes made of mesh or woven fabric that lets air circulate.

◆ Use over-the-counter antifungal cream or powder.

**Shingles,** or herpes zoster, is a disease of the nervous system that affects the skin. The disease is caused by the same virus that causes chicken pox. Small amounts of the virus sit dormant in the nervous system for years and then, because of a weakened immune system, stress or illness, the virus is revived. It travels along the nerves toward the skin, causing fatigue, headaches and chills several days before the disease is visible—symptoms which can lead to misdiagnosis. Then, as with chicken pox, small blisters appear, but usually only on one patch of the skin, not over the whole body. When the blisters open, shingles can be extremely painful, and the skin can continue to be sensitive for two to four weeks after the blisters have healed. In older people, scarring may take place.

Corticosteriods and aspirin will often ease the symptoms. Doctors sometimes wrap the skin in gauze soaked in a medicinal solution, and prescribe the drug acyclovir.

**Skin infections** are common in older people who are ill and quite frail, especially those who have poor circulation, diabetes or edema. The two most common skin infections—cellulitis and erysipelas—often start at the site of a scratch or wound, and grow into a red rash that is tender and warm to the touch. Erysipelas is often found on the face, has well-defined borders, can cause flu-like symptoms and can lead to serious eye problems as well as blood poisoning or clotting. Either type of infection requires a doctor's immediate attention.

**Skin reactions to medications** include swelling, burning, itching,

## ON THE ALERT FOR SKIN CANCER

Blemishes, warts, freckles, skin tags (tiny, flesh-colored or brown flaps of skin), red dots, moles and other markings are part of old age. Most are harmless results of the sun and the aging process, but keep a watchful eye, especially if there is no spouse around who can check your parent's body. Any moles or other markings that grow rapidly, are larger than one-quarter of an inch across, bleed or look unusual (for example, pearly round spots, gritty red patches or irregularly shaped dark moles) could suggest skin cancer and should be seen immediately by your parent's doctor or her dermatologist.

A skin exam should be part of every physical, but since some doctors overlook this it's worthwhile to ask if he or she will inspect your parent's skin. If anything seems suspicious the doctor will refer your parent to a dermatologist. If your parent has a history of skin cancer, she should be seen regularly by a dermatologist.

If you provide any hands-on care (and therefore routinely see her skin), be sure to keep an eye out for suspicious moles and bring them to the attention of the doctor.

blisters, allergic reactions such as hives or rashes, and a heightened sensitivity to the sun (unusual burning or staining after being in the sun). The doctor may be able to change the medication, lower the dosage or, at the very least, treat the reaction. Such reactions may occur after your parent has stopped taking a medication, so keep those medication records handy.

Whether or not she is using medications, your parent should forgo lengthy sunbathing and should wear a strong sunscreen (SPF 15 or higher) anytime she is in the sun for more than a few minutes. (Of course, this precaution applies to everyone, no matter what their age.)

## PREVENTING BEDSORES

Bedsores are a threat any time your parent is confined to a bed or a chair. The elderly are particularly susceptible to bedsores because their skin is thin and their circulation weak. Continuous pressure on a bony area, such as the heel, elbow, the back of the head or buttocks, blocks the flow of blood, which damages the skin and tissue below and causes redness, blisters or open sores. Here are some ways to prevent them:

◆ If your parent is bedridden, he should be repositioned every hour or two, or should shift himself regularly if possible. Move him gently because even being pulled across the sheets can harm his tender skin. Use pillows to raise his heels or elbows off the bed, or to relieve the pressure on his buttocks, hips and knees.

◆ Get your parent to stand up, sit in a chair or move about if he can. If he can't, get him to wiggle his toes, flex his arms, jiggle his legs and rotate his neck—whatever movement is possible—to keep the blood flowing. This should help prevent not only bedsores, but also blood clots, which can form when the body is kept still.

◆ Be sure your parent's skin is clean and dry, as moisture adds to the risk of bedsores. His sheets should be changed regularly, especially if he is incontinent or sweaty.

◆ Elevate his head only slightly, because when the head is raised high it puts pressure on the back.

◆ Use an egg-crate foam mattress on top of the existing mattress to cushion your parent's body and relieve the pressure of his own weight. More elaborate options include waterbeds and air-filled mattresses.

◆ Pads of sheepskin will help protect elbows, heels and other vulnerable areas. You can also buy small trapeze-like gadgets that hold the feet up off the bed. (Avoid doughnut-shaped cushions, which cut off the blood supply to the skin that's suspended in the center of the cushion.)

◆ Gentle massage will stimulate circulation (and is wonderful for physical and emotional comfort).

But don't massage areas that have become slightly red, because the friction can damage the skin even more.

◆ At the first sign of any redness, alert a doctor or nurse. Untreated, bedsores can become infected and life-threatening.

# Arms, Legs and Feet

**Stasis dermatitis.** When a person has poor circulation, fluids often accumulate in the limbs and slow the usual back-and-forth flow of nutrients and waste, causing swelling. The skin becomes cracked and discolored with reddish-brown patches or itchy purple dots, and varicose veins may appear.

If your parent has these symptoms, she should see her doctor because the problem can become severe. Treatment involves reducing pressure in the veins by using support stockings, elevating the legs, and, in some cases, using ointments to reduce the itching.

◆ **Varicose veins.** The bulging, blue veins that squiggle down your mother's leg can be painful. They are not, however, dangerous. Veins become distended because the valves that are supposed to keep uphill-flowing blood from draining downhill don't work. Instead, blood headed for the heart flows back down the leg. Your mother should avoid standing for long periods of time, and try to lie down whenever

## TLC FOR LEGS AND FEET

❖ Rest with the legs elevated. Avoid long periods of standing upright or sitting with the legs crossed or folded.

❖ Keep feet warm, dry and comfortable.

❖ Be sure your parent is wearing the right size shoe, as feet often expand with age. Shoes should have low or no heels, firm soles and preferably a wide cut across the toes. Shoes should be made of a material that lets air flow and feet move (cotton, mesh or real leather). Stick to cotton or wool socks— no synthetics, please.

❖ Walking or other exercise, foot and leg massages all improve blood flow.

❖ A warm foot bath is soothing for the soul as well as the soles.

❖ Keep toenails neatly trimmed, straight across, to avoid ingrown nails.

❖ Have your mother occasionally rub dead skin off with a foot file or pumice stone after a shower or bath, so calluses don't build up. Or do it for her. A pedicure is a welcome treat.

❖ Corns will disappear with over-the-counter medications (never shave them off). If they reappear, consult a doctor. Small, doughnut-shaped pads can relieve some of the shoe pressure on corns.

❖ If your parent has diabetes, her feet will require special attention, as diabetes affects blood flow and puts the feet at extra risk of infections. Consult the doctor about how to protect her feet.

possible with her feet elevated. Support hose (available from a medical supply store) should also help.

◆ **Foot troubles.** After 70 or 80 years of pounding, stamping and stomping, feet get pretty worn out, but they are often neglected by caregivers and doctors alike. Goodness knows, they aren't much to look at. But without proper care (see box), the various calluses, corns, bunions, infections and other sores that develop can become severe and make it difficult and sometimes impossible for your parent to get around on his own two feet.

# Oral Hygiene

Just because your father is old does not mean he has outgrown the dentist's chair. In fact, older people are at more risk than ever of oral cancer, and studies show that

**MEDICAL ALERT**

Red or white spots, sores in the mouth or bleeding that does not go away within two weeks should be checked by a dentist, as they can be an early sign of oral cancer.

people over 65 have more tooth decay than other age groups. Elderly people produce relatively little saliva, which cleanses the teeth. And they can have problems brushing properly and flossing if they can't see well or have difficulty moving their arms, hands or wrists. Lastly, with age, the gums shrink, exposing vulnerable areas of each tooth to potential infection or decay.

Your parent needs to see the dentist at least once a year. Dental problems are not only painful; they can also make chewing difficult, which can lead to poor nutrition.

Tell him that wearing dentures is no excuse for skipping routine checkups and ignoring dental hygiene. False teeth, like glasses, need to be checked and refitted, and the gums, tongue and the insides of the cheeks still need some brushing to kill bacteria and keep the breath fresh.

Here are some tips on caring for your parent's mouth:

♦ See that your parent visits the dentist at least once a year. If he doesn't have a good one, find a dentist with experience in treating elderly patients (some medical schools have postgraduate training in geriatric dentistry).

♦ If your parent is having trouble managing a toothbrush, elongate the brush by taping a sturdy wooden or plastic stick to it, or enlarge it by attaching a rubber or plastic foam ball to the handle.

♦ An electric toothbrush is sometimes easier to use, but have the dentist or dental hygienist show your parent the best way to use it.

♦ If your parent's mouth is dry, ask his doctor or pharmacist if medication might be causing the problem. Maybe the dose can be lowered or the prescription changed. (Diuretics, antihistamines, antihypertensives, anti-anxiety drugs, antidepressants, antipsychotics and drugs for Parkinson's disease all slow the flow of saliva.)

♦ Dry mouth can be relieved temporarily with sugarless candies or gum. Lip lubricants are a must, and chips of ice or sips of water will also help. Citrus fruits wet the mouth but also rinse it in harmful acid, so limit the oranges.

♦ If you are going to brush your parent's teeth, ask the dentist or dental hygienist to show you how. (Again, using an electric toothbrush is easier.)

♦ If your parent has trouble swallowing, or if he is confined to bed, skip or limit the toothpaste because he may choke on the foam. Just use a wet brush, or simply wipe his teeth and gums with a damp cloth.

If you're gasping for air because your father has bad breath, you need to decide just how big a problem it is. Be sensitive. The odor may be caused by his medications or illness, so he may not be able to do anything about it.

If you can tactfully broach the subject, let your parent know that better oral hygiene can help kill some of the germs that cause bad breath. Your parent should brush the roof of his mouth, his tongue and the inside of his cheeks, in addition to his teeth. Most breath mints and mouthwashes merely cover up odor, but gargling should help as it loosens mucus lodged at the back of the throat.

# Chapter Six

# THE BODY
# IMPERFECT
## PART II

*Bones and Joints • Incontinence • Constipation
• Other Digestive Disorders • Depression
• Delirium • Anxiety*

S OMETIMES EVEN SERIOUS HEALTH PROBLEMS DO
not get the full attention of a busy doctor. Or they may not
be mentioned to the doctor if your parent is embarrassed
about them or believes they can't be treated. Your father may assume
that achy, stiff joints are a condition he has to learn to live with.
He may not be aware that his depression is treatable. Or out of
shame, he may keep his incontinence a secret. Again, most of these
ailments can be treated, and adjustments to his house and daily
habits should make any remaining symptoms more bearable.

Learn the warning signs. If you suspect anything is wrong, urge
your father to talk with his doctor. If he denies there's anything
wrong, let him know that if he ever had such a problem, he is not
alone and there are treatments. When the problem is severe or affects
others (paralyzing depression, immobilizing arthritis or incontinence
that caregivers can't handle), consult the doctor yourself. Your
parent may not care if his illness is treated, but you do.

## ON THE LOOKOUT FOR SYMPTOMS

| | |
|---|---|
| ❏ Osteoporosis | Few symptoms until a bone is broken; women at most risk have a family history of the disease, are thin, smoke, have had their ovaries removed, did not take hormones after menopause |
| ❏ Osteoarthritis | Painful joints; achy, stiff movement, especially first thing in the morning |
| ❏ Incontinence | Stains or odors, wet sheets, reluctance to go out |
| ❏ Diabetes | Fatigue, weight loss, blurred vision, itchy skin, frequent urination, thirst, sensations of tingling or numbness, confusion, depression |
| ❏ Depression | Withdrawal, apathy, crying, hopelessness, changes in weight or sleep habits |
| ❏ Delirium | Inattentiveness and severe confusion that usually come on suddenly, often accompanied by grogginess or anxiety |
| ❏ Dementia | Confusion, chronic forgetfulness and other mental lapses. (Symptoms may be benign or they may be signs of serious illness, such as stroke or Alzheimer's disease. See Chapter Fifteen for a full discussion of cognitive loss and dementia.) |

# Bones and Joints

The human skeleton may look like a fixed, immutable frame, especially when it's hanging in a biology classroom, but skeletons are living organs that change with diet, exercise, body chemistry and, yes, age. Just like softer body parts, bones and joints peter out if they are not well cared for.

No matter what else ails your parent, you need to be aware of his body's scaffolding, because when it breaks, the rest of the structure can quickly collapse. Older bones don't heal easily and your parent may be laid up for months, putting her at risk of circulation problems, bedsores and pneumonia. Even a minor fall can damage your mother's confidence and make her afraid to go out or walk without support.

## OSTEOPOROSIS

Osteoporosis turns healthy bones into what look like termite-eaten pieces of driftwood that can

## MEDICAL ALERT

Get your parent to a doctor immediately if she has a fall, all-over body achiness, numbness in part of her body, severe pain, immovable joints or mild joint pain that lasts for several weeks.

break easily. It is primarily a woman's ailment because after menopause, when the production of estrogen slows, bones lose calcium (which provides them with hardness) and collagen (which provides elasticity). But your father is not immune to osteoporosis. Old age, and the inactivity that typically accompanies it, whittles away at the bones of all older people. Over time, the body's frame can become so brittle that tumbling off a step or tripping on a bathroom rug is all it takes to break a wrist, a pelvis or a hip. The bones of the spinal cord can also collapse and compress, causing crippling back pain. Thirty-two percent of women and 17 percent of men break a hip by the time they are 90, and osteoporosis is largely to blame.

### Spotting Osteoporosis

There are few symptoms of osteoporosis until a bone is broken, although stooped posture and a decrease in height often accompany spinal osteoporosis. A number of factors increase a person's chances of having the disease: early menopause (before age 45), the absence of es-

trogen replacement therapy soon after menopause, a family history of the disease, a thin frame, habitual smoking and drinking, a diet low in calcium and a sedentary lifestyle. For reasons that are unclear, Caucasian and Asian-American women are far more prone to the disease than are African-American women.

Risk alone merits preventative steps, but if your mother needs convincing, have her talk with her doctor. A look at her medical history and a physical exam, along with some professional advice, should help her understand the importance of prevention and treatment. In some cases, doctors will do a bone density test using low-level X rays. (This test is not recommended as a screening tool for the general population, but it is useful to pinpoint an individual's risk if there is some question about hormone treatment.)

### Combatting Osteoporosis

The best time to fight osteoporosis is long before it sets in, by exercising regularly, getting plenty of calcium and vitamin D, and taking hormone supplements when indicated. But the battle is not over at age 70. People can strengthen their bones even late in life.

◆ **Exercise.** Frail people, especially those worried about falling, tend to stay sedentary, safely propped up in the living-room chair. But that is the worst thing your parent can do. Bones, like all body parts, need to be used. Walking, swimming, riding a stationary bike, lifting weights and other exercise all strengthen muscles and bones; the bones actually get thicker and stronger. Exer-

*"My mother started going downhill after she fell three years ago and broke her hip. Before that she had been very active, going up to Maine for the summers and going into the city on weekends. But the fall slowed her down tremendously. She lost her gusto for life. It's a constant effort to restore her confidence."* —KEVIN B.

cise also enhances balance, coordination and reflexes, which further reduces the risk of falling.

An exercise regime should involve muscles throughout the body, and if possible should include weight machines and weight lifting, both excellent ways to fight osteoporosis. In one study, very frail nursing home residents put on an exercise regime dramatically increased their muscle strength and bone mass in just ten weeks. Practicing tai chi has also been shown to help reduce falls. (For more on exercise, see page 155.)

♦ **Calcium and vitamin D.** A regime of calcium supplements late in life decreases the rate of bone loss, but studies have yet to find any consequent reduction in the rate of fractures. Still, doctors strongly recommend that women past menopause take up to 1,500 milligrams of calcium a day (1,000 milligrams a day for men and younger women).

To meet this requirement a person would have to drink about a quart of milk each day, so before your mother goes on a milk binge, buy her some calcium supplements with vitamin D (600 to 800 units), which

the body needs so it can absorb the calcium effectively. Of the many calcium supplements available, calcium citrate causes fewer problems and is more easily absorbed into the body. (For more on calcium and a list of some high-calcium foods, see Appendix D, page 407.)

Recent research suggests that a slow-release form of calcium citrate combined with sodium fluoride is effective in treating spinal osteoporosis in elderly women.

♦ **Smoking.** Easier said than done, but nevertheless, your parent should give up cigarettes, which weaken bones.

♦ **Hormones.** The question of whether a woman who never used hormones should start at 80 or 90 baffles even the experts. Beginning hormone therapy within the five or six years following menopause prevents bone loss, but there is little solid data on the benefits of starting later in life. Some evidence indicates that it slows bone loss and lowers the rate of fractures. It also decreases the chance of heart disease, which is the number one killer of women. There are risks, however. Estrogen used alone may increase the risk of endometrial cancer.

Your mother should talk with her doctor and make a decision based on her family history, health risks and personal preference.

♦ **Drugs.** A number of new drugs, some of them not yet on the market, seem to combat osteoporosis. The field is evolving rapidly. Your parent should talk with her docctor about these options.

◆ **Fall prevention.** Even people without osteoporosis can stumble and break a bone. Regardless of your parent's bone density, her house should be made "fall-safe." That means ample lighting, well-secured rugs, marked stairs, sturdy handrails, and some nonskid shoes, among other things. (See page 141 for tips on safe-proofing the home.)

## MEDICAL ALERT

If your parent faints, nearly faints, or has dizzy spells, get her to her doctor. While fainting may be caused by something simple, such as reduced blood flow to the brain due to advanced age and/or medications, it can also indicate more serious conditions.

## ARTHRITIS

Arthritis is not a single disorder, but a general term referring to sore or swollen joints. The word actually encompasses about a hundred different diseases, all of which should be treated early, so look for the warning signs: swelling, redness and pain at the joint; stiffness, especially in the morning; and restricted range of motion. If any of these symptoms last for more than two weeks, your parent should see her doctor.

### Managing Arthritis

Most types of arthritis cannot be cured, so the aim of treatment is to alleviate pain and increase mobility. If your parent's arthritis is severe, she should talk to a specialist, such as a rheumatologist or orthopedic surgeon.

◆ **Non-medical treatments.** Before considering drugs or surgery, your parent should try non-medical treatments. Warm baths and heat pads can relieve the pain and stiffness, while cold packs can reduce the swelling and numb the pain. (Your parent should try both and see what feels best.) Also, gentle massage can help. While rest is important during a painful attack, exercise in the interim can prevent joints from stiffening and increase mobility. Any exercise program should be comfortable, not too challenging and, preferably, recommended by a doctor or physical therapist. Exercising in a warm pool is often easier on stiff joints. (Check with the local Arthritis Foundation for special classes.) If your parent is heavy, losing weight will also ease the burden on her joints. People with gout or pseudogout should avoid alcohol, poultry and organ meats, such as livers and kidneys.

◆ **Handy gadgets.** Canes, walkers and splints will give your parent support and a little more mobility. Shoes with shock-absorbing insoles can reduce pain. Jar openers, toothpaste dispensers, large-handled flatware, faucet grippers and other such devices can be found in many large pharmacies and in medical supply stores, or they can be ordered by mail. (See the list of catalogues in Appendix E, page 416).

# ARTHRITIS: THE COMMON VILLAINS

**Osteoarthritis,** or degenerative arthritis, is almost universal after age 65, particularly among women, although some people have few or no symptoms. The cartilage in joints, which allows bones to glide easily back and forth without friction, becomes thin, cracked and frayed. Movement is painful and the joints swell. It is most common in the joints of the hands, back, feet, hips and knees. In severe cases, a hand may curl and twist into a deformed shape, and will sometimes develop knobby lumps, called osteophytes (which actually look more painful than they are).

Severe osteoarthritis can make everyday life exasperating and discouraging. Every movement hurts, and simple tasks, like buttoning a blouse or holding a fork, are challenging if not impossible.

**Rheumatoid arthritis** also affects women more than men. The body's immune system launches a misdirected attack and injures healthy tissue in the joints. The disease usually begins with an all-over achiness and fatigue. The joints become stiff, swollen and painful, especially first thing in the morning. The hands—particularly the fingers—and the feet are often the first joints affected, but over time, the disease can spread to elbows, knees, hips and other joints. In some cases, pea-size lumps grow under the skin and the joints become deformed. Rheumatoid arthritis is one of the most difficult types of arthritis to control.

**Gout and pseudogout,** two of the most excruciating types of arthritis, occur more often in men than women. In gout, uric acid, which usually drains out of the body with urine, builds up (because too much is produced or too little is excreted) and forms crystals in the joints.

In pseudogout, it is crystals of calcium pyrophosphate that collect. This assault on the joints—usually the big toe and often the knee, ankle, wrist, hand or foot—happens suddenly, lasts for about two or three days, and then slowly fades out over a week or two. The person often has another attack within a year and may experience several more episodes in following years, although some people have just one or two attacks and are never bothered by symptoms again. These bouts are so painful that even a light brush with the bed sheets can be agonizing.

◆ **Drugs.** Aspirin and its relatives, ibuprofen and acetaminophen, are typically used to relieve the aches of aged joints and muscles. (By the way, "extra-strength" or "arthritis-strength" aspirin are simply larger doses of plain aspirin.) Recent studies suggest that acetaminophen (e.g., Tylenol) is the best choice as it works just as well as aspirin, but causes fewer side effects. Your parent should not begin a regimen of this or any other medication, however, without the approval of her doctor.

When these over-the-counter remedies aren't enough, doctors often prescribe more powerful nonsteroidal anti-inflammatory drugs. These NSAIDs block the production of prostaglandins, the source of pain and swelling. While they may provide some relief immediately, it usually takes several weeks for these drugs to have a full effect. NSAIDs can produce side effects, including ulcers, heartburn, vomiting, diarrhea and headaches.

When NSAIDs don't work, corticosteroids, which are a form of cortisone, a hormone produced naturally by the body, also reduce swelling and pain. Corticosteroids, however, are potent and are usually prescribed only for brief periods.

Rheumatoid arthritis is treated in a number of ways: by administering gold compounds, which take two to six months to work; antimalarial drugs, which relieve swelling but can cause eye damage; penicillamine, which also takes two to six months to work; or, in unusual cases, drugs that suppress the immune system.

Gout and pseudogout are treated with NSAIDs, corticosteroids, or the drug colchicine. Doctors also try to reduce the level of uric acid in the body (with drugs like allopurinol, sulfinpyrazone and probenecid).

◆ **Physical and occupational therapy.** Physical therapy increases movement and strengthens muscles. Occupational therapy trains people to manage everyday tasks. Both are often helpful in conjunction with other treatments.

◆ **Surgery.** If your parent is otherwise healthy, a doctor may recommend surgery to replace a badly damaged joint with an artificial one. Be aware that such surgery is a major undertaking, especially if your parent is old or very frail. Ask the doctor about arthroscopy, a less

 **FOR MORE HELP**

For more information about various ailments, symptoms, exercises, support groups, treatments and the latest research on joints and bones, contact:

**Arthritis Foundation Information Line 800-283-7800**

**National Institute of Arthritis and Musculoskeletal and Skin Diseases Information Clearinghouse 301-495-4484**

**National Osteoporosis Foundation 800-223-9994**

invasive procedure that requires only local anesthesia and usually no hospital stay.

# Incontinence

You've just noticed a large yellow stain on your father's pants or a distinctive odor coming from your mother's bedroom. There is a moment of shock. A wave of sorrow. Then the question: *What do I do now?*

It's understandable if you're upset, but try to shake off any disgust or embarrassment, because you need to talk with your parent about this. Though you may meet with resistance or denial, talking is the only way to ease the humiliation and find solutions. Be gentle, sympathetic and tactful. Find a time when others will not overhear or interrupt you. Let your parent know how common the problem is (up to 30 percent of people over age 60 are completely or partially incontinent), and that help is available.

Once the problem is acknowledged, get your parent to a doctor who will give the situation the attention it deserves. You may have to advocate with special persistence here. A recent report showed that 35 to 50 percent of doctors did nothing when told that a patient was incontinent. If your parent's doctor is not helpful, she should see a urologist, gynecologist or geriatrician. Some geriatric care centers have special clinics devoted to incontinence.

Urinary incontinence is almost

**“***My mother got up from her chair in the living room to go into dinner and I noticed this spot on the cushion. She is a fastidious woman, and I think she was unaware that anything had happened. She had developed fluid in her abdomen from the cancer and it was putting pressure on all of her organs, so maybe that triggered the incontinence.*

*I thought, 'Am I going to have to tell her, or will she notice it herself and try to hide it from me?' I wasn't offended by the problem. I was more worried that it would be just one more encroachment on her dignity. I really hurt for her.***”***      —RUTH S.

always treatable with exercise, bladder training, surgery and other techniques. Bowel incontinence is a somewhat more difficult problem, but it too can be treated in many instances, and it can always be made more manageable.

Although incontinence can cause infections and depression, it is not as much a medical crisis as it is a social one. You and your parent will fare a little better if you each have a thick social skin and a ready sense of humor.

## URINARY INCONTINENCE

Normal bladder routines run amok for all sorts of reasons—infections, prostate troubles, hormones, diabetes, dehydration, immobility, surgery, weakened or damaged muscles, and medications. Constipation can cause urinary incontinence if it

# TYPES OF INCONTINENCE

**Transient incontinence** comes on suddenly and acutely. A person who has never wet his pants starts having accidents, often because he can't physically get to the toilet, or because of an infection, a new medication or constipation. The incontinence is almost always reversible and may even disappear on its own.

**Stress incontinence** primarily affects women. They laugh, cough, strain, exercise, sneeze or pick up a heavy box and, oops. The culprit: the ring of muscles around the urethra (the passageway for urine), which usually holds in urine, is loose and stretched out, often as a result of bearing children and the hormonal changes that take place after menopause. As a result, small amounts of urine leak out when the woman exerts even the smallest pressure on the bladder.

**Urge incontinence** is characterized by a sudden urge to urinate and not enough time to get to the toilet. For a variety of possible reasons, including stroke or infection, the bladder contracts and releases the urine uncontrollably. In *reflex incontinence* the bladder releases with no warning at all.

**Overflow incontinence** is often seen in men with prostate troubles. When the prostate gland, which surrounds the urethra, is enlarged, it can block the passageway so urine can't drain out normally during toileting. Instead, the bladder holds on to urine, and it eventually overflows and dribbles out, causing minor leaks throughout the day. Overflow incontinence is also seen in people who have other disorders or infections that block the urethra or prevent the bladder from contracting normally. The buildup of urine can cause bladder or kidney infections if the disorder is not treated.

**Functional incontinence** has nothing to do with the bladder and urethra. What is at fault here is the brain. Because of dementia, a head injury or stroke, the brain no longer hears the bladder screaming, "Hurry up and find a toilet!" With no such message, the person not only leaves the floodgates open (often at the worst possible time and in the worst possible place), but he may not have any idea that something odd has occurred.

People are sometimes misdiagnosed as having functional incontinence when the real problem is that they can't get to the toilet quickly enough or they haven't been given a bedpan or commode.

puts pressure on, or otherwise irritates, the muscles of the bladder. Stroke, dementia and delirium can also lead to incontinence if the brain isn't sending or receiving bladder or bowel signals normally. How incontinence is treated depends in part on what type of incontinence your parent has.

## Managing Urinary Incontinence

Incontinence disappears on its own in about 12 percent of women and 30 percent of men. When it doesn't, a doctor's first task is to treat the underlying problem. After that, the best attack is a non-medical one—bladder exercises, bladder training and regular toilet scheduling. These techniques require commitment and practice, but they are quite successful in treating stress and urge incontinence in particular. About 20 percent of patients are cured and almost all the rest are helped significantly.

♦ **Kegel exercises.** These exercises require no gym outfit and no sweating, just commitment. Kegel exercises strengthen the ring of muscles around the urethra, the exit tube from the bladder, and are particularly useful in treating stress incontinence. The exercises entail squeezing the muscles of the vagina and anus. Your mother can get the feel of where the muscles are by stopping the flow while she is urinating. (She should not be tightening the muscles in her legs, fanny or stomach, which are not involved in bladder control.) She should do these squeezes (holding each for several seconds) through-

out the day, for a total of 100 to 200 squeezes each day. For stress incontinence, your parent should get in the habit of squeezing these muscles before lifting, sneezing, coughing or, if possible, laughing.

Kegels can be done discreetly while watching television, reading, lying in bed or even sitting in a restaurant. However, like other workouts, they require dedication. It usually takes at least one month of Kegeling before any real effect is noticed. Once there's some improvement, be sure your parent continues the routine to maintain bladder control.

♦ **A schedule.** Scheduling bathroom trips can help stress and urge incontinence. Have your parent keep track of when she urinates for a day or two, and then make a schedule that gets her to the toilet just before she typically needs to use it. She might sit on the toilet, say, every hour whether she thinks she needs to or not. (Bathroom trips shouldn't be scheduled too frequently, as that can actually cause urge incontinence if the bladder learns to hold only small amounts of fluid.) Your parent should also stick to a schedule of fluid intake—a glass of orange juice at 7 A.M., a glass of water at 10 A.M., and so on.

♦ **Bladder training.** Your parent can learn to extend the time between bathroom trips. In bladder training, a person gets on a schedule of going to the toilet every 30 to 60 minutes, and then slowly lengthens the time between visits. Your parent should increase these intervals until she can wait two or three hours. To practice, your parent should empty her bladder completely, and then suppress any urge in between scheduled trips by relaxing or diverting her attention. ("Holding it" during these intervals is a great way to strengthen the muscles around the urethra.)

♦ **Biofeedback.** Usually used in conjunction with exercises, this technique can be very helpful. The patient is hooked up to a device that informs him how well he is contracting and relaxing his sphincter, detrusor and abdominal muscles—all involved in bladder control. With this information as a guide, he practices ways to manipulate these muscles and gradually gains better control over them.

♦ **Bedpans and commodes.** If your parent has trouble getting to the bathroom because of a physical disability or urge incontinence, put a commode, bedpan or urinal by his bed or chair. Or, if it is possible, have him sit or sleep near a bathroom that is not used by anyone else in the family.

♦ **Dietary changes.** Limiting caffeine and alcohol should improve continence, and some studies suggest that avoiding spicy foods, tomatoes and imitation sweeteners may help too. Obesity also plays a role in some cases, so you might urge your parent to lose weight.

Do not let your parent drink less in order to urinate less. This will cause dehydration and can make her incontinence worse, as highly-concentrated urine may result in infections.

♦ **Medications.** In conjunction with exercises and training programs, certain drugs (and there are quite a number of options) can be used to stop bladder contractions or strengthen the resistance of the urethra. They are most helpful in cases of urge and stress incontinence.

Some medications can worsen incontinence, so be sure the doctor checks your parent's drug list to see if it needs adjustment. Drugs to watch for include diuretics, tranquilizers, sedatives, drugs for Parkinson's disease, psychotropics, antihistamines and calcium-channel blockers.

♦ **Surgery.** Usually a last resort, surgery is sometimes necessary to clear obstructions (for example, an enlarged prostate), to reposition the bladder or to repair or replace the urethra. A number of devices can replace or augment weakened muscles and control urination, and new studies suggest that injections of collagen, silicone or other materials into or around the urethra may narrow the opening and help control urination. Doctors have also found some success in using a balloon to open the urethra when an enlarged prostate has forced it shut.

♦ **Pads, diapers and catheters.** These should be used only when all else fails, or for trips and other occasions that require extra security. Besides being uncomfortable, demoralizing and inconvenient, diapers and catheters can worsen incontinence if the person learns to rely on them and stops exercising his bladder muscles. Over time, the body can become desensitized to its own messages. (This is especially true when a person is in the early stages of dementia.) Diapers and catheters, used incorrectly, can also lead to infections.

Nevertheless, when necessary, diapers and catheters can be lifesavers. Which of the many varieties to use depends on your parent's own situation and comfort.

For minor leaking, a menstrual "maxipad" or a similar pad that's made to absorb urine may be adequate. It is less bulky than a diaper, but also offers less protection.

Disposable adult diapers that are "super-absorbent" are thinner than others but still hold quite a bit of fluid. Washable diapers are often cheaper, but don't hold as much fluid and are not as convenient to use. Disposable liners or pads that fit into a washable outer pant may offer the best of both worlds.

Whenever your parent wears diapers, special attention is required to avoid skin infections and rashes. Your parent should not sit in wet or dirty pants for any longer than absolutely necessary. The crotch must be thoroughly cleaned at every diaper change with mild soap and water and then dried with a cotton towel. A small amount of moisturizer—no powders—helps prevent irritation. Boxes of "wipes," which are handy, along with diaper rash ointment, can be found in the baby section of grocery stores, department stores or pharmacies. Use diaper rash cream if necessary, and call a doctor if the irritation doesn't go away in a day or two.

A catheter is basically a tube that runs from the bladder into a storage bag that hangs from a bed or is attached to the leg and hidden under pants or a skirt. Your parent is most apt to need a catheter while confined to a bed or wheelchair.

A catheter can be inserted into the bladder permanently by a nurse, or inserted according to a schedule by your parent. There are also catheters that attach to the genitals (a condom-like device for men and a somewhat less useful suction gadget for women). But beware of infections. Catheters need to be changed regularly.

 **FOR MORE HELP**

**Help for Incontinent People (HIP)**
800-252-3337

**National Institute on Aging**
800-222-2225

**Simon Foundation for Continence**
800-237-4666

## BOWEL INCONTINENCE

Bowel incontinence is a less common problem, but it can be a far more troubling one. If your parent is immobile, bed-ridden or mentally impaired, and you have to change diapers yourself, it may become more than you can handle. Changing diapers and protecting the house against damage is an enormous task, both physically and emo-

## BETTER BATHROOM HABITS

❖ Clear a path to the toilet. If possible, make sure your parent has a private bathroom, so it's never occupied by someone else.

❖ Place night-lights and/or reflector tapes along the path to the bathroom to avoid any stumbling around at night.

❖ Make sure your parent can use the toilet with ease. Install grab bars, buy a raised toilet seat and put the toilet paper within easy reach.

❖ Get your parent to wear clothing that's easily removable (skirts or elastic-waist pants, Velcro or snap enclosures instead of buttons, knee-high stockings instead of pantyhose).

❖ If the toilet is far away or shared, buy a commode, bedpan or hand-held urinal. Get a portable urinal for traveling.

❖ Make sure your parent empties his or her bladder before going to bed.

❖ When in a new place, locate the bathroom immediately. Avoid situations where there are no bathrooms, such as buses or shops without public facilities.

❖ Choose seats in restaurants, airplanes, theaters, etc. that are near a bathroom. Call in advance and plan the seating so you don't have to make a fuss when you arrive.

❖ Use waterproof liners (disposable or washable) under bedsheets, in the car, and on your parent's chair. You can find these at a medical supply store. Or buy waterproof crib sheets, which are sold with other baby supplies, or place a plastic shower liner inside a folded sheet and lay it across the middle of the bed. (A shower liner alone is too slippery and may cause your parent to fall.) Never put rubber next to your parent's skin. It's not only uncomfortable; it can cause reactions and severely irritate the skin.

❖ To reduce odors, have your parent deposit soiled clothing in a small pail, equipped with a lid and a deodorizer, that you've placed in an inconspicuous spot in the bathroom.

❖ A fan and an open window, whenever possible, will reduce odor problems. So will an open box of baking soda. Baking soda will get rid of odors in carpets and upholstery too. Believe it or not, a cut onion left in a room will absorb odors without leaving its own smell—try it!

tionally. Don't be hard on yourself. If the treatments discussed here don't work, get outside help or begin to look into assisted-living or nursing home care.

Oddly enough, the most common cause of bowel incontinence is constipation. When the bowel is blocked, liquid leaks around the obstruction. Diarrhea can also cause incontinence in elderly people, as they are less able to hold on to soft or liquid stools. Bowel incontinence is also caused by surgery, medications, illness, childbirth, injury to the anal muscles or nerves around the rectum (often from straining or prolonged laxative use), dementia and severe depression.

### Treating Bowel Incontinence

Any severe constipation or diarrhea needs to be treated immediately. If the incontinence remains, the doctor needs to search for other causes. Torn sphincter muscles can be repaired surgically. Nerve damage that numbs the normal sensations of an approaching bowel movement can be treated by using enemas or suppositories to empty the bowels on a schedule. When muscles aren't working properly—the person feels the need to go but can't hold on or get to a bathroom in time—electrical stimulation (using painless electrical currents to "exercise" muscles) can help strengthen the sphincter muscles. Stool-bulking agents can firm up loose stool. A method of biofeedback, in which a balloon is placed in the rectum and the person learns muscle control by watching the results of his efforts on a monitor, is

also very successful in treating bowel incontinence.

A high-fiber diet can often help control bowel incontinence by restoring regularity. Also, try the suggestions for treating urinary incontinence—setting schedules, exercising muscles, using commodes—as many are useful in treating bowel incontinence as well.

# Constipation

After about age 70, many people become concerned about their bowels. If they don't go to the bathroom for a day or two, they worry that they may explode. The truth is, not everyone needs to move his bowels every day. In fact, once every three days will get your parent through the week just fine. So if he constantly complains of constipation, but has no symptoms other than irregularity, urge him as gently and tactfully as you can not to

*"I guess we all wish for the same thing—that our parents will be independent until they die. Then you could help them with a few practical things, like going shopping or taking care of the house, and you would include them in family affairs, and that would be it. You wouldn't have to hear about every bowel movement, which is the level I am at with my mother. I don't really want to take care of my mother's bowel movements. I'd rather just take her shopping."*  —BARBARA F.

## MEDICAL ALERT

Blood in stools, dark or oddly-colored stools, a sudden change in bowel habits or pain in the lower abdomen should be reported to the doctor immediately. Also, be sure that your parent has an annual colon exam.

worry so much about it.

True constipation—when bowel movements are difficult, dry or painful, and a person has gas, bloating and a sore, tender belly—is miserable. And if left untreated it can become extremely serious (and may be a sign of some other disease). A doctor should be consulted if the home remedies listed later in this section fail to work.

Your parent should avoid laxatives, as they not only don't solve the problem, but can worsen it. Contrary to what the ads suggest—with laxatives, your parent will stroll along breezy seasides or bound across tennis courts—laxatives used routinely can interfere with nature so severely that, over time, the body forgets how to operate on its own. So, use them sparingly or with a doctor's advice. (Stool softeners are okay to use, although their lubricants may hinder vitamin absorption. Sugarless candies that contain sorbitol are also a relatively safe "laxative" worth trying.)

Constipation may be the result of a number of underlying and treatable conditions. Hormonal problems, such as a thyroid disorder, can disrupt normal habits. Irritable bowel syndrome (also known as spastic colon or irritable colon syndrome) can cause both constipation and diarrhea. Hemorrhoids or any other sore near the anus can make a person resist the need to go to the bathroom, as can surgery in the abdominal area—though this is usually a temporary problem. Damage to the digestive system from cancer, nerve disorders, Parkinson's disease, diabetes and other illnesses can harm the digestive tract in such a way that bowel movements become difficult.

Severe constipation, when bowels become impacted, requires medical attention as toxins can seep into the blood stream. If enemas or suppositories don't work, doctors may have to remove the obstruction manually or, in extreme cases, surgically.

### Treating Constipation

◆ **Fiber, fiber, fiber.** A good diet, for bowels and everything else, is packed with green, leafy vegetables, fresh fruit and whole-grain breads, pasta and cereals. Fiber, particularly wheat bran, is great for treating and preventing constipation. A high-fiber cereal eaten regularly is a quick fix, but it shouldn't replace more varied and natural sources of fiber. (See Appendix D, page 412, for more on fiber and diet.) If your parent decides to eat high-fiber cereal or use fiber supplements, she should begin slowly, as taking a large amount suddenly may leave her doubled over with stomach cramps.

◆ **Water, water, water.** Fiber works to aid regularity by absorbing fluids and thereby softening feces. But it can't work on a dry stomach. Eight glasses of water a day is the standard recommendation, but even four to six will help keep things moving. Soda, juice or herbal tea work as well as water, but drinks containing alcohol or caffeine won't help at all.

◆ **Movement.** Exercise helps keep bowels regular, along with its many other benefits. Your parent needs to get out for a walk, do some stretching, or, if she is laid up, at least try to stand upright or move to a chair. Talk with the doctor about exercises and movement that your parent can do, even from a bed or chair, or call a physical therapist who specializes in the care of the elderly. Any exercise, no matter how little, is better than none.

◆ **Bathroom routines.** When it's time to go to the toilet, it's time to go. Make sure your parent doesn't "hold it," ignore the urge, or wait for a more convenient time and place. If your parent is in a new place, which can upset her daily ritual, she should try to go at the same time of day she normally does and also try to stick with her regular diet as much as possible.

◆ **Medications.** Narcotics, antacids, antispasmodic drugs, antihistamines, antihypertensive agents, antidepressants and tranquilizers can all cause constipation, as can some dietary supplements and a host of other drugs. Talk with the doctor about lowering the dose of any drug you suspect is causing a problem, or about changing or stopping the medication.

# Other Digestive Disorders

◆ **Difficulty swallowing.** Dry mouth is the most common reason for swallowing difficulty, but the problem can also be caused by weakened throat muscles or disorders such as dementia, cancer or stroke, which disrupt the signals to and from the brain that control swallowing. If the problem becomes severe, it can lead to malnutrition, choking or pneumonia (because fluid gets into the lung).

Keep an eye out for clues such as gagging noises, drooling, coughing, belching and the like, while your parent eats. Check to see if he has trouble swallowing only certain types of foods (for example, liquids and not solids).

Soft, moist foods and those accompanied by sauces may go down more easily than dry foods or thin liquids like juice or water. They slide down the throat easily, and yet still have enough substance to trigger the swallowing reflex. Urge your parent to sit upright while eating, to eat slowly rather than wolfing down food, to take tiny bites, and to avoid chatting while eating or gulping a drink before a bite of food is chewed and swallowed completely. If the problem is severe, consult a doctor (and see page 150 for more tips on helping your parent eat).

# RX FOR CHOKING

If your parent has trouble swallowing, be prepared with a little first aid.

If he is choking on food or another object, do nothing as long as he is able to speak, cough or breathe at all.

If the choking person is unable to breathe (in which case he may be silent, appear panicked or grab at his throat), perform the Heimlich maneuver. First, stand behind him, wrapping your arms around his chest. Make a fist just below the rib cage and above the navel, and clasp that fist with your other hand. With a quick, strong thrust of your hands, pull inward and upward four times. Repeat this thrusting motion until the food is dislodged.

If the person is unconscious or horizontal, place one hand just above the navel in the middle of the abdomen. Place the other hand on top of the first hand and press in with a quick thrust. Repeat.

If this fails, call for emergency help and begin artificial respiration. For more information on the Heimlich maneuver and other first-aid techniques, call the local chapter of the American Red Cross.

♦ **Heartburn.** Medications, chocolates, fried foods, spicy foods, rich foods, tobacco and alcohol may all contribute to the burning pain in your parent's chest, a searing just behind the chest bone that is sometimes mistaken for heart disease. The pain may become worse when your parent leans forward or lies down, as the esophagus fails to close completely and acid flows upward from the stomach.

If certain foods trigger the trouble, your parent has to avoid them. Also, eating smaller, more frequent meals, avoiding tight clothing, eating several hours before bedtime and elevating the head at night can all help. Antacids can be helpful but if symptoms persist, your parent should see a doctor.

♦ **Indigestion.** Indigestion, or dyspepsia, is often a Thanksgiving Day problem, caused by overindulgence at the dinner table—eating too much or too fast, or eating rich or spicy foods. But persistent indigestion can also be a sign of a digestive tract disorder, like an ulcer or gall bladder disease. It is usually characterized by heartburn, nausea, vomiting, bloating and discomfort. Again, a change in diet should solve the problem, but if it doesn't go away, consult the doctor.

♦ **Ulcers.** When the protective lining of the stomach fails to do its job, digestive acids, which break down food in the stomach, can eat away at the stomach lining and create raw, painful sores called peptic ulcers. Ulcers run in families and in most cases are caused by bacteria in the digestive tract. They are also caused (or worsened) by tobacco, alcohol, aspirin and other nonsteroidal anti-inflammatory drugs. Other medications, spicy or highly acidic foods and stress may also play a minor role. Ulcers, which can cause internal bleeding and other complications, can be more serious in the elderly than in younger people. If you think your parent may have an ulcer, call her doctor.

The first line of attack should be to ban smoking, caffeine, alcohol, aspirin and NSAIDs. Meals should be small, bland and frequent. Antacids are helpful, but must be used with care as some contain large amounts of sodium, and they can interfere with the absorption of other drugs. Drugs that decrease stomach acid production also help. Treated this way, ulcers generally heal within two or three months (large ulcers take longer to heal), but because they often recur, your parent should take precautions even after the symptoms are gone. Antibiotics also can cure most ulcers.

◆ **Diverticular disease.** Diverticula are small sacs that develop along the lining of the intestine for reasons that are not clear, although lack of adequate dietary fiber seems to play a role. The presence of these sacs is called diverticulosis, a very common ailment in elderly people. Half of all people over 80 have it, but only about 20 percent of them have any symptoms—cramps, bloating, constipation or diarrhea and pain in the lower abdomen. Usually the symptoms disappear with some rest,

a diet high in fiber, plenty of liquids, and if these don't succeed, antispasmodic drugs or antibiotics.

Diverticulitis is a far more serious problem that requires immediate medical attention. The sacs become inflamed, often because stool gets stuck, causing infection or a perforation. Diverticulitis causes pain, fever and stiffness of the abdomen and can lead to a number of complications. It is treated with antibiotics, intravenous fluids and, in some cases, surgery.

◆ **Hemorrhoids.** Hemorrhoids can ruin an otherwise good day. Straining puts pressure on the veins of the anus, which distend outward and form small, painful protuberances that feel a little like grapes. Hemorrhoids are often itchy and may be bloody. Older people may be at greater risk if they sit for long stretches of time, are constipated, or vomit, cough or sneeze fiercely and repeatedly.

Usually fiber, fluids and time will relieve the problem. Over-the-counter hemorrhoidal creams, warm baths, petroleum jelly, ice packs and cold witch hazel can ease the pain and itching. A doughnut-shaped pillow may make sitting more comfortable, but it should be used only for short periods as it can cause pressure sores. If hemorrhoids persist and are severe, they can be treated by a minor surgical procedure.

◆ **Gas.** Intestinal gas can be unpleasant for both you and your parent, but it is normal and not life-threatening. As with constipation, older people sometimes become overly concerned about gas because they have some preconceived notion of what is "normal." (Tell your parent that a study has shown that men ages 25 to 35 pass gas 10 to 20 times a day.)

Where does gas come from? Usually from swallowing air while eating, or from the production of bacteria in the bowels. It can be eased by avoiding dairy products, as lactose intolerance is common among the elderly. Other dietary culprits include beans, legumes, raisins, broccoli, cauliflower, Brussels sprouts, bran, cabbage—all those high-fiber, low-fat foods that are so healthful. Rather than cut out these good foods, have your parent cut down on them, and put up with a few bad odors.

While gas certainly can cause stomach pains and bloating, it is the ego that usually gets hurt. Elderly people often have little or no control over when or how gas is released. Your parent may embarrass herself, and you, but try to ignore it, cover for her or joke with her about it.

◆ **Diarrhea.** Severe or chronic diarrhea always requires medical attention (see box). But an occasional bout of diarrhea is not a serious problem, though psychologically it can be very upsetting. Diarrhea is the body's way of getting rid of toxins in the digestive tract, and can be caused by bad food, laxatives, antacids, diuretics, antibiotics, anxiety or intestinal disorders. Milk and other dairy products can also cause diarrhea in people who are lactose intolerant. Most of the time, the

## MEDICAL ALERT

If diarrhea is severe or lasts for more than a week, contact your parent's doctor. In the meantime, it is important that your parent's body be replenished with salt and water. Mix one quart water, a teaspoon of salt and four teaspoons of sugar (the sugar helps the body absorb the salt). If this mixture is unpalatable, try adding fruit juice instead of sugar, or try a drink like Gatorade, or some plain water along with something salty, like pretzels. Your parent should, if possible, drink up to a pint of this liquid every hour (but ask the doctor, as some elderly people should not drink as much of it) until the diarrhea has subsided. Over-the-counter anti-diarrheal medications are not always advised, as diarrhea is a sign that the body needs to rid itself of bacteria.

problem disappears fairly quickly on its own.

If it is severe or chronic, or if there is blood in the bowels, diarrhea may be caused by colon cancer, infection, diabetes, severe constipation (when liquid flows around the blockage) or other serious problems that need immediate medical attention.

◆ **Anemia.** Anemia, which is common in the elderly, is not really a digestive tract disorder, but a blood disorder, though some forms of the illness are caused by digestive or dietary problems. When a person is diagnosed as anemic it means that the red blood cells that carry oxygen around the body are damaged or in short supply. Anemia can make a person feel old and tired—even older and more tired than he already feels—and it can cause headaches, shortness of breath, chest pains, swelling, confusion, dizziness, depression, and, in the case of iron-deficient anemia, a sore tongue.

Iron-deficient anemia, the most common type of anemia found in the elderly, is usually caused by internal bleeding, which could mean something serious and must be checked by a doctor. (The bleeding often happens in small amounts over time, so the person is completely unaware of it.) Once iron becomes dangerously low, diet alone cannot restore it. Your parent may need iron supplements or iron injections, in addition to treatment for any underlying disorder.

Other types of anemia may be caused by chronic infection or inflammation, kidney or liver disease, or folate or vitamin B-12 deficiency.

◆ **Diabetes.** Non-insulin-dependent diabetes (also known as adult-onset or Type 2 diabetes) is more common in older people who are overweight and inactive. Eight percent of people over 65 and up to 25 percent of people over 85 have diabetes, a condition in which the body loses its ability to regulate the level of glucose, a simple sugar which acts as fuel. Early signs of the disease include fatigue, weight loss, blurred vision and itchy skin. While younger diabetics experience thirst and frequent urination, these symptoms may or may not be present in older people. Instead they may notice other symptoms, such as tingling in the feet or numbness, confusion or depression.

If your parent has such symptoms he should see a doctor right away, because diabetes must be carefully managed. Untreated, it can lead to serious trouble, including stroke, blindness, heart disease, kidney failure, nerve damage, unconsciousness and coma. The first line of treatment is a controlled diet (devised by a dietitian), exercise and, when necessary, weight loss. Insulin therapy is often necessary, as is medication—sulfonylurea agents—which stimulate insulin secretion.

For more information about diabetes, contact the American Diabetes Association (800-232-3472).

# Depression

Your father doesn't want to play bridge anymore. He turns down his favorite mint chocolate Girl Scout cookies. He dresses in the same clothes every day and won't go out. "What's the point?" he says, staring vacantly at the television set. "I'm just an old man. Nobody wants a decrepit old man around." Then he calls you by the wrong name and goes to bed.

It may seem that he's just being ornery, causing you untold anxiety or exasperation, but in truth he may be suffering from depression. Estimates suggest that up to 20 percent of the elderly are depressed, and in hospitals and nursing homes that rate jumps to 25 percent. And it is apparently on the rise. The suicide rate among the elderly is up, as is the rate of alcoholism.

What's really alarming is not the number of elderly people who are depressed, but the number who are never treated—nearly 75 percent of them! Elderly patients ignore depression because they were brought up at a time when depression was considered to be a weakness, some sort of character flaw (not that times have changed all that much). Doctors and families are often preoccupied with other medical problems, or think that malaise, weight loss, change in appetite, irritability and apathy are all just a normal part of growing old. They don't need to be.

This neglect is a shame because depression is almost always treatable with medication, counseling or both. Untreated, it saps an already weak immune system, reduces a person's incentive to care for himself, lowers his energy level, exacerbates dementia and makes your parent's

## SIGNS OF DEPRESSION

If your parent has several of the following symptoms for more than two weeks, press his doctor for action or get him to a psychiatrist:

❖ Dejection and sadness without any apparent cause

❖ Lack of interest in activities that were once considered enjoyable

❖ Change in appetite or weight

❖ Insomnia or change in sleep habits, including waking early in the morning

❖ Fatigue and lethargy

❖ Lack of concentration, trouble thinking clearly, indecisiveness

❖ Talk of suicide or death

❖ Feelings of hopelessness

❖ Excessive feelings of guilt and worthlessness

❖ Irritability or hostility

❖ Vague complaints of chronic aches and pains that seem to have no physical basis

❖ Poor grooming and personal hygiene

❖ Weeping or tearfulness

❖ Change in bowels, usually constipation

❖ Increased use of alcohol, drugs or tobacco.

late years miserable for him as well as for you. Studies show that depression increases the risk of stroke and reduces a person's ability to recover from surgery, infection and other illnesses.

Know the signs of depression and if you see them, get your parent medical help immediately. But you have to be on your toes because depression can be marked by perceptions of physical illness—your parent may complain of an upset stomach, back pains, insomnia, headaches or even vaguer aches and pains—or it can seem like early dementia or coincide with dementia itself.

## TREATING DEPRESSION

Depression is not a mood; it is a biological illness. The chemistry in the brain has changed and needs rebalancing. Why it comes on is not clear. Loss, fear, boredom, worry, loneliness and stress all play a role, but it is more complicated than that. Some people inherit a genetic vul-

**DEPRESSION AND DEMENTIA**

Your father may be confused and forgetful, leading you to fear the worst. But before you call the Alzheimer's Association, have him evaluated by a doctor. Depression is often mistaken for dementia and therefore left untreated.

Depression can also be coupled with dementia, particularly in the earliest stages of dementia. Between 20 and 40 percent of people with dementia also suffer from depression. It is important to treat the depression, since treatment can alleviate the confusion dramatically (albeit not permanently). For more on dementia see Chapter Fifteen.

nerability to depression, and some are more vulnerable because of poor or unresolved relationships with their parents early in life. Medications, illness, hormonal and biological changes, inactivity and poor diet can also contribute to depression.

The mere suggestion that your parent see a psychiatrist, or even his own doctor, about a mental health problem may be pooh-poohed or it may make your parent furious. Make it clear to him that depression is a biological illness that can be treated. Tell him that even if he has no interest in getting help, it would be

*"My father had to be hospitalized twice because of severe infections in his feet. We were all so concerned about his diabetes and his infection that at first we failed to see the real problem: depression. Because he was depressed, he wasn't taking care of himself. He wasn't controlling his diabetes, he wasn't eating well, and he didn't call anyone when he first noticed trouble. I guess he figured it didn't matter."* —KATHERINE S.

a great relief to *you* if he at least talked to a doctor about it. Tell him that you won't stop hassling him until he does it. Or get a trusted doctor or member of the clergy to initiate a discussion with him about his depression.

If the prospect of seeing a psychiatrist makes your parent uncomfortable, a family doctor who is savvy in such matters can treat the depression. But be sure the doctor he consults is one who takes the depression seriously; don't be deterred by a physician who tells you "it's natural at his age." No one should have to live with the deep misery of clinical depression, and a number of treatments can be tried.

♦ **Antidepressive drugs.** A variety of antidepressive drugs work well to relieve depression with only minor side effects. (Certain drugs, like nortriptyline and desipramine, are better for elderly people as they are less apt to cause confusion, drowsiness or dizziness.) Antidepressive drugs generally take two to three months before they are fully effective and, because recurrence is common, they are often continued at a low dose for six to twelve months after the symptoms of depression have subsided.

♦ **Psychotherapy.** Drugs are more effective if they are coupled with counseling. The drugs relieve the severity of the depression, bringing a person out of the pit of despair, but they do not resolve the issues that might have led to or contributed to the depression. Therapy, individually or in a group, will help your parent address these prob-

"*After my father moved into the retirement home, he didn't want to do anything. Nothing seemed to please him. He stayed in his room most of the time, refused to see people, and just didn't care about anything. When I suggested that he get help, he became angry.*

*Finally, I couldn't stand it anymore. I marched into his room and told him to get in the car, and I took him to the geriatric psychiatry unit at our local hospital. I've never been forceful with my father, but something just got to me. I couldn't bear to see him like that.*

*He had ECT [electroconvulsive therapy] for several weeks and now he's in a day program where he meets with the psychiatrist and goes to a support group. I have to say, it's made a difference. He's not jumping about, all excited about life, but he's definitely better.*" —ELEANOR R.

lems. If he is not open to the idea of psychological counseling, you may have to do some cajoling.

♦ **Electroconvulsive therapy.** When the depression is severe and antidepressants and counseling don't help, electroconvulsive therapy, or ECT, is helpful for certain patients and seems to be particularly successful in treating the elderly. We've all heard horror stories about ECT, but the procedure has been fine-tuned and is now considered to be an effective and relatively safe way to reverse depression. It usually works faster

## AN ILLNESS, NOT A MOOD

When a person is depressed he cannot "snap out of it" any more than he can snap out of cancer or Parkinson's disease. This is not "just the blues," it is an illness. Although your impulse may be to try to help propel your parent out of this despair, avoid urging him to "cheer up" or to "look on the bright side." Attempts to convince him that life isn't so bad, or to help him see that others are worse off than he is, will only send the message that these feelings are something he is capable of controlling and that because he is not controlling them, he is a failure.

Instead, acknowledge his fears and his misery. Give him lots of support and understanding. *I know you feel horrible. I'm here to help you and we're going to get through this thing together.* And be sure he gets immediate medical care.

than drugs, but the effects don't last as long. (Medications will sometimes help lower the rate of recurrent bouts of depression.)

In the procedure, a patient is given an anesthetic and a muscle relaxant. A padded electrode is then placed at the temple. A small machine sends an electric pulse through the electrode and into the brain until the patient has a minor brain seizure. People often need up to a dozen of these treatments.

The procedure is not painful, but there is a risk of mild memory loss, which is why it is used only when other treatments fail. ECT is a poor choice for a person with dementia or certain other medical conditions. Your parent or you should discuss all the pros and cons with the doctor. Understandably, the idea may frighten your parent (or you), so by all means, get a second opinion.

◆ **Lifestyle.** Exercise, social activities, sleep, a good diet, and an understanding and loving family are all important in keeping depression at bay. Don't think that just because your parent is taking desipramine you can sit back and wait for him to get better. Depression is a complex illness that

 **FOR MORE HELP**

**National Institute of Mental Health's Depression Awareness, Recognition and Treatment Program 800-421-4211**

**National Foundation for Depressive Illness 800-248-4381**

must be attacked on many fronts. Patients need lots of support and encouragement.

# Delirium

Delirium can resemble depression and dementia, but it differs from them in that it typically comes on suddenly and severely—and usually lasts hours or days—and the most notable symptoms are extreme confusion and inattentiveness. A person with delirium may not be able to follow even a brief discussion, or he may fall asleep in the middle of a conversation. He may suddenly have no idea what is happening, may not recognize familiar faces or know where he is. While most older patients with delirium become quiet and sleepy, some become anxious and restless. In severe cases, they hallucinate and panic.

Delirium is common in elderly people who are hospitalized. It can occur as a result of illness, medications, the change to a new environment, dehydration, infections and, more than anything else, surgery. People who are already compromised by dementia, Parkinson's disease, stroke or tumor are at the greatest risk, as are very frail elderly people, who do not have the reserves to deal with illness or surgery.

## DIAGNOSIS AND TREATMENT

As with depression, if delirium goes unrecognized and untreated,

**❝** *While my mother was in the nursing home, she became very confused and started to act oddly. She refused food and water and would wander about like she didn't know where she was.*

*I was more concerned than the nurses were, and so I was the one who called it to the doctor's attention. He said she was delirious, and he put her through dozens of tests. They found that she was dehydrated, had a urinary tract infection and was taking too much of an antipsychotic drug. As soon as they adjusted the dose and dealt with her other problems, she returned to normal, or at least to what was normal for her.* **❞** —GLORIA C.

the cost is high. (Delirium is most frequently overlooked in elderly people who are taking medications, particularly antidepressants, benzodiazepines, drugs for Parkinson's disease and sedatives, because it may come on more slowly in these cases.) As the person who best knows your parent, you may be the first to spot these symptoms. Anytime you notice a significant change in your parent's behavior, alert a doctor or nurse immediately. Unchecked, delirium can become a medical emergency, and the sooner it is identified the easier it is to treat.

Since it's often not possible to identify a single cause, doctors attack delirium on all fronts. Any infections or illnesses need to be treated and over-the-counter drugs should be stopped or, if that is not possible, the dose reduced.

You play an important role in the treatment of your parent's delirium. A calm and supportive environment is essential in easing the symptoms, so assure your parent that he is safe and try to keep him calm. Help reorient him by speaking softly, and by surrounding him with familiar objects. Keep movement at a minimum, lighting dim and the noise level low. Night lights are sometimes helpful so your parent doesn't become confused if he wakes up in the dark. (Physical restraints are neither necessary nor advisable.)

# Anxiety Disorders

Has your mother always been a worry-wart, or have her anxieties reached new heights? About five percent of the elderly suffer from a psychiatric illness known as generalized anxiety disorder.

The most prevalent symptom is excessive worry about several issues, particularly about the future. Worry is accompanied by a number of physical reactions, including agitation, shakiness and trembling, as well as dizziness, shortness of breath, nausea, hot and cold flashes, frequent urination and an exaggerated response when startled. A person with anxiety disorder is also apt to be extremely vigilant and edgy, and may have trouble concentrating and sleeping.

As you may know by now, nothing to do with the elderly is simple. There are several ailments that are often mistaken for anxiety, including hyperthyroidism, and heart or lung diseases that cause palpitations and shortness of breath. Also, anxiety may be a symptom of delirium, depression or dementia, not an illness of its own accord. It's possible, too, that your parent does not have a psychiatric disorder, but is reacting to justifiable fears (for example, running out of money or getting into a car accident).

Generalized anxiety is caused by some combination of true anxiety, disease and the effects of medications, caffeine, vitamin B-12 deficiency or withdrawal from alcohol or sedatives. Treatment includes counseling to deal with specific causes of concern, family support, biofeedback to learn to control some of the body's reactions and relaxation techniques. Antianxiety drugs (preferably short-acting ones) should be used only in severe cases because they aren't highly successful and they often cause side effects such as depression, speech trouble and memory loss. Valium, Dalmane, Librium, Nembutal, Seconal and related drugs should not be prescribed at all for older people.

# Chapter Seven

# ON THE
# FIFTH FLOOR

*Entering the Hospital • Tests, Treatments and Surgery*
*• Dealing with Staff • Your Role as Visitor*
*• When You Are Far Away • Preparing for Discharge*

H OWEVER HOSPITALS TRY TO LOOK MORE WELCOMING and genial—with large plants in the lobby, colorful prints on the walls, friendly volunteers at the door—it never seems to work. Hospitals are scary places. For your parent, entering the hospital means risk and loss of control. He may be dreading a diagnosis or fearful that he won't be able to return to his own home again.

Your parent needs your comfort and reassurance now. He also needs an advocate, someone to stay informed about tests, treatments and other procedures, and to keep in touch with the doctors and nurses. If your parent is confused or too sick to speak for himself, then your involvement is even more essential. You should be aware of the problems that can occur in hospitals and the mistakes that can be made by an overworked staff.

This doesn't mean, however, that you have to sit at your parent's bedside around the clock. Quite the contrary, if you've been caring for him on a regular basis, this hospital stay may be the first chance you've had in months to get a full night's sleep or to spend time with friends. Visit and support your parent, but take advantage of this break in your duties. Get others to fill in for you sometimes, and then, when you are not at the hospital, try to get your mind off your worries. You deserve it.

# Choosing a Hospital

A doctor can work only in those hospitals where he or she has admitting privileges, so there may be little choice in selecting a hospital if your parent is already committed to a doctor. If there is a choice about which hospital to use and some preparation time—if your parent is having elective knee surgery, for example—he, or you, should visit nearby hospitals.

Generally, large medical centers associated with a university have high-caliber specialists and more sophisticated technology than community hospitals. Thus, they are better equipped to treat unusual ailments and perform risky procedures. But it also means that people with common problems sometimes get less attention than they might in a smaller hospital. Teaching hospitals train young doctors, using patients as teaching models, which can be disconcerting and embarrassing. But sometimes physicians-in-training, who ask a lot of questions, bring important matters to the doctor's attention.

Smaller community hospitals are generally suited to handle routine problems and are often richer in TLC. (Surgery at a not-for-profit community hospital may also be as much as 25 percent cheaper than at a private hospital.)

*"My father always went to the same hospital, but when I called 911, the ambulance took him to Riverside Hills Hospital. Here my father was in a strange place, with a new doctor who didn't know him at all, who didn't have any personal relationship with him.*

*It took me more than a week, but I finally got them to move him. They kept saying that he was too weak to make the move, that he was fine where he was. But I knew that he wasn't. I knew that this was an unfamiliar place for him.*

*He was moved and he died about two weeks later. But I know that he was more comfortable in a familiar place, with doctors and nurses who knew him and where his friends could visit him more easily. He couldn't tell me so, but I believe that I did the right thing.*"
—CHRIS D.

Veterans Affairs hospitals are sometimes unwieldy and top-heavy with bureaucracy, but since they are often associated with a university hospital, the medical care may be quite good. In any case, they are inexpensive. (The Department of Veterans Affairs, 800-827-1000, can tell you about eligibility and benefits.)

In an emergency, your parent may have to go to the nearest hospital—one where her doctor may not be able to treat her. But once she is out of danger, she can usually be transferred.

# Entering the Hospital

Unless there is an emergency, the hospital will want a variety of information before your parent is admitted, including name, address, social security number, phone number, birth date, name of next of kin, and Medicare, Medicaid and other health insurance numbers. Staff should also ask about advance directives, which are critical if your parent is seriously ill or if she is headed for surgery. Many older patients become briefly delirious after surgery and need family members to act on their behalf.

## WHEN ONE PARENT IS WELL

If one parent becomes chronically or dangerously ill and the other is well, your attention naturally turns to the patient, but in fact your primary focus should be to support your healthier parent. If your father is sick, it is your mother's responsibility to take care of her mate; it is yours to nurture her so that she can do her job well. Express your concern about your father's condition, step in when necessary, but be sure to support your mother.

The person who is well, or relatively well, is often ignored in these situations, but her life has taken a dramatic turn and she may be dealing with profound anguish—she stands to lose her mate and may already have lost many vital aspects of their relationship together. She also has taken on enormous responsibilities as the primary caregiver and decision-maker.

She may be faced with duties that she never had before, such as paying bills or handling home maintenance, that are not easy to learn.

Encourage your well parent to talk about her needs and hurts. Find out how she is managing and how you can help. Monitor her health, as she may be neglecting it now. Get her to eat well, exercise and see the doctor when necessary. Nudge her away from her duties occasionally and urge her to see friends or do other things that she enjoys. Otherwise, her health may dwindle rapidly, and you may find yourself with two ailing parents.

The Well Spouse Foundation (212-644-1241) can offer help. It hooks members up with support groups and pen pals and issues a newsletter six times a year.

If you know in advance about the hospitalization, ask if the paperwork can be done early so your parent doesn't have to deal with a lot of questions on an already tense day. Also, see if someone can drop you and your parent off at the hospital so she doesn't have to wait while you park.

Among the forms your parent, or you if you are acting on his behalf, will be asked to sign is a blanket consent form, which basically says that the hospital can do whatever needs to be done while he is under its care. Don't be alarmed. These forms are routine. The staff still needs a patient's consent before undertaking any measures beyond emergency procedures, but most hospitals won't admit patients unless they sign this form. If signing it makes you uncomfortable, add a note before the signature that says, "I'm signing this only so that my parent can be admitted to the hospital."

Ask right away if there is a choice in rooms, because once your parent is assigned to a room the staff will be reluctant to move her (it requires a lot of paperwork). If there is any choice, ask for a bed near a window. Natural light and a view—

---

## PACKING THE BAGS

There is little that your parent really needs in a hospital and anything valuable should stay at home. A hospital bag might include:

❖ hearing aids, eyeglasses, dentures, cane or walker

❖ a supply of her regular medications along with a list of her medications, their dosages, any allergies and medical history

❖ copies of pertinent legal documents, such as a living will, a health care proxy form or other advance directive

❖ slippers with rubber soles

❖ a couple of pairs of socks, preferably with rubber soles

❖ robe and pajamas or nightgown (short-sleeved or sleeveless, for easy access)

❖ toiletry items including toothbrush, razor, lip balm and moisturizer. Check before packing electrical devices, as some hospitals don't allow them.

❖ a clock and a calendar

❖ magazines, books, games, knitting, puzzles, a small inexpensive radio or tape player

❖ crackers, dried fruit, cereal or other non-perishable foods

❖ a box of ear plugs

❖ a telephone credit card number and a small amount of cash for vendors—no more than $20.

**❝**When the two of us brought my father to the hospital, my sister asked about the room selection and I was completely embarrassed. It didn't occur to me that there would be a choice, and I thought she was being frivolous and pushy. But just as I was searching for something conciliatory to say, the woman at the admitting desk said that she could arrange for Dad to be in a corner private room with windows on two sides, even though his insurance covered only a semi-private room. It had to do with their occupancy level. Boy, I learned my lesson that day.**❞**

—KATHERINE S.

even if it's just a rooftop—boost the spirits. You should also ask about roommates, privacy and anything else that concerns your parent. She may not be given a lot of choice, but it's certainly worth asking.

At the same time, inquire about a telephone and television, as it can take a day or two to get these services up and running. Find out about other amenities as well, such as newspaper delivery, barber and hair stylists, book and magazine carts. Patients often don't know about these services unless they ask for them.

## PREPARING FOR DISCHARGE—EARLY

As soon as you know your parent's prognosis, talk with the hospital's discharge planner, especially if your parent may have difficulty returning to her former life after she leaves the hospital. The discharge planner will help you prepare for your parent's return home, lining her up with community services, in-home care and medical equipment, or helping to make arrangements for her to move into a rehabilitation center, a nursing home or another living situation, if necessary. All of this planning takes time and you want everything to be in place when your parent is ready to leave the hospital. (See page 134.)

# Tests, Surgery and Treatments

Studies suggest that up to one-third of medical procedures are unnecessary, but it also has been found that older patients often receive too little treatment. On the one hand, doctors tend to over-probe and over-scan because they are fearful of malpractice lawsuits, enamored of technology, or baffled by a profusion of unusual symptoms. On the other hand, doctors also fail to order certain tests or procedures for the elderly and to investigate certain complaints because of ageism, concluding that certain ailments aren't worth treating in older patients.

How are you to know whether your parent is getting too much treatment or too little? Honestly, you can't, but you can impose safeguards by asking plenty of questions, making informed decisions and getting a second opinion whenever you are unclear about the best course of treatment.

## QUESTIONS TO ASK

Be tactful and considerate, but be sure to ask (and write down the answers you are given):

• Why is this test/treatment/ surgery being recommended?

• Is it absolutely necessary?

• What will this test tell us and where will we go from there? (For example, if the doctor is going to do surgery in either case, why bother with the test?)

• What other options are there and what are the potential risks and benefits of each?

• What happens if this is not done?

• How much will it cost? Is it covered fully by Medicare or by my parent's private insurance?

• Can other doctors who are treating my parent use the results from this test or blood sample so it doesn't have to be repeated?

• Are there other measures my parent might try first before undergoing this treatment or procedure, such as changes in diet or exercise, to correct what ails her?

• Are any experimental treatments available, and what are the risks and benefits of those?

## PREPARING FOR SURGERY

If your parent is going to have surgery, you or your parent should meet with the surgeon her doctor has recommended and find out his or her credentials and experience—in particular, how often he or she has done this particular procedure (be leery if it is less than 20 times in the past year, unless the operation is extremely unusual). Find out how soon and how often the surgeon or your parent's doctor will vis-

## GUILT, AGAIN?

Remember that your parent is not in the hospital because of something you or anyone else in the family did or failed to do. Don't torture yourself with guilt. *I knew I shouldn't have left him alone all afternoon. . . . I told her Dad was having chest pains. She should have had him come in for an exam days ago.*

Life is so clear in hindsight, but there really was no way you or anyone else could have predicted this accident or illness. And doing things differently might not have changed the outcome; in fact it might have led to a worse problem. This hospitalization is not anyone's fault, so focus your valuable energy on taking care of your parent now, and leave the guilt and blame behind.

it your parent after the surgery and note how to reach each of them if there is a problem or question. Learn about the anesthesiologist's qualifications and expertise, and make sure he or she will meet with your parent before surgery.

If the surgery is exploratory, find out what the doctor expects to find and what he might do about it. (Does your parent need to sign a consent form now so the surgeon can do what may need to be done?)

Ask the surgeon about possible complications and their symptoms. Elderly patients who undergo surgery are generally at high risk of heart and lung complications, blood clots and delirium, a state of extreme confusion.

In some teaching hospitals, residents (doctors-in-training) perform surgery, which should be acceptable as long as your parent's surgeon is close at hand to monitor every move. If the idea doesn't sit well with your parent or you, ask the doctor to perform the surgery personally.

If your parent is having one-day, or ambulatory, surgery it is best if the procedure is done either in a hospital or in a clinic or office that is near a hospital, in case there are unexpected complications. Be sure that she has an escort to and from the clinic and that you or whoever will care for her at home knows what sort of attention she will need during her recovery—what medications she needs to take, what potential problems to be on the watch for, and how the doctor can be reached if something seems wrong.

# At the Nurse's Station

In the hospital, a doctor will continue to oversee your parent's medical care, but it is the nurses who will tend to his needs and, to a large extent, monitor his health. The nurses are usually the ones to notice if a medication is having bad side effects, if your parent has a new symptom or if his mood or mental abilities have changed. Nurses know a lot about medicine and often understand a good deal (often more than the doctor) about individual patients. The nurse also acts as a liaison to the other hospital personnel, including social workers and escorts for medical tests.

Unless your parent is in the hospital for only a very brief stay, make a real effort to get to know

> **"**Sometimes we encourage families to help do things, like feed the patient—either because the person eats better when someone familiar helps, or because the family is going to take this person home and will have to do these things there. We want them to get comfortable with it.
>
> But some families feel put out by that. They feel like they are being asked to do the nurse's work. It's a challenge for the nurse to say, 'No, I'm not trying to get out of work. This is really better for the patient.' It's a very fine line.**"**
>
> —GAIL W., R.N.

the nurses who care for him. Learn their names and the times they work, and try to build a rapport with them. In the hospital, they are your best allies, and you need them on your side in order to assure that your parent receives the best care and comfort.

◆ **Respect them.** No matter how urgent your concerns may be, no matter how unraveled you feel, avoid the urge to bark orders. *I don't want my mother waiting for her pain medication. She was supposed to get it at two o'clock!* Protect your parent, guard her rights and advocate firmly on her behalf, but treat the staff as friend, not foe. Recognize the pressures that the nurses and other staff are under, carefully choose the matters you want to raise with them, and then work with them to find solutions. When you treat them with respect, they will be far more willing to treat you and your parent with respect.

If you do lose your cool, and most likely you will, be sure to apologize later.

◆ **Ask questions.** Don't withhold important questions and comments for fear of "bothering" the nurses. Most nurses do not consider questions or comments from family members a bother. They are often helpful at explaining things that the doctor didn't make clear. And your questions may bring an error or an oversight to their attention.

◆ **Provide information.** Be sure the nurses know about your parent's allergies or sensitivities, the other medications she is using or

any symptoms she may have. If you are worried about something in particular, tape a large note by the bed—"Mrs. Parker is severely allergic to all seafood." Also, be sure the nurses know about any particular habits, quirks, food preferences or special needs that might help them care for your mother. They will usually respond positively to any reasonable requests.

If your parent has dementia, is paralyzed from a stroke or has become extremely crotchety in her old age, tell the nurses. Let them know what she used to be like, or bring in a photo of her in her younger

*❝The rehabilitation therapist got very frustrated with my dad because he wasn't cooperating. But he wasn't cooperating because he didn't know what the hell he was doing. He has dementia and he gets anxious and ornery when things are new or when people push him to do things he doesn't want to do.*

*I learned that at some point, it's the habit of the rehab people to stop trying. I guess they deal with people like this all day long and it gets to them after awhile. I told the therapists that I understood it probably was demoralizing for them, but also how grateful we'd be if they could keep trying with my dad. I had to cajole and encourage and push to get them to keep working with him, but they did stick with it and Dad did, finally, go along with it.❞*

—Jacqui L.

## PRIVATE-DUTY NURSES, AIDES AND COMPANIONS

If you can't be with your parent as much as you would like, or if he needs more supervision than the hospital staff can provide, hire a companion or find out if there is a volunteer program in the community or the hospital.

If your parent needs more elaborate care—if he needs more nursing care than the staff can provide, for example—you can hire a private-duty nurse or a nurse's aide, but this is expensive. The hospital staff can refer you to the nurse's registry, or you can call a local home-care agency or a visiting nurse association.

Licensed practical nurses and nurses' aides have less training, but are also less expensive, than registered nurses. A health aide has even less expertise, but he or she can monitor your parent's medications, help feed her, bathe her, get her to the bathroom and do some minor medical tasks. (Some health insurance policies may cover the cost of a registered nurse and not a nurse's aide or health aide, so check first.)

Two guidelines to follow if you decide to hire additional help for your parent in the hospital: First, be sure the person you hire knows what responsibilities you expect him to perform, as the hospital is not supervising their work, you are. Second, make it clear to the hospital nurses and other personnel that this is no reflection on their work.

days—skiing, lecturing, dancing or doing whatever she used to enjoy. Let them get to know the person behind the illness.

♦ **Lend a hand.** Your assistance, even with little tasks, makes life easier for everybody—your mother gets better care, you feel useful, the nurse or aides are relieved of another chore. If your mother needs water or tea, if the floor near her bed needs to be wiped up, if she needs help bathing or feeding herself or getting out of bed, see if you can take care of it. Then ask if there are other things you can do to be helpful. You will win points for asking, even if there is nothing you can do to help.

♦ **Kindness counts.** Anxiety can make you forget all the usual social customs, but thoughtfulness can be enormously important to an overworked nurse, aide or housekeeper. When things are done well, when an extra task is undertaken, don't forget to express your thanks to the staff.

If your parent is going to be in for a long stay, go another step. If

## WHO ARE ALL THOSE PEOPLE IN WHITE COATS?

Who is checking your parent's stitches? Who is that new young man reading his chart? Who are all those other people in white coats who go by the name "doctor"? *Attending physicians* are doctors with admitting privileges to a hospital, like your parent's personal doctor. *House staff* have medical school degrees but are still in training and are not yet certified in a specialty. The house staff is comprised of *interns*, who are one year out of medical school, and *residents*, who are two, three, four (and sometimes more) years out of medical school. Residents may at times oversee your parent's care or perform medical procedures, including surgical procedures, while interns perform less technical tasks and are usually overseen by residents.

Teaching hospitals also have *medical students* who watch the house staff for the most part but also perform certain minor tasks. They, too, wear white coats and, in some hospitals, are called "doctor," although they do not have medical degrees.

There is no way for you or your parent to know who's who just by looking, but you should feel free to ask.

you bring cookies to your parent, bring some extra for the staff. If the care has been especially thoughtful, send a fruit basket, some flowers or an assortment of nuts.

Kindness to the staff is especially important if your parent is withdrawn, confused or a bit of a curmudgeon. It's hard for nurses and aides to be pleasant or helpful when a patient is uncommunicative or rude. You have to make up for your parent's behavior by being especially kind. Remind the staff that your parent's attacks are nothing personal and keep letting them know that you appreciate what they are doing.

# Problems and Disputes

If you or your parent has a problem with a hospital doctor, nurse or other staff member, talk with that person first, if at all possible. Do it privately, so as to not cause embarrassment, and do it at a time and place where you won't be interrupted. Be specific about your concern and try to cite an example of the problem. Many problems are due to a lack of communication—the nurse didn't know that your parent is allergic to aspirin because it hadn't been entered in her chart, or you didn't realize that the doctor had ordered her pain-killers stopped.

If the problem isn't resolved and you believe that it is serious, go up a step on the ladder, to the head nurse on the unit or floor, for example, or the hospital's director of nursing. If you are still not satisfied, try these other channels:

◆ **Patient advocates.** More than half of all non-government hospitals and nearly all veterans hospitals hire patient representatives or patient advocates who serve as a link between patients and the hospital system. Their job is to represent the patient, making sure that questions are answered and that any problems are resolved. Your parent or you can ask a patient advocate to help with practically anything—disputes with staff, lost hearing aids, billing questions, faulty plumbing, late lunch trays, roommate problems or inadequate insurance coverage. Of course, some patient advocates are more helpful than others, but the good ones are godsends.

Patient advocates should be listed in the hospital brochure or directory, or their phone number may be posted on the hospital room wall. If you don't see it, ask the nurse.

◆ **Hospital committees.** If a dispute is over a medical decision— you and the doctor disagree about when to withhold treatment or you believe your parent has received the wrong treatment—many hospitals have medical or ethics committees that review such dilemmas. Ask the hospital's patient advocate about how to appeal a decision.

◆ **Peer review organizations.** If you believe that your parent has received inadequate care or unnecessary treatment in the hospital, if she is refused admission, if she is being discharged too soon or if you believe Medicare coverage is being denied unfairly, you or your parent should contact the state Peer Review Organization (PRO) as soon as possible. A PRO is a group of physicians contracted by the federal government to ensure that Medicare patients receive proper care. For the address of the PRO in your parent's state, call the local social security office, the Office of Medical Review in Baltimore (410-966-6851) or your state agency on aging.

Hospitals are required to give your parent a pamphlet about Medicare, patient's rights, and the PRO appeals process. (See Appendix C, page 404 for "A Patients Bill of Rights.") Sometimes the hospital's patient advocate will even contact the PRO on behalf of your parent.

◆ **Last resorts.** When the trip gets really rough, if the nurse is abusive, the doctor reeks of alcohol, or your parent's Do Not Resuscitate order is being violated and the patient advocate is not helpful, there are still a few places where you can go for help or at least to lodge a complaint. Call or write the hospital administrator (if you mention that you have talked with your lawyer about the problem, you will get more attention). Report the problem to the local medical society and to the state board that licenses nurses or doctors. The state may also have a separate agency that oversees "medical quality assurance."

When a health professional is unprofessional, or a patient is otherwise treated poorly, the People's Medical Society in Pennsylvania (610-967-2136) will be able to tell you how to file a complaint in your parent's state.

# Your Role as an Advocate

Unfortunately, hospitals are not always safe havens. Because doctors and nurses frequently work at, or beyond, capacity, mistakes are made and patients are sometimes neglected. You can't expect to eliminate all the risks, but you can reduce them significantly by your persistent (yet pleasant) vigilance. The information given here is not intended to frighten you, simply to alert you.

## CONFUSION, DELIRIUM, DEPRESSION

Elderly patients who show no signs of confusion at home may become disoriented, argumentative and forgetful in the hospital, and those who already suffer from dementia very often become only more muddled. Illness, the foreign environment of the hospital, medications and surgery all take a toll on the mind as well as the body. The confusion and anxiety typically appear or grow worse at sundown, when the body is tired and the light is dim. This phenomenon is so frequent among elderly hospital patients that doctors have a term for it—"sundowning."

To ease confusion, bring in familiar objects and family photos, and leave on low lights at night. Lots of visits and physical contact will also reassure your parent and reduce any confusion.

If your parent becomes confused or agitated, remain calm no matter how it upsets you, because your mood will affect his. Reassure him that he is safe and that you are taking care of him. Do not argue or disagree with him; try to take your

*❝My mother started talking about a high-school friend of hers, a woman she hasn't seen in at least fifty years. Here I was, thinking my mother was very sick and these might be our last moments together. I wanted her attention. I said, 'Mom, why are you doing this?' But she looked up at me as though she didn't have any idea who I was.*

*I was so crushed that I left. I walked the halls for a while and tried to calm down. I was so hurt and angry. I felt betrayed. Then I spoke to this wonderful nurse who helped me realize that I had to take what I could get, that being angry or trying to force her wouldn't help either of us. So I went back in and I just sat there and stroked her hair and listened to her ramble. I learned to meet her wherever she was, not where I wanted her to be.❞*

—CAROL P.

cues from what he offers. *(Yes, it is nice here on the beach.)* Keep conversations simple and don't ask a lot of questions. And gently offer lots of reminders. Tell him patiently what day it is, where he is and why, and say the name of anyone entering the room. *Dad, your daughter, Sally, is here to see you.* (See Chapters Fifteen and Sixteen for more on dementia.)

If confusion is acute, if your parent suddenly becomes agitated, inattentive or unable to recognize familiar faces, or if he hallucinates, bring this to the doctor's attention immediately. He may be suffering from delirium, which can be a medical emergency. It often follows surgery, but illness, infection, medications and changes in the body's chemistry can also trigger it. Treatment includes reducing or discontinuing certain medications and creating a calm environment. One of the best ways to prevent severe postoperative delirium is to anticipate the possibility and talk about it before it occurs—studies show that people who expect postoperative confusion fare much better than those who are taken by surprise.

Be on the lookout, too, for depression, which is common in hospitalized elderly patients, especially if they stay in the hospital for more than a few days. Because you know your parent best, you are in the best position to notice personality changes or mood swings. If you suspect depression, talk with his doctor or a hospital psychiatrist. (For a list of symptoms of depression, see page 107.)

## FALLS AND RESTRAINTS

Whenever you visit your parent, take a look around the room for things she might trip over—furniture on wheels, chairs without arms, waxy floors. Try to fix what you can (for example, buy a rubber runner for the stretch between the bed and the toilet, or take the faulty chair out of the room) and, if she is well enough, make her aware of the dangers. (See page 140 for more on preventing falls.)

*"My father spent so much time in bed that the nurses and I thought it would be good for him to sit up in a chair for a while each day. But he was so weak that he would just fall onto the floor unless he had some support.*

*This strap, it's a seat belt really, works quite well. He doesn't stay in the chair long, but at least it's a change. I don't think it's dangerous or confining for him—I think it's freeing in a way because it allows him to get out of bed."* —SASHA L.

To guard against falls and to keep patients from pulling out tubes, meandering away from life-saving monitors or crushing a delicate injury, hospitals sometimes restrain patients either physically, with arm bands, vests or full body straps, or chemically, with sedatives, tranquilizers and other drugs. Be aware of restraints because in many cases they are not necessary and in some cases they are dangerous.

Be sure you know what sedat-

## CONVALESCING: UP AND AT 'EM

When your parent is recuperating from illness or surgery, your instinct may say, "rest," while the doctor is saying, "move." Trust the doctor here. In most cases, people need to walk to get all the bodily systems functioning again (for example, to avoid constipation after surgery), and they need to do simple tasks, including feeding themselves or combing their own hair, to regain movement and other abilities.

It may seem as if the nurses and therapists are being cruel if they are forcing your mother to move in ways that she doesn't want to move, or being lazy if they leave her to do certain things for herself, but actually they are just practicing good medicine.

The process may be painful to watch, especially if your parent is struggling, complaining of pain or spilling her food. But restrain yourself from helping her. Let her do it herself and encourage her to keep going. It will help her recover faster and more fully.

ing drugs your parent is being given and why. Likewise, if your parent is being physically restrained, ask the doctor if it is absolutely necessary. Discuss risks, benefits and alternative solutions. If restraints are unavoidable, you can usually get permission to remove them while you are visiting, or the staff may free your parent if you hire a companion to sit with him.

## BEDSORES

Although the nurses will try to prevent bedsores, you should be watchful for any red or raw spots. Pressure on a bony area impedes the flow of blood, creating a tender area that can develop into an open wound if not treated immediately. Be sure your parent is being routinely repositioned to alternate the pressure on vulnerable areas and alert the nurses to any suspicious-looking marks. (See page 82 for more on bedsores.)

## HOSPITAL-BORNE INFECTIONS

Some studies have found that five to ten percent of patients develop infections while in the hospital (these are called nosocomial infections). The combination of hospital bacteria and patients with weakened immune systems, open wounds and tubes inserted in their bodies is a volatile one.

Hand-washing is the best weapon against hospital infections. Doctors, nurses and staff are supposed to wash before touching or examining a patient, but they sometimes neglect to do it. If you think this is the case, ask the person handling your parent to please wash his or her hands first and, preferably, to wear gloves.

Unfortunately, asking a health professional to wash his hands is a little like asking someone not to smoke back in the days before secondary smoke was known to be carcinogenic. So be tactful, but ask anyway, because this simple request will reduce the risk of infection significantly.

You should wash your own hands frequently as well when caring for your parent, as neither you nor he is immune to the bacteria you routinely encounter in a hospital or that you might have encountered elsewhere.

Urinary tract infections are one of the most common nosocomial infections. Older women, in particular, are prone to contract them because menopause leaves the urethra, the exit channel for urine, more susceptible to infection.

Your parent should drink plenty of fluids and get to the bathroom at least every two hours. Her genital area needs to be kept clean, and if she has a catheter it needs to be changed regularly and checked to make sure that it is draining smoothly.

If your parent (and men get them too) has symptoms of a urinary tract infection—a persistent urge to urinate, burning during urination, and pain in the lower abdomen—alert the doctor or nurse. Urinary tract infections are treatable with medications, but they can lead to serious problems if ignored.

## IATROGENIC DISEASE

Iatrogenic diseases, those that are caused by doctors, are a serious hospital problem. An injury or ailment may be caused by a doctor's neglect or incompetence, or it may be the result of acceptable medical care. For example, a necessary treatment for one illness may cause another, less serious illness. The elderly are at high risk of iatrogenic disease because their medical care tends to be complex.

The single most important step you can take to avoid iatrogenic disease is to ask questions, which forces the doctor or nurse to think about what he or she is doing.

## INADEQUATE PAIN RELIEF

In most situations, your parent should receive as much pain medication as he needs to be comfortable. This provides relief that goes beyond the medicine's physical properties. Studies show that people actually use less medication when it is at their disposal because they aren't worrying about getting the next dose and tensing up at the thought of the approaching pain. Also, pain is much easier to fight when it is treated before it sets in rather than when it has become well established.

If your parent is in pain, talk to the doctor. If it turns out that the doctor has approved medication but the nurse is slow in bringing it, talk to the nurse or nurse supervisor about how to speed things up. Many hospitals now allow patients to dispense their own pain medication by pushing a button on a pump that delivers a dose through a needle under the skin.

## STAFF OR DOCTOR NEGLECT

Most doctors are responsible and compassionate, but some are not, and almost all are carrying heavy patient loads. Furthermore, Medicare allows doctors to bill per visit. Make sure your parent's doctor is not spending either a dangerously or an insultingly short time with your parent during these visits.

Nurses and other staff may also give your parent short shrift. If your parent is left sitting on a bedpan, or if no one responds to her request for one until she is distressed, chances are that the hospital unit is understaffed and under extreme pressure. If your questions to the unit supervisor don't immediately improve the situation, consider hiring outside help to supplement your parent's care.

*"After the operation, I tried to help my father get his teeth back in. I struggled for a time and they finally went in. Then I looked at him and thought, 'Pop, you look weird.' I called home to see if anyone knew a better way to get his teeth in. I tried that cushion stuff, but nothing made it better.*

*Finally I realized these weren't his teeth. They were someone else's! I went traipsing to the room he used to be in, and to the doctor's office, and even to the operating room, all over the hospital looking for the right teeth, but I never found them. It was really kind of funny because here I am looking around for a set of teeth and realizing that somebody else must be wearing Pop's teeth. Luckily, he thought it was funny too and we had a good laugh about it. He had another set at home, but he never did use them again. Once old people take their teeth out, they don't like to put them back in."* —JACQUI L.

# When You Are Far Away

Absence sometimes makes the heart grow fonder, but in this case the heart usually just grows more anxious, and understandably so. If you can't act as your parent's advocate, try to find a nearby relative or friend who can, or if you can afford it, hire a geriatric care manager, private health aide or companion to monitor your parent's care.

In any case, when you are far away, call the head nurse on your parent's floor and explain your dilemma. Find out if there is a regular time when you can call, perhaps each morning, when the nurse has a moment to talk to you about your parent's progress and care.

Check with the doctor too. Use only one family spokesperson to call the nurse and doctor, and get that person to relay information to others who are concerned. More than one spokesperson can lead to misunderstandings and miscommuni-

## "WHY DON'T YOU EVER COME TO SEE ME?"

If your parent doesn't remember that you have visited or doesn't seem to know who you are while you are there, try to remember that your visits are very important nevertheless. They are comforting, and they allow you to make sure that your parent is being well cared for. They also show the staff that your parent's family is concerned about his condition and the quality of his care.

cation, and it can hurt your family's standing with hospital staff who have to field repetitive calls. (See page 235 for more on sharing responsibility with siblings.)

Try to make sure your parent has some company, as it gets lonely on the fifth floor. Ask others who are nearby to visit occasionally. (Most people don't mind doing this once or twice, even though it may feel to you like an imposition.) If you don't know anyone well enough, call a local church, synagogue or other community organization to ask about visiting volunteers.

Be sure to call and write. Send your parent a big, colorful card, a photo of yourself, an audio cassette (and inexpensive tape player) of you and others talking about what you are doing with your day and how you miss him. Mundane, day-to-day things—what happened at the bus

stop, what the kids did in school, what the dog brought home—may seem trivial, but for someone alone in the hospital, these are wonderful stories that temporarily bring him home and help him forget his pain.

# Comfort on the Fifth Floor

Don't get so caught up in your role as an advocate that you neglect the more important comfort and care that your parent needs now. Visit and recruit others to visit. Not only can they cheer up your parent, but they will ease some of the burden on you.

## VISITS

Visitors are the best first-aid going. However, they should plan their trips so they come one at a time or in very small groups, and for only a brief interlude—less than 30 minutes may be enough—as your parent may tire easily now. They should also call first, as an unannounced visit can be awkward for everyone.

At times, your parent may be too tired for visitors, but may not be willing to tell people for fear of hurting their feelings. It's your job to tell them, as tactfully as possible, to come another time. In fact, there may even be times when your parent doesn't want you to visit. Don't take it personally.

Some things to keep in mind when visiting:

◆ **Be prepared.** If your parent has had a sudden and severe illness or accident, you may be shocked by his appearance on your first visit. He may not only look different, he may be confused, weak or in pain, or he may be attached to a lot of machines. If possible, talk with the nurses on your way to his room and find out what to expect. Brace yourself so you don't gasp in horror or burst into tears as you first enter the room.

Understand that if your parent is in the intensive care unit, it doesn't mean that he is close to death, only that he is being watched closely. Elderly people are often put in ICUs after surgery, stroke or accidents. Try to remain calm. Your parent needs your confidence and warmth.

> " *Quite often we'll see a family come, six or seven of them at one time. They all cram into the person's room and chat with each other, and the grandchildren run around and there are a lot of gifts and food and flowers. It's all very hectic, and very exciting.*
>
> *And then they all leave. And no one comes to visit for two weeks. That's very sad.* "
>
> —LORRAINE N., R.N.

◆ **Be yourself.** Hospitals and illness breed awkwardness. *What do I say? Should I be cheery? Should I talk about what the doctor found or avoid mentioning her illness?* Relax. Your embarrassment will only make your parent ill at ease—and she is already ill enough. It's okay to ask about her ailments, her pain and her feelings, if that's something you want to know about. In fact, she may welcome such honesty and an opportunity to talk about her situation.

◆ **Arrange for some privacy.** Interruptions are a way of life in hospitals. Someone comes in with medication, then it's time for a blood sample, and just as you and your parent start talking, her temperature must be taken.

If your parent shares a room, pull the curtain around his bed and turn on some music to drown out your voices. If his condition allows it—ask the nurse—get him into a wheelchair and move the conversation into a lounge or hallway.

◆ **Silence is golden.** If your parent can't speak or if she is too confused or tired for conversation, you might simply read to her or tell her a story and let her sit peacefully. Or just sit quietly with her; your presence alone will relieve her fear and ease her loneliness.

◆ **Get physical.** Don't let tubes and monitors or illness deter you from touching, stroking and holding. Human contact is good medicine. Hug him, hold his hand, stroke his cheek, caress his arm. It says more than any words can say and it's healing.

◆ **Pamper her.** Do something to make your parent feel dignified and pampered—wash or comb her hair, offer a foot massage or paint her nails. (Be sure to ask the nurse first. A massage, for example, might be inadvisable if there is a circulation problem.) You can also help with other tasks around the room—replace the water in flower arrangements, read letters aloud and then, if he wants you to, write his responses as he dictates to you.

♦ **Respect the rules.** Enforcing visiting hours allows patients—not just your parent but others in the room and down the hall—to get some rest. Try to stay within the rules whenever possible. You may need to stretch them if the only time you can visit is after hours, or if your parent is nervous about a procedure or is extremely ill and needs your presence. In these cases, talk with the nurse or other administrator.

When it's really important, they will usually adjust the rules.

If your parent is in an intensive care unit, the rules will be stricter, and need to be obeyed. Patients here need all the rest they can manage and the staff needs precious space if an emergency arises.

♦ **Don't forget the children.** In most cases, a child is a welcome visitor, adding vitality and sparkle to a dreary hospital day, singing songs, asking funny questions, stroking Grandpa with tiny fingers. Children also tend to see beyond the ugliness of illness and don't notice the things that adults find worrisome (they may

## REST FOR THE WEARY

While it was suggested earlier that you might use this hospitalization to get away from your caregiving duties, it may turn out to be anything but a break. In fact, it may well be a rigorous test of your endurance. Deeply worried about your ailing parent, you return to the hospital at every free moment you have. Then, after several warnings that visiting hours are over, you drag your tired, hungry body home only to be deluged by messages and phone calls from concerned relatives and family friends. There isn't a minute when you aren't living and breathing your parent's hospital experience.

Protect yourself. Ask a sibling or another relative to relay information to others in the inner circle so you aren't handling all the phone calls.

When other people are visiting your parent, get away, even if that means just going down to the hospital coffee shop and flipping through a magazine. Ask one of the nurses if there is a lounge or an empty room where you can lie down and get some rest. Take a day off and go out with a friend and talk about something else.

It's vital to take care of yourself now. Your parent will need your strength when he returns home. (Be sure to read—or reread—Chapter Three, "Caring for the Caregiver.")

be more absorbed by the bag of urine by the side of the bed than by a grandfather's paralysis).

For your child, such a visit is equally important. Your instinct may be to protect children from seeing Grandma ill, but children learn from seeing life and death, and all that falls between.

If Grandma doesn't seem pleased at the prospect of a child's visit, or if your child is afraid or hesitant, however, don't press the matter.

## GIFTS

Flowers are always nice, but a framed photo, notepaper, a small pine-scented cushion and even cheerful cards are also great gifts. The smallest thing can mean a lot when one is facing the four walls of a hospital room. You don't have to spend a lot of money. In fact, some of the best gifts are a story, a song, a special poem or prayer, or if the proper equipment is available, a videotape from someone who can't visit in person. Anything at all that is made by a grandchild is wonderful—a child's drawing brings color and life into an impersonal hospital room.

If your parent is relatively alert, his hospital stay will seem awfully dull, so you should look for gifts that are entertaining—games, books, puzzles, playing cards, materials for a hobby, knitting supplies, music (an inexpensive radio), books on tape and a tape player (which you can get free of charge through the Library of Congress if your parent can't read for himself).

If your parent is going to be in the hospital for some time and you are able to spend a little more money, buy a bed jacket or robe, new slippers, a pouch that attaches to a walker or wheelchair, or a soft, downy pillow.

## MEALS

Although hospitals are sprucing up their menus, hospital food is still notoriously tasteless. It's also served at odd times and sometimes left to grow cold in front of a patient who is unable to feed himself. Your parent's diet isn't simply a matter of comfort; the rate of malnutrition among the hospitalized elderly is estimated to be as high as 50 percent. A poor diet will make your parent's recovery more difficult and may contribute to new ills. But you can help.

*When my mother was in the hospital after her stroke she turned to me and said, 'Pizza.'*

*I said, 'What?!'*

*And she said, 'I really want some pizza. And a chocolate milkshake. It's all I can think about.'*

*My mother is not a pizza-eater. She usually eats like a bird. So I drove around town looking for pizza and a chocolate shake. She didn't eat much of it, but she ate enough. I guess it was just a craving. Her body was crying out for something caloric and filling, and I was glad to see her eat something with such gusto.*

—FRAN M.

When possible, visit during mealtimes so you can check up on your father's eating habits. Bring him a home-cooked meal occasionally and help him to eat. Simply having company may encourage him to eat more. If you can't be there, ask another visitor to be a guest at mealtime, or ask the patient advocate about volunteers who might help your parent eat.

Although hospitals don't advertise it, most offer an array of foods and special meals—kosher, vegetarian, low-salt, and even sandwiches. You can call the kitchen and order special meals, or ask that meals be brought at different times.

## RELIGION AND COUNSELING

Whether or not your parent was religious before her hospital stay, she may have some spiritual thoughts now. Hospital clergy will gladly stop by a patient's room, or a representative from your parent's church or synagogue may be willing to visit her in the hospital. Hospitals also have counselors, social workers or psychologists who will talk with your parent about particular issues—fears about dying, family relationships, a diagnosis of cancer, as well as practical matters like housing, finances and community services.

## DIGNITY

Like the military, hospitals tend to strip people of their dignity and independence. Patients walk along public hallways in flimsy nightgowns that are open in the back. They uri-nate into bedpans and receive enemas from strangers, as yet other strangers sometimes look in the open door. And their condition is discussed among doctors and residents as though they were not in the room or not even still alive.

Depending on the severity of your parent's condition, be sure that he is involved in all decisions about his health care and that he is kept up-to-date. Even if he cannot speak for himself or his mind is in a fog, assume that he still can hear and understand what is being said. He very well may understand and he will feel that respect, in any case.

When hospital staff care for him, they should always tell him what they are doing and why—this is especially important if your parent is not aware of what is happening and may be taken by surprise. *I am going to wash you with a warm washcloth. I am going to wipe your neck and then your arms.*

Ask the staff to address your parent by whatever title he is used to—Mr. Asher, Professor Madison, Doctor O'Neill, or just a nickname.

Protect your mother's modesty. Get her a nightgown or a robe, or have her wear a second hospital gown over the first, but in the opposite direction. If your father is mortified because medical students are circling his bed to peer at his prostate incision, ask the students to skip his room on the next tour. If the nurse gives enemas in public view, ask that the curtains or the door be closed. (Post a big reminder over the bed if the staff is forgetful, starting with the word, "Please.")

## ROOMMATES AND ROOMS

If a roommate or his visitors are keeping your parent awake, talk to the roommate or a nurse about setting up a schedule of "quiet time." Or get your parent some earplugs or a small cassette player with earphones to muffle any snoring or chatter. If the roommate is obnoxious, see if you can't leave a curtain drawn permanently between the two beds. If all else fails, request a room change. It involves a lot of paperwork and hassle, but sometimes it is necessary.

# Preparing for Discharge

Before your parent signs out, be sure that she has *written* information about medications, proper dosages and their timing, potential side effects, meals, exercise, precautions, symptoms to watch for and foods to avoid. The hospital discharge planner is responsible for planning your parent's return home, ordering any medical equipment she will need, or locating a nursing home or rehabilitation facility. The planner, who usually knows a fair amount about local nursing homes, can be helpful, but be aware that his or her primary job is to get patients out with speed. Take sufficient time to study the options and make a careful choice, if at all possible. (See Chapter Eleven for more on moving to a nursing home.)

If you do not believe that your parent is ready for discharge, talk with the doctor, the nurse, the hospital social worker or the patient advocate. Although Medicare and other insurance carriers like to get people out of the hospital as soon as possible—and so may stop payment after a certain date—there may be valid reasons why your parent shouldn't leave the hospital yet. Discuss your concerns. The social worker or you may be able to convince the insurance carrier that your parent needs coverage for a longer hospital stay, or that he should go to a separate rehabilitation facility.

# Expenses

Hospitals have perfected chaos when it comes to billing. They use so many codes, abbreviations and notations that it is almost impossible to figure out what a bill actually covers. And you receive not just one bill, but a seemingly endless series of bills—from the hospital, the surgeon, the anesthesiologist, the physical therapist, the laboratory—all of which may come from different billing offices. Then there are the insurance companies, Medicare and Medigap agents and claim forms to wrangle with. What does your parent's insurance cover? What does your parent owe? Which bills are redundant?

If you are handling your parent's finances and trying to sort out his medical bills, be patient. Even doctors and health policy experts have trouble deciphering and confirming their own hospital bills.

Whatever you do, don't assume that health-care providers are all honest and hospital billing departments know what they are doing. The U.S. General Accounting Office has found that nearly all hospital bills include overcharges.

If the bill your parent receives is confusing, call the hospital billing department and ask for an itemized bill, including explanations of all notations. Look through it for duplications, charges for services that your parent never received, unauthorized tests or procedures and anything else that looks suspicious. If anything seems out of place, ask for an explanation. If the explanation is not adequate, refuse to pay that portion of the bill.

If you have the energy and foresight, keep a record of all tests, procedures, medications and equipment that your parent receives and compare it to the bills.

## HELP THROUGH THE INSURANCE MAZE

Insurance claims agents can be hired to handle all your parent's medical bills and insurance paperwork. You can find one by calling the National Association of Claims Assistance Professionals (NACAP) at 800-660-0665, or by faxing 800-660-9228. See Chapter Thirteen for more on claims agents, Medicare and other government insurance, private insurance, medical bills and appeals.

# Chapter Eight

# TIPS FOR DAILY LIVING

*An Ounce of Prevention • Safe-proofing the Home*
*• Hygiene • Eating • The Question of Driving*
*• Exercising Body and Mind*

W HO CAN HELP BUT WORRY ABOUT AN ELDERLY parent getting through the day, or even part of the day, alone? *What if Dad doesn't bother to eat dinner on his own? I wish Mother would stop driving.* And yet, nearly 1.5 million people over the age of 85 live alone (nearly 10 million people over 65 live alone) and millions of others spend at least part of the day on their own.

If your father has arthritis, fuzzy vision, some residual paralysis from a stroke or mild dementia, it doesn't mean that it's time for a nursing home or that you have to follow him around tending to his every need. You don't want to do it and he probably doesn't want you to, either. What you can do is help him rearrange his house and revise his habits so that he can function independently in his own home for as long as possible.

Ask your parent about the details of his day or spend a day with him observing how he goes about his basic chores. Does he have trouble holding his razor, walking down stairs, heating up spaghetti or locking the door? Does he have a way to get groceries or visit a friend? Once you know the day's snags, brainstorm solutions with your parent. (Be sure to involve him.) There are a number of ways to make cooking more manageable, dressing more doable, exercise more feasible and free time more entertaining. If you need help with a specific problem and don't find a solution here, contact an occupational therapist, visiting nurse, carpenter or electrician, depending upon the situation.

# Safety First

Bad eyesight, dull hearing, arthritis, poor balance, multiple medications, illness and other health problems all put your parent at risk for accidents. Look through her house for hazards. Be particularly thorough if your parent suffers from any sort of confusion.

◆ Make sure that chemicals, harsh cleaners, insecticides, medications, paints, etc. are all labeled with big, clear letters. If your parent gets confused easily, put them out of sight completely.

◆ Check to see that smoke detectors work. Your parent's waning sense of smell makes a smoke detector that much more important.

◆ Check to see for easy escape routes in case of fire. Your parent won't be able to climb out of a window as easily as you can, so look for escapes she could use. Is the back door wide enough for your mother's wheelchair? Is there a back stairway that your father can manage? If possible, hold a fire drill. If your bedridden parent wouldn't be able to escape, call the local fire department and ask for safety instructions.

◆ Buy a small fire extinguisher that is easy to handle and put it in a convenient place, preferably near the kitchen, where fires may start. And instruct your parent in how to use it.

◆ Have at least two flashlights, with working batteries, ready to use and easy to find if the lights go out. Put one by your parent's bed and one on a kitchen table. If there is a blackout, several large flashlights are safer than candles.

◆ Make sure all bathroom and kitchen outlets contain working circuit interrupters to prevent shocks.

◆ In the kitchen, check to see that the burners and the oven work properly. Be sure that outlets are not overloaded, and that wires don't rest on a hot toaster, for example. Is your mother apt to reach for equipment located above the hot stove, in which case a sleeve or apron string might catch fire? If so, rearrange things.

◆ Because of their thinner skin and slower reactions, elderly people are at risk for scalding. Set the hot water heater so the temperature of the water doesn't rise above 120°F.

◆ If your parent gets cold easily, buy him some good long underwear and turn up the heat. Be careful with space heaters and electric blankets, as they can cause burns and fires.

◆ Keep a list of clearly-written, large-print emergency phone numbers by *every* phone, or program them into the telephone's memory. The list should include police, fire, ambulance, your home and work numbers and the phone number of a nearby relative or neighbor. Don't assume your parent will remember your number, or even 911, if she's injured, burglarized or in some other trouble. Even the keenest minds can go blank during moments of panic.

## MEDICAL EMERGENCY IDENTIFICATION

Slip a medical identification card into your parent's wallet so in case there is ever an emergency, medical crews will know who he is, who to contact and whether there are any medical conditions (dementia, diabetes, heart disease, allergies) that require special attention.

You can make one yourself or, in many locations, the area agency on aging distributes free identification tags which either hang on a chain or are placed in a wallet. Otherwise, some companies sell them (look under "Medical Emergency Information" in the Yellow Pages).

## MEDICAL ALERT SYSTEMS

"I've fallen and I can't get up" made for a funny ad, but the message was quite serious. Medical alert systems (or emergency response systems) are worth the investment if you are worried about your parent living alone. (Installing one makes a nice gift that says, "I care.")

With these devices, your parent is given a "help" button about the size of a pendant, which she wears on a necklace or bracelet. When she falls, has chest pains or needs help for any other reason, she pushes the button, which sends a signal to a receiver next to her telephone, which in turn dials a response center (most systems are set up so they can dial out even if the phone is off the hook). At the response center, your parent is identified by a code. The responder calls her house and communicates with her either over the phone or, if she cannot get to the phone, through a two-way intercom attached to the phone. If your parent doesn't respond to the call or says that there is, indeed, an emergency, the responder then calls an emergency crew.

Dozens of companies now sell emergency response systems. You can find them in the Yellow Pages under "Medical Alarms," or check with a medical supply store. Or you can ask your parent's doctor if the hospital he is affiliated with offers such a service. Prices vary, so call several companies. Some sell the system (for anywhere from $200 to $2,000) and then charge a monthly service fee, while others lease systems (for $20 to $50 a month, after an initial installation charge). Renting is usually preferable because you don't have to worry about repairs or the company going defunct or moving.

When comparing systems, ask for details about the staff receiving the emergency calls. Are they situated nearby? How are they trained? Do they speak your parent's native language, if it's not English? Find out the company's average response time (if they are not checking their response time periodically, they should be). Ask if your parent can try the system for a trial period or get a money-back guarantee. Be sure your parent can operate the buttons, and then test the system to see how well it operates within his house and how far he can venture into the backyard, for example, before the system fails.

Once your parent has an emergency response system, check the batteries regularly. It's no good to have it if it's not working.

## CRIME PREVENTION

The elderly are popular targets for criminals because they are easy prey. But your parent shouldn't lock himself in the house because he is afraid of being mugged. Even if he is physically frail, common sense can protect him from most dangerous situations.

Talk to your parent about the precautions he should take and what he should do in specific situations. Do some role playing. Going through the motions now will mean quicker and smarter reactions should there ever be a problem. Check with the local senior center or police department to find out about talks on crime prevention, or see if a police officer might speak with your parent individually about safety. In the meantime:

♦ Let the local police department know that your parent is elderly and living alone, especially if he lives in a small town where the

police might pay some special attention to him.

♦ Make sure your parent can properly operate all his home door locks and that he uses them. Get locks that can be opened from the inside without a key, in case he needs to exit quickly.

♦ Install a peephole in the front door. Your parent should not open the door for anyone unfamiliar—a salesman or repairman—unless he has asked the person to come. He can also invest in an intercom for the front door.

♦ If he doesn't already have one, install a security alarm system in your parent's house. You can also install "panic buttons," which alert the police or security guards to trouble, by his bed or favorite chair.

♦ Several companies now sell remote controls that operate house lights as well as a radio or a television from afar. When your parent arrives home at night, he can light up the house and even make it noisy several minutes before entering, allowing burglars time to escape. You can also install exterior floodlights that can be operated from the bedroom.

♦ Talk with your parent about where and when it is best for him to walk outdoors. There may be certain routes to the store or the park that are safer than others, and particular times of day when he should opt for cabs or buses.

♦ Your parent should leave diamond rings or expensive watches at home when traveling in cities or in any crime-ridden areas. They attract thieves and pickpockets.

♦ Money and credit cards should be carried in an inside pocket or money belt rather than a purse, which can be snatched. Nevertheless, your parent should always carry a little cash ($20 or $30) with him so he has something to hand over to a mugger.

## Preventing Falls

Everyone catches a toe or trips on a step occasionally, but now a minor tumble can have major repercussions. Older bodies break more easily than younger ones and they don't heal as quickly or as completely. Then, while they are trying to heal, enforced bed rest exacerbates previous medical ills and can cause new ones, such as pneumonia, infections, bedsores and other circulatory disorders. Half of all older people who fracture a hip end up needing canes, walkers or wheelchairs for the rest of their lives. Twenty-five percent of people entering nursing homes cite falls as the primary reason for the move.

Falls can also make an older person needlessly cautious. After a fracture has healed, even when the fall didn't cause any real injury, your parent may be afraid to move around. Sedentary, he may become dependent, isolated and depressed.

The bottom line: Prevent falls in the first place. Your parent needs good medical care, a safe house and exercise to improve mobility, coordination and strength.

*"My mother rode three miles every day on a stationary bicycle until she was ninety-six years old. She volunteered, she traveled, she read. But when she fell and broke her ankle she was immobile for a couple of months and I think that just killed her spirit. She could never really get around very well after that and her mood, her body, everything just went. She died a year later."* —MEL T.

While everyone with an older parent should be alert to the threat of falls, you need to be particularly cautious if your parent has osteoporosis, Parkinson's disease, dementia, poor eyesight or arthritis, or if your parent has any injury or disability in the legs, has fallen before, has had a stroke or is taking medications that might make him dizzy or faint.

### ROOM-BY-ROOM PREVENTION

If you request it, a visiting nurse or an occupational or physical therapist will examine your parent's home for hazards and show you how to reduce risks. If the inspection is done as part of a hospital discharge, Medicare or other insurance policies may cover the cost. But you can also tour your parent's house yourself and look for places where she has to bend, reach, stoop or step over something. Look for anything that might trip her up or get in her way. Here are the most important steps toward preventing a fall:

## PRACTICE MAKES PERFECT SENSE

Show your parent what to do in case he falls. If possible, get him to lie down and then roll onto his hands and crawl to a phone or to a piece of furniture that he can use for support while he hikes himself up. Such practice may sound a little silly, but when people fall they often become confused and disoriented. If they have practiced what to do in advance, it will come to them naturally when they need to do it.

### Floors and Pathways

• Check carpets for worn areas and rips. Tack down flaps or curled edges.

• Use low-pile, wall-to-wall carpeting wherever possible. Avoid thick-pile carpets.

• Get rid of throw rugs or make sure they have rubber, nonskid backing on them.

• Use nonslip wax or be sure that wax is buffed thoroughly.

• Make sure floors are even and level. Repair loose floorboards and remove thresholds at doorways.

• Clear hallways and other pathways of wastepaper baskets, footstools, magazine racks, electrical wires and other small objects.

• If your parent has any hanging plants, be sure she doesn't have to duck to get past them (or reach up on tiptoes to water them).

• Install handrails in hallways.

### Stairs

• Avoid stairs completely, if possible. This may mean turning a downstairs den into a bedroom or building ramps onto short stairways. You can also buy a lift which carries a passenger up and down stairs in a chair—expensive, but helpful if you can afford one.

• When stairs are unavoidable, be sure handrails are sturdy and extend the full length of the stairs. Handrails should be placed on both sides of the stairs. Don't forget stairs leading to a basement and those by the front and back doors.

• Ideally, each step should be no more than six inches high. Taller steps may be cause for concern.

• Mark the edges of steps—or any place the floor changes elevation even slightly—with brightly-colored adhesive tape.

• Use nonslip treads on stairs. Consider getting rid of carpeting on stairways, as it rounds off the edges of steps and shortens the depth of each step, making footing precarious.

### Furniture

• Make sure that chairs are high enough to get out of and into easily, and that they have strong armrests and high backs that can be used for support. If necessary, keep a walker or cane by the chair or look into electric-powered pneumatic chairs that lift a person up and lower him down.

• Likewise, make sure the bed is not too high or too low, so your parent can get in and out easily.

• Get rid of beds and other furniture with nonlocking wheels.

• Furniture legs that curve outward create a tripping hazard. Move such furniture out of any pathway or get rid of it.

• Avoid tripod tables which are not sturdy.

• Repair broken or wobbly furniture immediately.

**Bathrooms and Kitchens**

• Install grab bars near toilets and tubs, and get a raised toilet seat, which makes sitting and standing far easier.

• Attach a wall-mounted, liquid soap dispenser in the shower.

• Install nonslip strips on the floor of the tub or shower.

• Place nonslip strips or rubber-bottom bathmats on the bathroom floor. Keep a nonslip rug or runner, or a rubber mat, in front of the kitchen sink where the floor is apt to be wet and slippery.

• Avoid or be careful when using oils in the bath which make feet and hands slippery.

• A shower curtain may be easier to manage than a glass door, but make sure it's hung on a secure rod that is screwed into the wall, not a tension rod. If your parent slips, a cur-

*My father has this little, three-legged pine table in his living room, right by his favorite chair. Every time he got up or sat down, he would lean on the table, using it for balance. I told him a hundred times that the table was wobbly, and that one day he was going to lean on it, fall over and kill himself. I even bought him a new table one year, but he didn't use it. He's pretty stubborn. He said, 'I've had this table here for forty-five years and I haven't fallen yet. Why would I fall now?'*

*But I think my warning sank in a little, even though he would never admit it. I've noticed that he doesn't really lean on that table anymore. He puts more weight on the chair. He listens if I bother him enough about something. I just have to be a little more stubborn than he is.*
—SKIP R.

tain on a screwed-in rod will offer better support.

• Your parent or someone else in the household should clean up any grease, water or other spills right away.

**Lighting**

• Lighting should be bright and evenly distributed. Older eyes need more light. They also don't adjust quickly to changes in lighting, so avoid having dark hallways that lead into brightly-lit stairways, or vice versa.

• Reduce glare by aiming lights at a

wall or the ceiling, and use low-glare bulbs and lampshades. If there is a sunny window facing your parent as he uses the stairs, hang curtains or shades to block the glare.

• Install a light by the bed so your parent isn't fumbling around at night when she needs to get up. Make sure light switches are easy to use, easy to reach and accessible at the entrance of each room so your parent isn't walking through a dark room to get to a light.

• Use night-lights in the hallway, the bathroom, the kitchen, the stairway or anywhere else your parent might venture at night.

• You might want to install sound-activated lights which go on when your parent gets up during the night and go off after he has stopped moving around. Look for them in catalogues, medical supply stores, hardware or lighting stores.

## Other Measures

• Make sure your parent has comfortable, sturdy, nonslip shoes with low, broad-based heels. Sneakers with splayed soles provide a solid base. Avoid sandals and shoes with open heels or toes. Bedroom slippers should have rubber soles. If your mother likes to walk around in just her socks, get socks with rubber pads on the bottom.

• Teach your parent how to rise from chairs and beds gradually to avoid dizziness. She should get up in stages, with two hands planted firmly on armrests or other supports.

• Make sure the house is warm enough—the thermostat probably needs to be higher than it used to be. Low body temperature can lead to hypothermia and dizziness, which can, in turn, lead to falls.

• Organize things so that frequently-used items are within easy reach, to discourage your parent from exerting himself or climbing on chairs.

• Place telephones in those places where your parent spends the most time—next to the bed, by his easy chair—and within easy reach. Or get him a portable phone. (But he has to take it with him and not lose it or it will be more trouble than it's worth.)

• Install grab bars by the closet, so when your parent is dressing he has something to hold onto for balance.

• If it will help his mobility, encourage your parent to use a cane or walker. It should be fitted by a doctor and he should be taught how to use it correctly.

• If your father uses a cane, attach a loose wrist strap to one end. Then, if he drops it, it won't fall to the ground and leave him in the precarious position of having to stoop to pick it up.

• Get your parent to limit her drinking, as alcohol certainly will make her unsteady.

• In winter, your parent should keep a bag of rock salt or sand by the front door, so he can toss a few scoops on icy steps. He needs to beware of wet, slippery or uneven pavement. Tell him to walk on grass or loose snow instead of hard, wet or icy patches, and to step slowly over slippery surfaces, with his feet apart and his knees slightly bent. (And remember those rubber soles!)

### IF YOUR PARENT FALLS

If your parent falls and doesn't seem to have broken any bones (no severe pain or difficulty moving), help her up by supporting her and then lifting with your legs, not your back. This means bending at your knees, getting a good hold and pushing up with your legs. Don't twist your body to turn her around; pivot by taking small steps.

If your parent is heavy, you may have to push her, a little bit at a time. Get her to a sturdy table or bring a table or chair to her, so she can lift herself up with your help. Talk to her as you move her, telling her exactly what you are doing. If you cannot get her up, don't pull

### MEDICAL ALERT

If your parent has a serious fall and is in pain, don't move her unless you need to restore her breathing or get her away from fire, out of water or clear from some other danger. Call an emergency crew. Cover her with a blanket if it's cool and assure her that medical help is coming. Continue to talk to her in a calm voice until help has arrived.

your own back out trying. Wait for help to arrive.

Whether or not she is injured, have your parent make an appointment with her doctor so he can determine what caused her to fall and can talk to her about ways of preventing accidents in the future. Falls are sometimes indicators that a drug is causing problems or that your parent has an illness such as dehydration, heart disease, stroke, infection, pneumonia or internal bleeding.

# Bathing and Grooming

In addition to preventing falls, grab bars in the bathroom and raised toilet seats make life easier for aching knees and backs. Also, lever-style faucets, rather than knobs, are easier to use for arthritic hands. They are a good idea for door and cabinet handles, as well.

Beyond these items, medical supply stores and mail-order catalogues (see Appendix E, page 416) sell a mind-boggling array of bathroom gizmos—some of them more useful than others—including a razor holder that attaches to the hand, a dental floss holder for people who have trouble winding the little thread around their fingers, and a wall-mounted soap dispenser. You can also find sponges with long handles, toothbrushes with thick handles and a variety of nail clippers, toothpaste dispensers, mirrors, shower-head attachments and urinals that are simple to use. Even if you don't buy anything, it's worth flipping through

## MORE THAN CLEAN—BEAUTIFUL

Good hygiene is important not only for good health (poor hygiene can lead to skin infections), but also for self-esteem. People feel better when they look good. A new hairdo and some makeup may improve your mother's outlook, energy level and, to some extent, even her health. Your father will feel more dapper and proud with a clean shave and combed hair.

Make sure your parent has the proper tools not only for basic hygiene but also for preening and primping. Your father may be able to use the toilet safely but can he clip his nails, shine his shoes and open his after-shave? Can your mother manage a powder puff, a mascara brush or hair curlers? (She may say that she doesn't care about makeup anymore, in an effort to hide her problems. So you have to play sleuth.) If easy-to-open lids and other handy devices don't help, find out about local barbers and beauticians who make house calls. Some offer discounts to senior citizens.

*"When my mother's hair started to fall out after the chemotherapy, I didn't think much about it. We all knew it would happen, and she's never been terribly concerned about her appearance.*

*A friend of hers suggested that she buy a wig. I thought, 'Mom? In a wig? Never!' But sure enough, she bought one and she wears it all the time. She looks pretty good in it and it's made a big difference in how she feels. She has a lot more confidence."*
—DIANA M.

a few catalogues for ideas about things you can make yourself. For instance, simply wrapping a strip of foam around a toothbrush handle makes it easier to hold.

If you or someone else is helping your parent bathe and brush:

◆ Buy a chair made for the shower or use a regular plastic chair as long as it's stable and won't slip. You can also buy a rubber device that deflates to lower a person gently into the tub and then inflates to get them out again.

◆ If your parent is completely immobile, a sponge bath is as good as a regular bath. Typically a home health aide will bathe your parent, but if you are doing it yourself, prepare a bowl of warm, slightly soapy water and with a soft washcloth wipe her down, top to bottom, being sure to get into all cracks and under every fold of skin. Dry thoroughly. You can also buy a rubber basin for hair-washing in a bed or in a chair, or a full-body tub for the

**In my mother's era you took baths. She never used the shower. Ever. But I couldn't get her into the tub. And if I did, she couldn't get up once she got down. I said to her, 'A shower is so wonderful. You don't know what you're missing.' But she absolutely would not do it.**

**Finally, she did try it, not long ago. She had her first shower at ninety-some-years old. I said, 'Isn't this wonderful?' You know, I'm standing outside and she's in there, but I'm holding her and I'm getting all wet. She wouldn't say that she liked it. But she accepted it.**
—MARGARET F.

bed (which may be a little unwieldy).

♦ It is easier to brush someone else's teeth with an electric toothbrush. Use very little toothpaste or avoid it altogether. When your parent is quite sick, simply use a wet, soft toothbrush or damp washcloth or disposable mouth cleaner (available in medical supply stores) to wipe the teeth, gums and tongue.

# In the Dressing Room

If your parent has trouble reaching the zipper on the back of her dress or managing the tiny buttons on her sweater, explore the latest line of "easy clothing"—dresses with large zipper handles, pants with Velcro closures, shirts with snaps, shoes that slip on and skirts that pull on. There are also gadgets that make dressing easier, such as metallic arms or "grippers" that help pull socks and pants on and devices that pull buttons through their holes. (See the list of catalogues in Appendix E, page 416.)

But before you order a new specialized wardrobe for your parent, peruse the racks of the department stores or make adjustments to clothing your parent already owns—it will be a lot cheaper and probably more attractive. Buttons can be replaced with zippers or Velcro; elastic shoelaces turn a tie-up shoe into one that slips on; jersey dresses with wide necks slide over the head, and wraparound dresses pull on like a coat. Sweatpants and tops are often the easiest (and most comfortable) outfits to wear, and many stores now sell dressier elastic-waisted pants.

Don't forget the little touches that make your parent feel attractive and proud. Buy a clip-on tie for your father, if he's a tie-wearer with tired fingers. Give your mother a colorful silk scarf, which hides humped shoulders, surrounds the face with color and makes her feel special. (You can tie it permanently so all she has to do is slip it over her head.)

# What's for Dinner?

Does your parent skip breakfast, dine on a corner of yesterday's sandwich, or return meal trays that have barely been touched? Is he growing thinner by the day, or maintaining his weight entirely on cookies and chips? If so, it's time to act. A poor diet will worsen his health and deprive him of energy.

Studies suggest that nearly a quarter of the elderly in this country are malnourished—not starving, but failing to get the vitamins, minerals and other nutrients that their bodies need. But the problem is typically overlooked by doctors, who examine heart function and brain waves, not lunch plates, so it's up to you to monitor your parent's eating habits. You can make some simple changes that will vastly improve your parent's meager diet. (See Appendix D, page 407, for information on diet and nutrition.)

## IN THE GROCERY STORE

♦ Once a month—on a shopping trip with you or someone else who can help with heavy bags— your parent should stock up on frozen and canned foods, pasta, rice, beans, cereal and other staples that keep well. (Bread, butter, cream and meats can all be frozen and used at a later date.) Interim shopping trips can be used for getting light loads

## NOT TOO FAT FOR ME

If there's anything wonderful about old age, it's that thin is not always better. Studies suggest that older people who are a little bit overweight fare better through illness and surgery because they have some extra reserve to call on. So unless your parent has arthritis, osteoporosis, heart disease, diabetes or another condition that requires weight control, she shouldn't worry about a little plumpness.

**When the weight should go.** If your parent needs to lose weight for health reasons, forget the fad diets, which tend to fail and usually aren't very healthful. Have a doctor or registered dietitian work out a meal plan for her, or use your common sense to teach her more healthful eating habits. She shouldn't aim for a large weight loss. Losing five to ten percent of her weight, a more attainable goal, is enough to lower her blood pressure, reduce her cholesterol levels, improve her diabetes or relieve the pressure on her joints.

**When the weight should not have gone.** Sudden and unintentional weight loss can signal a number of serious problems, including depression, cancer, heart failure, worsening dementia and malnutrition. If you notice such a weight change, urge your parent to talk with his doctor about it.

of fresh fruits, vegetables and dairy products.

◆ Your parent should read the labels, looking for products with the lowest sodium and fat content. (Canned vegetables often contain sodium and syrup or butter sauces; frozen ones are usually a better choice.) Frozen and prepared dinners are more healthful than they used to be and can be supplemented with a salad, steamed vegetables or a piece of fresh fruit.

◆ "Long-life," or UHT, milk (heated at ultra-high temperatures), costs a little more but can be stored on the shelf at room temperature for up to six months. (Once it is opened, it must be refrigerated and lasts about ten days.) It is perfectly safe, quite tasty if chilled before drinking, and just as nutritious as regular milk.

*In the weeks and months after my father died, my mother didn't eat much. She couldn't be bothered to make a real meal just for herself. She said she hated eating alone. So she lost a lot of weight, which was bad because she was thin to start with.*

*I taught her how to sauté vegetables in a wok and showed her a few easy pasta and rice recipes—all things she can do in one pot with very little work. Whenever I visit I load up her shelves and refrigerator with food. She protests a lot, but she eats it. Maybe only because she can't stand to see things go to waste.*

—ALICIA B.

◆ Some dietary supplement drinks, like Ensure, or powdered breakfast drinks are useful on those days when your parent doesn't feel up to cooking or eating.

◆ Buy in small quantities. If your father is shopping for one, he should ask the grocer to break open large containers and give him just two potatoes or a half-dozen eggs. Most will do this readily. He can also buy small portions of cheese, cooked meat, a pint of milk, a half pound of hamburger—so unused food doesn't spoil.

◆ If your mother walks to the corner grocery or has to transport her bags from the bus stop, get her a hand cart for toting them.

◆ If you can't help out with the shopping, find out if a grocery store in her neighborhood delivers, or see if a local volunteer or a friendly neighbor will take her shopping occasionally.

## IN THE KITCHEN

◆ Update the kitchen equipment. Small toast-and-broil ovens, microwaves and woks are convenient for single-serving meals, and small food processors are helpful for chopping and slicing.

◆ If your parent uses a gas range, make sure the dials are easy to read. If she has poor vision or suffers from any confusion, mark the "off" position clearly with a strip of colored tape.

◆ If your parent has stiff joints or weak muscles, there are dozens

## KEEP IT CLEAN

While most of us can tolerate hundreds of germs without any ill effects, the elderly are more vulnerable to food poisoning and less likely to recover easily once they get it. So take special precautions.

❖ Get your parent to throw out food that is past the expiration date, moldy or smelly. If his sense of smell isn't what it used to be, he should mark foods with a date when he buys it.

❖ Food that is susceptible to bacteria—salads, meats, sauces—should always be refrigerated and never left sitting on the counter. (It's okay to put warm food directly into the freezer.) Thaw frozen foods in the refrigerator or the microwave, not on the counter.

❖ When handling raw meat, especially chicken, your parent should rinse it well and then wash everything it has touched before moving on to the next stage of cooking. Bacteria from the raw chicken can easily travel to the salad if the two are chopped on the same surface, and unwashed hands are common carriers of bacteria.

❖ Cook meat thoroughly. Rare meat is a poor choice for anyone who is frail or elderly.

❖ Wash the kitchen sponge in the dishwasher and throw the dish towel into the washing machine every few days—both gather germs.

❖ Use a wooden cutting board instead of a plastic one; bacteria don't live as well in wood.

Call the Department of Agriculture's Meat and Poultry Hotline (800-535-4555) or the Food and Drug Administration's Seafood Hotline (800-332-4010), for more information about food storage and safety.

---

of aids that can be bought—jar openers, spoon holders, lightweight cookware, stirring devices, etc.—to make cooking easier. (See Appendix E, page 416.)

◆ Put Lazy Susans in cabinets that are full of small items so your parent has easy access to them.

◆ Move utensils, plates, food, pans and other frequently-used items to lower shelves or onto the countertop so your parent doesn't have to reach to high shelves or stoop to get things from low places.

◆ Buy your parent some (large-print, if necessary) cookbooks with easy recipes that serve just one or two people. Some cookbooks cater to special diets, with low-salt or fat-free dishes. Or show your parent how to make a few easy dishes. He can add vegetables, beans, tofu or rice to a can of broth or other soup; toss some tomatoes, cheese, vegetables or left-over meat into a helping of pasta or fold it into a small omelet; or sauté an assortment of favorite foods in a wok.

◆ If you bring food to your parent, make sure that he can easily open and heat whatever you bring. He may just toss it out, not wanting to admit that he couldn't undo the twist-tie on the bag or unwrap the foil.

◆ To perk up food, rather than adding more salt or sugar, your parent should throw in some herbs, spices, extracts, lemon or garlic, and he should heat food whenever possible, so it gives off more aroma. A variety of textures on the plate—crunchy vegetables, creamy sauces, crispy crusts—also makes a meal more appetizing.

◆ If you are cooking for your parent, prepare the foods she prefers. She may be much happier with meat loaf, baked beans and rice pudding than with fancier fare.

## AT THE TABLE

◆ Make dining social. Elderly people often fail to eat well purely because they don't like to eat alone. Join your father for meals occasionally, and when you can't be there urge him to get together with friends. He might enjoy a regular potluck dinner, to which each person brings one simple item, or a regular dinner date with a friend.

◆ Make it special. When your mother dines alone, encourage her to put her dinner on a plate, rather than eating it out of the pan, and to sit down at the table to eat. She might also have a glass of wine, if that makes dining more enjoyable.

## MEAL PROGRAMS

Congregate meals offered at local community centers, churches and senior centers are nutritious, social and inexpensive (or free). Even if your parent goes only once or twice a week, you'll know that he's eating well at least some of the time. (Some senior centers also provide transportation to meals.) If he can't or won't go out, find out about meal-delivery services, which are also inexpensive or free. (See page 174 for more on these meal programs.)

◆ If your parent has trouble handling utensils, buy him forks and knives with longer, heavier, thicker or bent handles; glasses with built-in straws; and plates with rims.

◆ Food that doesn't have to be cut up is easier for less dexterous hands, and finger food is often easier for people with dementia, who can be confused by utensils.

◆ Portions should be small so meals don't look overwhelming. The sheer volume of food may spoil your parent's limited appetite.

# AT HOME, IN THE BEDROOM

If your parent is in bed or in a bedroom most or all of the time, you need to set up his room for days of dining and entertainment, as well as safety. If you don't live with your parent, many of these things can be done during a visit.

❖ Make sure your parent is situated on the same floor as a bathroom, preferably close to his room. Otherwise, buy a commode for his room. (Medicare will often cover the cost.)

❖ If you have any choice, select a room for your parent that has a large window and a view, or bright, cheery pictures on the wall.

❖ Arrange the room so there is a sitting area for your parent and for visitors—a chair or two, a reading lamp and a table near a window or in front of a television set, for example.

❖ Place a table near the bed where you can store all the day's needs—magazines or books, pills, a water glass and pitcher, lamp, telephone, radio, writing paper, clock, calendar, remote controls, etc.

❖ Set up a television so your parent can watch it easily, and make sure he has a remote control.

❖ Buy a large pillow for sitting up comfortably in bed (most department stores sell cushions for reclining, and medical supply stores have large triangular-shaped foam cushions for propping people up), and supplement this with lots of regular pillows.

❖ If the house is large, put a bell or a baby monitor by the bed so your parent can call for someone if necessary. Or buy a telephone with an intercom so he can summon help.

❖ Stock some crackers and other nonperishable foods by the bed so you don't have to come running every time your parent wants a snack. You might even buy a miniature refrigerator for his room or load up a cooler with food each morning.

❖ You can buy or rent all sorts of equipment to make bed rest more manageable—for example, an electric or manual hospital bed, side-rails for getting up or turning over; a trapeze above the bed to grab and pull up on; a hospital-style table that slides over the bed; wheelchairs and walkers. These items are expensive, but some may be covered by Medicare.

❖ If your parent is bedridden, you or whoever is caring for her should be on the lookout for bedsores.

◆ When your family dines together, let your parent eat at her own pace. Have her start before the others sit down, or let the children leave the table while she finishes. If she feels that others are waiting for her, she may quit in mid-meal, or worse, hurry and choke on something.

◆ If your parent lives with you, don't enforce "normal" mealtimes. Sometimes, as people grow older, the established routines don't work anymore. Your mother may eat six small meals a day instead of three larger ones. For her nibbling, have healthful snacks on hand such as chopped vegetables, raisins and other dried fruit, popcorn, cole slaw, yogurt, cheese, humus, meat slices, apples and other fresh fruit, or peanut butter and crackers.

## WHEN EATING IS DIFFICULT

If your parent has trouble chewing and swallowing, is confined to bed or unable to feed herself, you or some other caregiver will be more involved in her dining habits.

◆ Anyone who's had a baby knows that most food can be pulverized into a gruesome-looking but healthful mush. A mini food-processor or blender (or even a hand-held masher) will grind meat, mash potatoes and puree vegetables and fruit. Also, try scrambled eggs, oatmeal (banana, cinnamon or raisins add flavor), egg salad, custard, applesauce or flavored gelatin. When you have no time, baby food straight from the jar is soft, nutritious and perfectly good for adults—the fruit selections are actually tasty.

◆ Sauces help dry food slide down more easily, and there is no end to the possibilities—cream, apple, barbecue, gravy, lemon, wine, tomato, cheese. And thicker liquids are easier to swallow than thin ones, especially if your parent is trying to drink while lying in bed.

◆ If you are feeding your parent, never hurry her or thrust oversized bites at her. If you don't have the time (and one meal can take an hour or two) see if a home health aide or a local volunteer can help.

◆ To avoid choking, your parent should eat sitting up, if possible, take small bites and avoid talking while eating.

# In the Driver's Seat

Anyone who has followed a snail-paced car or one that darts past stop signs knows that plenty of older drivers shouldn't be on the roads. Studies show that the elderly have more car accidents per miles driven than other age groups. As we age, our reflexes slow, our peripheral vision narrows, our night vision dims, our eyes can't follow moving objects well and we become less coordinated. Medications and illness only compound the hazards.

And yet, driving is a way of life. Who can forget the exhilaration of turning sixteen and getting a driver's license? It was a ticket to freedom and a sign of maturity. To give up this mobility, and the independence it still represents, can be devastating for your parent. Even if she has no place to go or if ample public transportation is available, her driver's license and the car keys are a vital part of her life.

## SAFETY BEHIND THE WHEEL

Depending upon the extent of your parent's limitations, you may be able to help improve his skills and keep him at the wheel a little longer. He won't take your advice readily: In fact, he is likely to be offended by it. But do it anyway. See if you can find a driving refresher course for senior citizens because that takes the hard work out of your hands (see box). If there is no such course in his area, tell him that you are concerned about his losing his license if he gets into an accident or gets a ticket—say that you know of other people his age who are no longer allowed to drive—and that in order to help him keep his license you need to address some issues and review a few matters together.

◆ Get your parent to wear his seat belt—both at the shoulder and at the waist. (Let him know that airbags and shoulder straps are not a replacement for safety belts that go around the waist.) Be sure that he can fasten and unfasten the belt easily. Automotive shops can adjust the shoulder strap so that it is comfortable or reset the belt so it can be more easily hooked and unhooked.

◆ Has your parent had his eyesight and hearing tested recently? If not, urge him to make the necessary appointments at once.

◆ If your parent suffers from dizziness, confusion or blurred eyesight, all of which affect driving, ask

## A DRIVING REFRESHER

Your parent can take a refresher course in driving (which, as a bonus, will qualify her for a lower insurance premium in most states). The National Safety Council (800-621-6244) and the American Association of Retired Persons (800-424-3410) offer such courses. Senior centers, local AAA offices, driving schools and the Department of Motor Vehicles should have information about other driving courses in your parent's area.

Some of these groups also issue information and brochures that you might obtain and then casually leave on your parent's coffee table. The AAA Foundation for Traffic Safety (800-305-7233) offers several good publications, including a guide for families, a self-exam for older drivers and a fitness booklet aimed at improving the driving abilities of older people.

the doctor about ways to reduce these symptoms. They may be caused by untreated illness or inappropriate medications.

♦ Urge your parent to exercise, which will improve his reaction time, his range of motion and his attentiveness. Simply stretching the neck each day by rotating the head side to side and up and down, and circling the shoulders can help people twist around to parallel park or check oncoming traffic with greater agility and safety.

♦ Make sure that the car is in good working order—including brakes, defroster, defogger, battery, wipers, dashboard light and exterior lights and turn signals.

♦ Install large mirrors and add extra mirrors if your parent is having trouble turning his head to see what's behind him.

♦ If your mother cannot see clearly over the dashboard, buy a seat cushion at an automotive store. (Don't use a pillow because it might slip.) Automotive stores also sell gadgets to raise the pedals.

♦ If your parent is buying a new car, opt for power everything— brakes, seats, steering, locks, etc.

♦ Once on the road, your parent should avoid driving:

• at night, dawn or dusk
• during rush hour
• on unfamiliar routes
• in city centers or busy streets
• long distances
• in bad weather
• when he's not feeling well.

♦ Throughout all this, begin to wean your parent away from his automobile. Introduce him to carpools and public transportation or offer to drive him yourself, if possible. Do it in such a way that your parent can save face. Make it possible for him to bow out without feeling embarrassed.

## WHEN IT'S TIME TO QUIT

When your parent is too ill, crippled or disoriented, or when you decide that it's not safe for your children to be in the car with Grandpa, you need to act. Get him off the road. Unfortunately, you can't rely on the state to monitor his driving because most states, reluctant to alienate a large population of elderly voters, refuse to retest or otherwise restrict older drivers. Don't put this off. It's a matter of your parent's safety as well as the safety of others. It truly is a matter of life and death.

If you can't do it yourself, ask your parent's doctor to tell him that it's time to stop driving. It will be easier for your parent to hear *and* heed this, if it comes from a doctor or another professional. If you decide to take it on, brace yourself, because your parent is bound to be hurt if not irate. Be sensitive to the gravity of what you are suggesting, to the implications, both practical and emotional, but remain firm in your resolve. And be ready with solutions to his travel problems—look into public and senior transportation programs, and ask family and friends if they can provide some transportation. If your parent uses his driver's license for identification, call the Department of Motor Vehicles to request a photo ID card.

If you don't make any progress, you can report an unsafe driver to the DMV or your state licensing agency. It's a difficult step, but it may be your only choice. Before you report your parent, ask that your name be kept confidential and find out in advance what happens when someone is reported. The states have varying procedures.

# Pumping Iron

Even if your parent can't hobble across the hallway or push herself out of a wheelchair, she can still benefit from a little heave-ho, one-and-two. Don't be overprotective here. *But my parent is really too old and too sick for this.* If she can't lift weights or go to a senior swim class, maybe she can walk to the mailbox, sway to her favorite music or sweep her own front step. If she is confined to a wheelchair or a bed, she might do a series of neck rotations, arm stretches and foot flexes each day. Pretty much everyone can do something. Yes, even *your* parent.

## BEFORE HE BEGINS

If your parent embarks on any exercise regime, he should first talk with his doctor, a physical therapist or a sports medicine specialist. Any weight training should be done with an experienced trainer.

## WHY BOTHER?

Much of the physical decline that we attribute to old age is actually due to inactivity. By exercising, your mother can slow and maybe even reverse the effects of time, making her feel years younger, and giving her greater mobility, independence and energy. Exercise can reduce arthritis pain, boost immunity, enhance sleep and even improve memory.

A number of recent studies have demonstrated the vast benefits of flexing, lifting and stretching, even very late in life. In one study, a group of frail nursing home residents in their 80s and 90s worked out for ten weeks in a highly-supervised program of weight lifting. These patients, many of whom had been written off as barely mobile, dramatically improved their strength, muscle mass, walking speed and stair-climbing abilities. Some gave up their canes and walkers. Others found they could climb stairs or get out of a chair without help for the first time in years. A second study of more than two thousand elderly people found that exercise reduced the risk of falls by 13 percent. Tai chi, a Chinese martial art that emphasizes balance, was found to be the most helpful. Those practicing tai chi lowered their risk of falls by 25 percent.

Once again, the old adage proves true: Use it or lose it.

## THE RIGHT EXERCISE PROGRAM

A good exercise regime has three components: aerobic, strength

## WALKING FOR LIFE

Walking is a great form of exercise for an elderly person. It's easy on joints. It's entertaining. It's cheap. And it can be social. It requires no special skills and can be done virtually anywhere. Your parent might just walk to the end of the driveway and back. Or for more serious walking, schools often have outdoor tracks and some malls are open during certain hours just for walkers. (Scenic routes are more enjoyable, but he should avoid wooded paths where rocks, roots and stumps can trip him up.)

Get him to start with a short walk, which may be a few paces or a few miles, depending upon his abilities, three times a week, and then add a little more each week. If possible, he should pick up the pace from a leisurely stroll to a more determined stride. As he walks, he should stand straight, with his head erect and arms swinging loosely at his sides. Tell him to lift his feet rather than shuffle, so he doesn't trip on cracks and bumps.

Your parent should drink plenty of liquids so he doesn't dehydrate. And he should drink *before* he's thirsty; once he's thirsty his body is already seriously low on fluids.

Buy your father comfortable sneakers with arch supports and thick rubber soles. Find sneakers made of nylon, mesh, canvas or other material that lets the air circulate. He should wear layers of clothing that he can shed as he warms up. If he needs to carry things with him, get him a fanny pack.

Someone should always know where he is headed, and he should keep to well-populated, safe areas.

and flexibility exercises. If your parent is able to move about (and remember those frail nursing home residents were lifting weights, so don't sell her short), she should alternate, doing aerobic exercise one day and strength-building exercises the next. Before or after each session she should do some stretching.

♦ **Aerobic.** Aerobic exercise strengthens the heart and lungs and improves endurance. It requires working the muscles without interruption for at least 15 minutes. Walking, riding a stationary bicycle, swimming or water exercises (which are especially good for people with arthritis, osteoporosis or back, knee or hip problems) are all good choices.

♦ **Strength.** Lifting light weights is a great way of increasing strength, but your parent can also stand in a doorway and push against the door jams, squeeze his palms together, let someone else act as an immovable barrier, or work against the weight of his own body, as in push-ups or sit-ups. If your parent is frail, he can keep repetitions simple—lift his shoulders slowly and lower them, make a fist and release it, and so on.

◆ **Flexibility.** Bending and stretching improve range of motion, alleviate arthritis and relieve tension. With the lack of use that comes with age, muscles and bones shrink, and tendons and ligaments fail to extend. As a result, older people often stoop over, have trouble with their balance and experience back pain. Your parent should take it easy, stretching gently until he

---

**"***When I was pregnant I did stretching exercises from a video, special exercises for pregnant women that were easy. My mother, who is in a wheelchair, would watch me. She enjoyed the music and energy of it. And it was something for her to do. I encouraged her to join in and, with some reluctance, she finally did. She did simple versions of what I was doing, or she would swing her arm out to the side when I was swinging my leg, that sort of thing. But she had fun with it.*

*After the baby was born and I wasn't using the tape anymore, I gave it to her. She says she still uses it most days. I know it helps her keep moving, and it's entertaining.***"**
—JANE D.

---

feels a slight pull, then hold it for anywhere from eight to thirty counts, depending on how it feels, and then release it. He can stretch his fingers, rotate his head, arch his back, reach for his toes, raise his arms upward, pull his elbows back, lift his toes off the floor, and so on. Yoga classes are a great way to improve flexibility, and some are geared for seniors.

## RULES OF THE GAME

No matter what exercise program is followed, an easy beginning, safe surroundings and a slow ending are especially important when the exerciser is aged. Your parent should be sure to observe the following guidelines:

◆ Rest whenever necessary. He should stop exercising immediately if he feels palpitations, chest pains or cramps, or if he becomes nauseated, dizzy, faint, light-headed, breathless or exhausted.

◆ Start slowly, and work up gradually, doing more each week.

◆ Begin and end with simple, easy stretches, warming up beforehand and then cooling down slowly toward the end.

◆ Stay in balance. Stand with legs planted slightly apart, back straight, body aligned and eyes focused ahead. Have something nearby that he can grab if he feels off balance.

◆ Don't exercise on an empty stomach or right after a big meal, but get ample fluids, especially if it's

## VIDEO EXERCISE

A number of new videos offer exercises for older people, even those with disabilities. Try your local library or video store, or order one of your own.

"Armchair Fitness" by CC-M Productions (800-453-6280). The one-hour tape features gentle, easy exercises set to big-band music. Twenty minutes are done seated, for those who are less mobile. $39.95 plus shipping

"55+ and Fit: A Life-Enhancing Stretch & Tone Program for Older Adults" by the University of Iowa (800-369-IOWA). This is for older people who are relatively fit and active. It's not aerobic, but requires the exerciser to get down on the floor and back up again for stretches. Fifty-five minutes long. $19.95 plus $3 shipping.

"Smile: So Much Improvement with a Little Exercise" by the University of Michigan, School of Public Health, Dept. of HB/HE, 1420 Washington Heights, Ann Arbor, MI, 48109. A thirty-five minute, low-intensity workout for frail elders. $15 for videotape; $7.50 for booklet.

"A Stroke Survivor's Workout" by Courage Stroke Network (800-553-6321.) An easy workout with lots of stretching for people who have had a stroke and have mild to severe mobility problems. $19.95 plus shipping and handling.

"Exercising with Dorothy" by Stuart Choate, (800-779-8491). An easy, slow-paced workout for all elderly people, including those who use walkers or wheelchairs. $69.95 to buy or $25 to rent.

a warm day (not ice-cold fluids, which can cause cramping).

◆ Avoid dizziness by not getting up too fast or changing directions too rapidly.

◆ Breathe regularly with each repetition. Inhale just before exertion and exhale at the maximum point of exertion. People tend to hold their breath when exercising.

◆ Choose a comfortable time of day, when it's not too hot or cold, and the sun isn't too strong. If ex-

ercising outdoors, remember to apply sunscreen.

◆ Wear loose, comfortable clothing that doesn't impede movement, and wear layers that can be shed as the body warms up.

◆ Make exercising part of a daily routine. It's also helpful to keep a daily record of exercise—how many minutes, what movements, how many repetitions, etc.

◆ Do it to music, if possible.

◆ Do it with friends. If none are willing or about, join a class or gym. Exercising with others is more fun and is more likely to remain part of a routine.

◆ If exercising in the house, clear plenty of space to allow for safety and freedom of movement.

## WHERE DO WE SIGN UP?

Find a community exercise program for elders which is oriented toward the special needs of your parent. It's apt to be a safe workout and it will add a nice social aspect to the sport. Call the local senior center, community center, department of recreation, Jewish center, YMCA or YWCA to find out about such classes. Ask local gyms and health clubs about exercise classes that might be appropriate. Don't forget to ask about yoga, tai chi and other forms of exercise that may be fun for your parent.

For those who choose to exercise at home, the American Association of Retired Persons (800-424-3410) puts out a free booklet called "Pep Up Your Life: A Fitness Book for Seniors," which describes a number of exercises with clear illustrations.

# Staying Involved

Once you know your parent is safe, well-groomed and well-fed, what about feeding her mind and spirit? Stimulation and a sense of purpose will keep your parent's mind off her problems, boost her immune system and, quite simply, make life worth living. And what a relief it would be for you to know that your parent is enjoying her afternoons without you!

In this day and age of accessibility, even people with poor vision, no mobility or another disability can do quite a bit. If your mother is in a nursing home, she can still take up a new hobby, listen to books on tape or volunteer to help others in the home.

Your parent's real obstacle to activity may not be disability, but ageism and boredom. If you've ever been laid up or between jobs, you know how boredom can lead to feelings of worthlessness. Having nothing to do, then feeling useless, leaves a person with no initiative to do anything. Over time, the idea of do-

*"My father lives in a nursing home and he gets very bored and lonely. When anyone visits him, it's as though he won the lottery, he gets so excited. The rest of the time he basically sleeps and roams the hallways and talks to the nurses. He's not interested in any of the games or activities at the home and says all the other residents are 'too old' or half-crazy.*

*I've tried a lot of things and I think my most successful effort was signing him up as a foster grandparent. This little boy, Tyler, not only visits, but sends him games and calls when he has homework questions. They've developed a really nice relationship."* —ELEANOR R.

ing something new becomes frightening. So if your mother doesn't want to do anything and is unhappy doing nothing, it's your job to push and prod. You may have to try a number of ideas before something strikes her fancy. Think about what she enjoys or used to enjoy in her earlier life. If she was always involved in local politics, for example, call local political offices to see if she can volunteer. Look through the newspaper, read bulletin boards and community calendars. Talk to her friends about what they are doing. Don't give up. You will find something. This section offers a few suggestions.

## VOLUNTEERING

Volunteering is a wonderful way for your mother to regain a sense of purpose, to meet new people of different ages, to take her mind off herself and to be involved in things —politics, the arts, children, medical care, women's issues—whatever interests her.

Even if she can't leave the house or her bed, she may be able to make phone calls, offer advice, stuff envelopes or help in other ways. If she is in a nursing home she may be able to give tours, answer visitors' questions, deliver meals or flowers, or visit patients in the infirmary. The local chapter of the American Association of Retired Persons should have ideas. The volunteer agency Corporation for National Service (800-424-8867) runs a Retired and Senior Volunteer Program. The National Council on the Aging (202-479-1200) can make referrals to a local Family Friends Program, which trains older people to work with seriously ill or disabled children, homeless children and rural families.

To find out about other possibilities call churches, synagogues, senior and community centers, hospitals, libraries, schools, foundations, grass-roots organizations, day-care centers, fund-raising groups, political campaigns, local museums, theaters, nature centers, the United Way and the Red Cross.

## WORKING FOR PAY

If your parent doesn't want to work for free and she is relatively healthy, she may be able to find a job that pays. More and more shops and restaurants, for example, are finding that older people are more reliable and harder-working than teenagers, and some senior organizations specifically look to hire older people. The area agency on aging should also know of local employment programs for seniors. Also, look through the want ads or call some businesses that interest your parent—a museum gift shop, a children's clothing store, a movie theater.

## LENDING A HAND

In earlier days you may not have wanted to bother or burden your parent by asking for favors. Well, now is the time to ask. If your parent is bored, give her a project—not a time-passer but something that would really help you. Ask her to sort through old photos, write addresses on all those holiday greet-

## SPIRITUAL NEEDS

As a person's life heads into its last stages, questions about mortality and the meaning of life take on a new importance. Whether or not your parent practiced a religion, she might like to go to church or synagogue, attend a religious discussion group, speak to a member of the clergy or have someone read to her from the Bible or other religious books.

It's quite possible that she may be embarrassed to bring this up with you, or she may not even think of it unless you suggest it.

ing cards, look something up in the library for you, or otherwise help you in your personal or business life. You get a task done and she gets to feel useful.

### EXERCISING THE MIND

It's never too late to learn new things. Call local colleges, community centers, high-school extension programs and art museums about classes and lectures. If your parent is relatively well, she might learn to paint with oils, cook Italian food or play the piano. Perhaps she wants to study classical music or learn about modern architecture. Through an organization called Elderhostel (617-426-7788), colleges, universities, museums, theaters and nation-

al parks offer special low-cost, short (usually about one week) courses for people who are over 60. (This usually involves travel so it's only useful for those elders who are relatively independent and mobile.)

Find out about tours of museums and art galleries, many of which have special programs and prices for the elderly. For her next birthday, buy your parent tickets to the ballet, theater or opera.

Chronic illness and bed rest can stifle your parent's mind and make her listless. If your mother is laid up in bed, but still mentally able, encourage her curiosity in the world beyond her. She can read about foreign places, study history or learn about anything that sparks her interest. If she can't read anymore, get her books and lectures on tape or videotapes from the local library. She doesn't have to take it all in— there are no exams—but learning gives a person optimism and pride.

### TRAVEL AND OTHER EXPLORATION

If he's mobile, your parent should find out about tours—senior citizen or otherwise—to foreign countries or nearby cities, colleges, botanical gardens and historic sites and monuments. You may even want to join him. (Some tours don't require any walking, if your father would rather ride.)

Most senior centers offer discount trips, from day trips to weekend foliage tours to full vacations. Colleges and special-interest organizations, like museums, environmental groups and history clubs,

## A RIDE IN THE COUNTRY

If your parent is very frail and doesn't get out much, he will benefit from a change of scene. Even if it takes some logistics to get him into the car, try it. Driving down a country road, by the sea or along a busy city street may cheer him up considerably. If you don't have time for pleasure trips, take him with you when you run your errands, just to get him out of the house.

often offer tours. And travel agents can book trips that are specially designed for older people or people with disabilities.

## VIDEOTAPES AND BOOKS

If your parent is laid up or just likes to stay at home, get her some books and movies. She may not have the initiative to do this for herself, but once she is involved in a good story, she may get lost in it. How about some of her favorite old films? If she is active, get her to start a book club, with friends gathering once a month to discuss a book they have all read, or she might get some friends together to see a weekly movie at home.

If your parent has trouble seeing or can't read for some other reason, get books with large print or books on tape. Your local library, the Library of Congress at 800-424-8567, the American Foundation for the Blind at 800-232-5463, or the National Association for the Visually Handicapped at 212-889-3141 can help. Or buy a closed-circuit television that magnifies words, or see if there are local volunteers who read to older people.

## PROJECTS AND HOBBIES

Maybe your parent isn't into making birdhouses, but what about other hobbies and projects, like gardening, bird-watching, collecting, model-building or painting? You never know what he will find fun. Think small-scale. If he doesn't want to take care of a full garden, he can have a few small planters in a window. It will give him something to tend to and learn about, and something that will grow and bloom. If he can't get about, put a bird feeder

*The thing my mother loved most was music. The Jewish home where she lived had concerts and even a 'music therapy' class, but she couldn't go because she was afraid of riding in the elevator by herself and the nurse said there wasn't enough staff to escort her. One day I ran into the woman who directed the program in the hallway. I told her about my mother and she said she would be happy to bring Mom to and from the class each day. It was such a relief. Her spirits seemed to pick up right away.* —BARBARA F.

near the window so he can watch the different birds from a comfortable seat. If his interest grows, buy him a pair of binoculars or a bird-guide for his birthday. Ask what sorts of things he used to do in his younger days; he might enjoy picking up an old hobby. If he doesn't want to do things on his own, ask at senior centers about hobby clubs and see if he doesn't have a few friends or neighbors who might like to explore a new subject or start a project with him.

## SPORTS AND GAMES

Sports and games are a terrific way to exercise, meet people and build some confidence. It might be bingo, bridge or shuffleboard, or it could be walking, golf, cross-country skiing or swimming. Your father may have to take it easy, but that doesn't mean he can't partici-

## SIMPLE PLEASURES

If your parent is severely ill, heavily medicated or suffering from dementia, it may take very little to entertain him. Children's games, like checkers or Go Fish, an otherwise monotonous task like sticking labels on envelopes, stroking a cat or listening to the jingle-jangle of children's songs may give his day a boost. What might seem silly to you may engage or even delight him.

pate. Some other activities to consider: fishing, horseshoes, darts, bowling, croquet, badminton, archery, miniature golf, camping or paddle tennis. Again, local senior centers may arrange or know of such events, or call the local department of recreation or community center.

## SENIOR CENTER ACTIVITIES

Senior centers and adult day-care centers offer elders a place to socialize, talk about the events of the day, attend lectures, go on trips, learn new skills, and, in some cases, find out about practical matters like estate planning and budgeting. If there is more than one center in the area, your parent is welcome to sign up for classes at any or all of them.

## SOCIALIZING

Calling other people is hardest when you need them the most, and if your parent is recently widowed, or just not used to socializing on her own, then initiating a new friendship or activity is difficult. She may need a little push from you. Urge her to call a potential friend or an acquaintance for lunch, a pot-luck supper, a movie, a ball game or a museum tour. It's often easiest to set up standing dates—a bridge game every Tuesday night, for example—so she doesn't have to think about creating new social events each week. If you don't get anywhere, maybe you can make the first effort, bringing your mother and one or two others together for

## CREATURE COMFORTS

What has come to be known in medical lingo as pet-facilitated therapy, or PFT—basically, having a dog or cat—seems to boost people's emotional state as well as their physical health, according to several recent studies. Animals make us feel loved and less alone, and also give us a sense of responsibility. And, since Rascal needs a daily walk, a pet provides a little exercise as well. For someone who is anxious or agitated, stroking a pet is calming. The findings about "pet-facilitated therapy" have been so conclusive that federal law now mandates that elderly people living in subsidized housing be allowed to keep pets, so don't let the landlord shoo Patches or Felix out the door.

Look into foster grandparent programs or talk to a child you know about adopting your parent as a grandparent. If your parent is going to day care, some programs are intergenerational, mixing seniors and toddlers. The Corporation for National Service (800-424-8867) runs a Foster Grandparent Program.

### REMINISCING

The next time your father drifts back several decades and tells you stories you've heard before, rather than shake your head in resignation or despair, encourage him to tell more. He's doing something that's healing. Reminiscing allows him to review his life, think through important issues and digest it all. More important, it returns him, temporarily, to a time when he was younger, stronger, more confident and more capable.

If you can get your parent to tell new stories or flesh out the old ones, reminiscing can be a wonderful experience for you too. Or your children might like to share this activity with their grandparent. Exploring these details gives you insight into your parent's life and background, and it may be one of the last chances you have to learn about your heritage.

dinner. They'd probably be delighted if you accompanied them, at least the first time.

### CROSSING THE GENERATION GAP

If your parent has always been good with children, he can still have them in his life. His involvement can enrich them and make him feel young again. Call local schools and day-care centers to find out about ways your parent might get involved.

Tape-record your father's tales because you are sure to forget important details or a tone of voice that made the story his. Ask about his own life as well as his views of historical events he witnessed. What was his childhood house like? What about the school he attended? What were his parents like? What girls did he

**"**Dad and I always had what I call a business relationship. We talked about finances and health and practical matters, but never emotions and that sort of thing.

Then one day I was visiting him in the hospital and running out of conversation and, for some reason, I asked him about a girl he dated in college. I guess I had heard her name somewhere. Well, his eyes got misty and he started telling me all about being in love for the first time and the college parties and how hurt he was when she left him. He got lost in his past, lying in that bed, with tubes all over the place. He told me about other women he dated, his friends, funny things that happened, and the day he met my mother.

He was like a kid, remembering all this stuff. And I was seeing, for the first time in my life, this very human and vulnerable and youthful side of my father.**"**         —ALICIA B.

date? How did he travel or dress or cook as a young boy? Why did he chose his career? Does he remember the first time he saw a car or a plane? What Presidential elections were most exciting to him and why? What was life like for him during the Depression? Where was he during World War I or World War II?

Get your parent to talk about your ancestors. Draw a family tree together, gathering the additional information you need from other relatives. Find out where you came from and what those long-ago people were like. This is invaluable information that you can call on in resolving your own life and relationships—are there familiar patterns?—and pass down to your children and grandchildren.

As your parent talks, let him ramble about the subjects that he feels comfortable with. Don't correct him or force him to stay within some chronological order. Just listen, encourage him and enjoy it.

# Chapter Nine

# GETTING HELP:

## Community and Home-Care Services

*What's Available • Where to Find Help • Geriatric Care Managers • Hiring and Managing Workers • Taking Advantage of Respite Care*

Y OUR FATHER NEEDS SOMEONE TO DRIVE HIM TO THE doctor's office, do his housekeeping and prepare his meals. Your mother needs someone to nurse her through chronic illness, guide her when she's confused and keep her company when she's lonely. You can't possibly do it all, which means that you have to find others who can do it for you.

Help is available, but it can be hard to find. You'll have to make a number of calls to see what is offered in your parent's community. Large cities generally have a greater range of services than small towns, but even in rural areas you should be able to find basic support for the elderly, such as meal programs, transportation services and adult day care. In almost every area, you can also hire home health aides, nurses and physical therapists. (Health insurance sometimes covers these costs.) If you don't have the time or the resources to locate the help you need and to coordinate your parent's care, you can hire a geriatric care manager to do it for you.

Learn about the programs and services available in your parent's community early on, preferably before your parent needs them. Don't wait until you run out of steam, your parent is entirely dependent upon you and resistant to change, or there is an emergency. By that point, the pressure of the crisis may keep you from investigating local services carefully. Do it now.

# Community Services

Communities establish services for the elderly in response to the demographics and specific needs of the local population. As a result, while all communities offer a handful of basic services to elderly residents, the details of those programs are as different as the communities themselves. Adult day care in one town will be very different from adult day care in the next. The funding sources, costs and sponsors are equally diverse, with services being offered by public agencies, private businesses, churches and synagogues, civic groups and non-profit organizations for seniors. In most cases, your parent or your family has to pay for community services, but a few are free and some are subsidized. (Insurance pays for little, if anything, in this regard.)

Before you sign your mother up for extensive and expensive care, determine exactly what she needs. Write them down and be specific. Does she need help first thing in the morning getting showered and dressed? Should someone shop and cook for her, or just give her a ride to the grocery store? Does she need some regular nursing care? You might discover that she doesn't require round-the-clock home health aides after all; maybe a homemaker in the mornings to get her dressed and fed, her dinner delivered, and two days a week of adult day care are sufficient. If you are not sure what help to get, the area agency on aging should have a social worker or case worker on hand who can guide you.

The following are general descriptions of the types of elderly services offered in most areas, but you will need to call to get the specifics on what's available in your parent's community.

## TELEPHONE REASSURANCE AND VISITORS

Most communities have a telephone reassurance program in which volunteers, often senior citizens, call once a day or once every few days to see how your parent is doing. Some programs will send visitors to her house to provide a little companionship and to check up on her. In either case, the volunteer will ask how your parent is doing and may

## COMMUNITY SERVICES AT A GLANCE

| TYPE OF HELP | SERVICES PROVIDED | AVERAGE COSTS |
|---|---|---|
| Telephone reassurance and visitors | Phone calls or brief visits to check on your parent's well-being | Free or minimal charge |
| Companions | Companionship, supervision and some help with meals and tasks | $5 to $15 an hour, some free through state-funded programs |
| Homemakers | Light housekeeping, laundry, cooking, errands, some help with bathing and dressing | $8 to $30 an hour, although some areas offer free or sliding-scale homemaker services |
| Chore services | Minor repairs and handyman chores | Free or based on a sliding scale, plus materials |
| Meal programs | Group dining at a community center or meals delivered to home | Free or minimal charge |
| Transportation services | Rides to day care, senior centers, shopping malls or specific appointments | Free or minimal charge |
| Senior centers | Clubs that provide social activities, information and a range of services | Usually free |
| Adult day care | Supervision, recreation, meals and some health care, and counseling | $30 a day; some are government subsidized |
| **HOME-CARE PROVIDERS** | | |
| Home health aides | Personal care (bathing, feeding, etc.), some medical care and light housekeeping | $50 per visit (usually anywhere from two to four hours), or $10-$15 per hour; may be covered by Medicare |
| In-home therapists | Training in communication, physical movement or doing daily tasks | $85 per visit (from a half-hour to two hours); may be covered by Medicare |
| Nurses | Medical care | $90 per visit (from a half-hour to two hours); may be covered by Medicare |
| Geriatric care managers | Management of some or all of your parent's care | $30 to $150 an hour |
| Respite care | A break for caregivers, from a few hours to a few weeks | Cost varies; some are subsidized and use volunteers |

remind her of some daily needs. *Did you take your medications this morning? What did you eat for lunch? Do you remember that you have a doctor's appointment this afternoon?* If anything seems askew, the volunteer will alert you or another person who has been designated as a contact.

Using such a service should help ease your mind, reduce the number of interruptions at work, and save you money if you routinely make long-distance calls to your parent.

The programs are usually run by senior centers, religious organizations and other public or non-profit agencies. Sometimes the services are offered by privately owned home-care agencies, in which case there will be a fee.

## COMPANIONS

Companions are basically elder-sitters who will keep your parent company, help him with minor tasks and generally watch over him. Some focus on the companionship aspect, while others provide more supervision and help. Some companions come for an occasional friendly visit while others fill in for a specified time—for instance, while you are at work or out for dinner. In general,

## DISCOUNTS AND SPECIAL SERVICES

The elderly are big business and everyone seems to be getting into the act. Shops and professionals of all types now offer special services and discounts to elderly customers. So when your parent needs something, call the supplier and ask about free delivery services, discounts and house calls—it can't hurt, and might help. Some popular marketing programs aimed at seniors include:

❖ Grocery stores—free deliveries, senior discount days

❖ Veterinarians—house calls, discounts and pet-walking services

❖ Pharmacies—free deliveries and discounts

❖ Hair stylists and manicurists—house calls and discounts

❖ Phone and utility companies—discounts and other services, including amplified phones, large-button phone pads and large-print bills

❖ Health clinics, hospitals and public health departments—free health screenings and shots, and some discounted services

❖ Dentists and hygienists—discounts and services for the homebound.

## WHERE TO FIND HELP

To learn about the services in your parent's community, here are some of the people and organizations you should contact:

**The area agency on aging.** The best place to begin a search for home care is your local agency on aging, which can direct you to services in your parent's neighborhood, send booklets and brochures on specific topics and, in some cases, let you talk to a care manager who will discuss the needs of your parent and refer her to appropriate help. Some agencies also offer legal, financial and family counseling free or at little cost.

Area agencies on aging go by a medley of names—bureau on aging, council of senior services, commission on the elderly, center for elder affairs—and are overseen by state units on aging. You can find them by calling the Eldercare Locator (800-677-1116) or by calling the state unit on aging (listed in Appendix A, page 377).

**Local senior centers.** The area agency on aging can direct you to a local senior center, which should be able to provide additional information about community services. Some centers provide services directly, such as volunteer visitors and companions, and some sponsor senior advocates, people who counsel elderly residents about what community services they need and how to locate them.

**Discharge planners and care managers.** Most hospitals employ nurses or social workers who arrange housing, home care and community services for patients who are leaving the hospital with disabilities. Although it is best to contact the planner while your parent is in the hospital (even if she is there for a one-day procedure that has nothing to do with her disability), some discharge planners may offer guidance even if your parent is not a hospital patient.

Geriatric care managers will guide you and oversee your parent's care for a fee. (See page 182.)

**Employers.** See if your workplace (or the workplace of a mate, sibling or adult child) has an employee assistance program. Some of these programs provide information, referrals and counseling to people who are caring for an elderly person. A few companies have contracts with eldercare information and counseling referrals nationwide (very helpful if you live in Tulsa and your parent is in Tucson). Some companies also offer flexible hours, counseling and stress management to employees who are caring for a parent.

**The local United Way.** The United Way, which funds a number of community services, is a good source for referrals. You can find the number of the local branch in the telephone book.

**Churches and synagogues.** Even if your parent is not affiliated with any religious organization, such groups often provide direct help to people of all faiths, or can refer you to programs and services in the area.

**National organizations.** For virtually every ailment or interest—from asthma to veterans—there is an organization that can guide you to services, refer you to professionals and provide information. Many, such as the Jewish Family Service, the Red Cross, the Alzheimer's Association and the Arthritis Foundation, have local chapters that provide services directly. A number of good organizations are listed in Appendix B, page 383; additional ones can be found in the phone book or in the *Directory of Associations,* available in most public libraries. You can also get referrals to national organizations by calling the National Health Information Center (800-336-4797) or the National Rehabilitation Information Center (800-346-2742).

**Government agencies.** The health department can inform you about free flu shots and health screenings. The department of protective services should be notified if you suspect abuse. The parks and recreation department may know about exercise classes for the elderly. The departments of housing and social services may also know about services and programs for the elderly. But before you call, gather your patience and persistence. Call in the middle of the morning when the lines tend to be freer and write down the names and telephone extensions of the people you talk with, so you can get back to them if necessary. If you get lost in the bureaucracy, ask for a supervisor. And don't give up. The help is often there, and your parent, as a taxpayer, is paying for it.

**The Yellow Pages.** If you haven't found the help you need, try the phone book. (If you live far away from your parent, bring home a copy from your next visit.) Look under such headings as senior, elder, aging or under the name of a particular subject (vision, depression, home care, diaper service, Jewish services, alcohol). And before you wedge the book back under the phone, look at the first few pages of the White Pages, where emergency numbers, hotlines and often-used community services are listed. You should also find information there about telephone services and products for deaf or disabled people, and utility discounts for senior citizens and people with disabilities.

**Home-care agencies.** If your parent needs care at home, such as home health aides or nurses, call a local home-care agency. Some of them provide other services as well, such as companions, homemakers and care managers.

*After his wife died my father-in-law went into hibernation. He didn't have many friends, so he stayed at home and watched television. My husband said he was fine, but I was worried. He aged so quickly and he seemed so lonely. I had him for dinner once a week, but we both work and we have two young boys, so we couldn't do much.*

*I learned about a companion program and convinced Dad to try it. I think it's really been great for him. Scott, the companion, is in much the same situation as Dad. He's alone and can't get around all that well. He visits two or three times a week now and they play rummy and have lunch together. Last week they went to a hockey game together, which is something Dad always loved but hadn't done in years.*　　—LUCY A.

companions do not do housework or chores, but they might prepare meals, help your parent get dressed or pick up a few groceries on the way over.

Many communities have free or low-cost companion programs run by a public agency or a private group. For example, the Corporation for National Service (800-424-8867) runs a Senior Companion Program in many communities, in which elderly people are trained to work as companions. Churches or other religious organizations also sponsor companions.

Volunteer programs are wonderful if your parent simply needs

company. But if she needs reliable and consistent help, you should find a paid companion.

Home-care agencies often provide paid companions (look in the Yellow Pages under "home care"), or you can find one on your own in much the same way you would hire a baby-sitter—by asking friends, putting a classified ad in the local newspaper, or posting a sign in a senior center or church. (If you run an ad, leave your telephone number, not your parent's. You don't want to publicize her vulnerability.)

Companions cost anywhere from $5 to $15 an hour, depending upon the area and the services provided. Live-in companions charge $100 to $400 a week plus room, board and often transportation expenses. If your parent needs a lot of care and there is a spare bedroom, this

## A REMINDER

Be organized even in a crisis, or before you know it, you'll have crumpled brochures tucked in kitchen drawers and illegible notes scribbled on napkins. As you learn about community services, develop a filing system with folders for each topic and a master list of all relevant agencies and representatives with their phone numbers and extensions. (Refer back to page 9 for a refresher on organizational techniques.)

## CREATIVE ARRANGEMENTS

If there is a spare bedroom in your parent's home, or a den that can be converted into a bedroom, find a college student, a struggling writer or a young couple who would like to live with your parent in exchange for some help around the house and companionship. Your parent loves Italian? What about a foreign-exchange student from Italy? Call a college housing office, put an ad in the newspaper or call the local shared-housing program (see page 202).

This type of arrangement may provide less constant or reliable care than a hired companion or homemaker, but if your parent is still relatively independent it is usually less expensive than hiring companions and aides. It will also make your parent feel less like an invalid (because no one is being paid to watch him) and it may provide greater continuity—it may even blossom into a friendship.

Another money-saving possibility is for your parent to share a companion or homemaker with an elderly person who lives down the block or in the same apartment building. A worker could get your mother up, bathed and dressed and go to the neighbor's house for two hours to help out there; return to your parent briefly to get her lunch; and then come back in the late afternoon to prepare her dinner. Be sure that the worker can be contacted quickly in case one person suddenly needs her assistance.

---

arrangement can be less expensive and more convenient, but it also means giving up some privacy.

## HOMEMAKERS

Homemakers shop, do laundry and light housecleaning, prepare meals, and usually will assist with other tasks, such as helping your parent to bathe and dress. Many homemakers, especially those hired through home-care agencies, are trained specifically in caring for elderly people, and some can teach your parent how to manage house-hold tasks on his own. But again, the quality of the service depends upon the individual worker.

In most cases, your parent has to foot the bill, paying anywhere from $8 to more than $30 an hour for homemaker services. In some areas, homemakers are available at no charge or on a sliding scale, and paid for by public monies, but there can be long waiting lists for such services. In some states, under certain circumstances Medicaid will pay for homemakers.

As with companions, if homemakers are not offered through community programs, you can hire one through most home-care agencies or on your own by putting an ad in the local newspaper or on a church or synagogue bulletin board.

## CHORE SERVICES

Chore-service programs enlist workers, often volunteers, who do minor repairs and odd jobs for elderly residents. Most won't tackle major repairs or renovations and they may not do regular chores like shoveling snow, but they will usually construct ramps for a wheelchair, weatherstrip windows, put up storm windows or install grab bars.

Chore services, like visitor and telephone services, are sometimes offered by local nonprofit groups, such as senior centers or churches. Your parent pays for the materials that are needed, but the labor is often free or charged based on a sliding scale. (Your parent may have to meet some minimum income guidelines to be eligible.)

## MEAL PROGRAMS

If your parent can't or won't cook for himself no matter how you simplify the kitchen, or if he isn't eating well for some other reason, look into congregate dining and meal-delivery programs.

Congregate meals are typically hot lunches served in schools, community centers, apartment buildings, churches and synagogues, senior centers, adult day-care centers or other community sites. Most programs are open to all elderly people and they often provide trans-

portation to and from the site. The meals meet federal nutrition guidelines and usually cost nothing—some programs request a voluntary contribution based on income, but the average donation is less than a dollar a meal, and many programs accept federal food stamps. The best part of all is that the meals are social occasions. If your parent doesn't know people in the neighborhood, the first few visits may seem a little awkward, but eventually he will meet people and become accustomed to this routine.

If your parent can't or won't leave the house, meal-delivery programs will bring a hot lunch and often a cold, bagged dinner to his doorstep. These programs, called by a variety of names but generically known as meals-on-wheels, are typically operated by senior centers, religious organizations or hospitals. The cost is nominal ($2 to $5) and sometimes the meals are free. As a bonus, the volunteers who deliver the food are often trained to look for signs of trouble.

If your parent isn't eligible for meal delivery—some limit eligibility to homebound or low-income residents—don't give up too quickly. Some meals-on-wheels programs are now designed for financially secure clients, offering gourmet menus. Some specialize in kosher and other special meals. To find out about meal-delivery programs in your parent's location, call the area agency on aging or the National Meals on Wheels Foundation (800-999-6262).

Beyond meals-on-wheels, some cooks and caterers will come to your

## WHEN YOUR PARENT BLOCKS THE PATH

You've found a reliable homemaker as well as a good adult day-care center, but your mother says no. She insists that she doesn't need help (she forgets that she has set off the smoke alarm three times in the past month), she refuses to go to one of those places for old people, she wants only you to help her, or she doesn't want strangers in her home. When you persist and bring the homemaker to see her, she fires her on the spot.

Before you blow your top, remember, her fears are pronounced these days. She may be confused about what is happening; she may feel vulnerable and be desperately afraid of being robbed or hurt by strangers. Or she may be worried that you are abandoning her. Telling her that her fears are silly won't erase them and may only magnify them; pushing her to accept services she doesn't want will only fortify her objections.

Encourage your mother to express her fears and concerns. Be candid with her about the risks and opportunities the situation presents. Has she read reports of home-care workers harming or abusing their elderly clients? Try to reassure her. Discuss her options and what could happen if she doesn't allow people to help her. (If she is con-

fused because of dementia, see page 319 for tips on hiring and working with companions.)

If the situation is not dire, proceed very slowly as you introduce her to new services and to the idea of receiving outside help. For example, get someone to do her shopping or to drop off a meal every afternoon, rather than sending a companion over her sacred doorstep. Find someone who is kind and patient, someone who can earn your mother's trust over time. Once she trusts one person to come into her home, she may be more open to others.

If this doesn't work or if the situation doesn't allow for such slow steps, you might have to leave your parent for a day without your help so that she understands the severity of the situation. A day without meals or an hour or two in soiled clothing may help her understand that she needs regular assistance, which you can't provide.

If the situation is dangerous or if you can't handle this yourself, consider hiring a geriatric care manager (see page 182) or a counselor from a family service agency who can guide your mother into this new way of life. Many such professionals are trained specifically to do just that.

parent's house and prepare a week's worth of meals. This may not be as expensive as you think, especially because the servings are apt to be large enough to be stretched into two meals. The senior center may know of such people in your parent's community, or look in the Yellow Pages for private caterers.

Another possibility is prepared food by mail order. Your parent chooses from a list of entrees, soups, appetizers, etc. and receives a shipment of frozen meals for the week. (The Extended Family, 800-235-7070, sends meals out nationwide, charging about $65, plus shipping, for a week's worth of prepared food.) Of course your parent has to be able to heat the food.

## TRANSPORTATION SERVICES

If your parent needs a ride to a doctor's appointment, the grocery store, day care or elsewhere, a number of public and private groups provide door-to-door transportation specifically to elderly or disabled people. The area agency on aging should know about vans, buses and private drivers who serve elderly residents. Some such services pick up groups of people on a set day and take them to a shopping center, for example. Some take elderly people door-to-door for appointments and errands on an on-call basis. Many of the vans are equipped to take people in wheelchairs. These community services are usually free, but some groups ask for a donation or charge a minimal fee.

In addition, the local department of public transportation can tell you about bus routes, discounts to seniors, and other special transportation services.

## SENIOR CENTERS

Senior centers were originally established as social clubs for relatively healthy, elderly people, but that focus is shifting. As the population grows older and more frail, senior centers are serving a more diverse and needy population. Some are still small social clubs that operate out of a church basement, but some are large, publicly-funded organizations, housed in free-standing buildings and offering an array of services, including help with chores, volunteer visitors, homemakers and adult day care, along with recreational programs, meals, health screenings, counseling, exercise classes, lectures and field trips. So call and find out what your parent's local senior center offers because it may do far more than run bingo games. Senior centers are usually free and open to all elderly residents of any age, income or state of health.

## ADULT DAY CARE

Your mother is weak and her memory is fading. She can't get her own meals and she needs help getting to the toilet. You take care of her two days a week, but what do you do on the other five days? One possible answer is adult day care, which provides care and supervision outside the home to elderly people who have physical or mental limitations.

In a typical adult day-care program, your mother would be picked up by a van at 9 A.M., taken to a center where she is fed and cared for by a trained staff, and then returned home at 5 P.M. At the center she would see friends, listen to music, have a hot lunch, go for a walk, and possibly receive some routine medical attention. Just as important as what she gets, however, is what you get—a break from the work and stress of her daily care.

Most centers accept people with dementia (half of all people using adult day care have dementia) and some care for extremely frail elderly people who would otherwise have to live in a nursing home. The latter sometimes provides a full range of services, including periodic in-home care, pharmacy and laboratory services, rides to appointments and errands, and, when necessary, alternate housing.

A typical center costs about $30 a day, although prices range from a few dollars up to $150 a day. Clients usually pay most or all of these fees themselves. A few states allow for some Medicaid coverage of adult day care, but usually only if the person would otherwise need nursing home care. And some centers are subsidized or publicly-owned and can charge a lower rate or assess fees on a sliding scale. Given the high cost of in-home care or elderly housing, adult day care is a bargain at almost any price.

Larger communities often have more than one center and some cities have dozens of them, so find out which one offers the level of care that your parent needs. Then, if there is still some choice, tour the centers. Ideally, a program should have a nurse and a social worker on staff, at least one "care provider" for every six clients (or one for every four if the clients are severely impaired and need a lot of assistance), and should provide some minimal training for the staff. (Day-care workers are not required to have any formal education, but may be required to take a few days of informal training within the center.) Check, too, to see that a center offers activities that your parent finds interesting but also manageable. Obviously, a center should be clean, well-vented, safe and arranged to meet the needs of its clients—no open door if someone with dementia might roam out, an amply wide bathroom if someone is in a wheelchair.

If your parent refuses to go, be persistent. Urge her to try it for a few days. People are often surprised at how much they enjoy adult day care once they get used to it.

**❝**My mother would just stay in bed, almost all day. I could not get her up to do anything. She would eat and that was it. Day care was the answer to my prayers. I still have a hard time getting her to go each morning, but once she's there she's fine. She does things and meets people. She's really started coming out of her shell. We've even started playing cards together in the evenings.**❞**
—LINDA K.

## HELP FROM FRIENDS AND NEIGHBORS

When your father needs help, some of his immediate family and close friends may volunteer their assistance right away. But what about more distant relations and less dear friends, and what about his neighbors? All of these people can supplement the work of volunteers and professionals, providing not only practical help but much-needed emotional support and assurance.

You may be reluctant to ask for help, but keep in mind that while people may not come to you to volunteer their services, they are often more than happy to help out once they are asked. Keep favors small. A friend might pick up a few groceries from time to time, get books or videos at the library, water the garden, walk the dog or drop by for a visit every now and then. A neighbor might take your parent's garbage out once a week, a neighbor's child might adopt your parent as a grandparent, or a local teenager might help with raking or snow-shoveling occasionally (perhaps for a nominal fee).

Also, ask the people your parent sees on a regular basis—the newspaper delivery boy, the apartment superintendent, a barber, a rabbi or a grocery clerk—to contact you if anything seems wrong, for example if your parent seems confused or hasn't picked up his newspaper for two days. (Of course, you should approach only those individuals you know your parent trusts. You don't want others to know that your parent is frail and alone.) Mail carriers and utility workers are sometimes trained to spot trouble—the mail hasn't been picked up, the lawn hasn't been mowed, the power hasn't been used. Call the local post office and utility company to find out if such a program exists in your parent's community.

Don't forget your own friends. People who are in the same situation might share some of the workload—you check out local day-care options while your friend investigates Medicaid eligibility and procedures. Those who aren't in the same situation might be willing to exchange duties with you in the name of mutual relief and a refreshing change of pace—a friend sits with your parent while you take her children to the mall.

If you don't have friends in the same situation, you can start a cooperative of Adult Children Caring for Aging Parents. Not an emotional support group, but a real cooperative—people working together, sharing tasks and trading information.

# More Care, at Home

If your mother is very frail, ill, injured or recovering from surgery and needs more than the services described so far, health-care workers will come into her home. Home-care workers include nurses, home health aides, physical, speech or occupational therapists, social workers and even physicians in some cases. The care is often arranged by a hospital discharge planner or doctor's office, but you can also make arrangements on your own.

You can hire home-care workers through an agency or directly, by looking through the classified ads or talking to friends. There are several advantages to using an agency. Most important, if your parent expects Medicare or Medicaid to foot the bill, she must receive her care from a certified agency (about half of all home-care agencies are certified). Certification also means that the agency and workers meet minimal standards set by the federal government. If she uses a government agency associated with the local health department, for example, or one operated by a Visiting Nurse Association, her care may be subsidized by public monies or donations, meaning that she will pay only what she can afford. Besides that, agencies make life easier. They find workers, screen them and monitor their work. If an agency offers a full range of services, the care tends to be better coordinated and more comprehensive than anything you can arrange on your own. Lastly, agencies have insurance in case of an accident, and they handle the paperwork, such as social security forms, for employees.

To find a home-care agency, look in the Yellow Pages, or call your parent's doctor, a hospital discharge planner, the area agency on aging or the Visiting Nurse Association of America (800-426-2547), which represents nearly 500 non-profit home-care agencies. Most libraries and senior centers also have the *Home Care and Hospice Directory*.

---

*"When my father left the hospital I took a leave from work and went home to help my mother care for him. It was the most grueling few weeks of my life. We had to be with my father, or within earshot of him, pretty much every minute of the day. We were lifting him, turning him, feeding him, cleaning him and helping him go to the bathroom. Mom was staying with him at night, too, and she wasn't getting much sleep.*

*About two weeks into it, we realized that we needed help. We were physically and mentally fried. We hired a home health aide who came every morning. But even with that we were still both exhausted. So we hired a companion who came five afternoons a week and stayed overnight three nights a week.*

*I'm not sure why it took us so long to get help. We should have had all that in place the day he came home from the hospital.*"*

—Alicia B.

If you choose to hire workers independently, you may pay less because there is no middleman, but use caution. Get a number of references and monitor the work carefully. Many of these unaffiliated workers are first-rate and provide excellent care, but there are scoundrels in the world. In some cases, a person known as a "registry" will provide you with names of freelance workers and then take a cut of the worker's fee. Know that these are not the same as home-care agencies and are not licensed or government regulated. While they can be useful, you need to screen workers carefully yourself.

## HOME HEALTH AIDES

Home health aides are trained to provide "custodial care," which means help with bathing, dressing, getting to the toilet and other personal tasks. They will prepare meals and do some light housekeeping (but only that which pertains to your parent, such as changing and laundering his sheets and tidying his room). Some are trained to do simple medical procedures such as change bandages, check catheters and intravenous lines, take temperatures or administer medications. Certified home health aides have slightly more basic medical training than noncertified ones.

Fees vary, depending upon the experience and training of the aide, and the cost-of-living in the area. The average cost through an agency is $50 per visit, which can range from two to four hours. Sometimes fees are charged hourly, at anywhere from $10 to $15 an hour. Medicare and other insurance will cover the cost of home health aides only when their services are needed in addition to nursing care or therapy.

## CHECK THE COVERAGE

Medicare and Medicaid will cover home care only when the care is provided by a certified agency, when your parent is virtually homebound, and when such care is prescribed by a doctor. Even then, the coverage is only for intermittent or part-time "skilled" home care—that is, care provided by nurses and therapists. Home health aides and social workers may be covered if their services are an integral part of the skilled-care package. However, once the nurse is no longer needed, the health aide will no longer be covered, even if your parent still needs such care. In other words, if a nurse comes in twice a week to change bandages and check catheters, and a health aide comes five days a week to bathe, dress and feed your parent, the aide will not be covered by insurance once your parent's wounds heal and the nurse is no longer visiting her.

## NURSES

Doctors stopped making house calls some time ago (although some are going back to the old ways and teaming up with home-care agencies), but nurses make house calls routinely these days, and do much of the work that a doctor would do. Nurses can monitor your parent's health, change dressings, insert catheters and intravenous lines, administer medications, give injections and perform other medical tasks. They can teach your parent or family members how to perform some tasks, and can provide counseling to families, especially in hospice situations.

**❝**I used to stay in the house the whole time the aide was there. It was a control thing for me. I felt that I had to oversee everything and that I couldn't trust anyone with my father. I was afraid that if I left, something would happen. Fortunately I've gotten over that. Now I leave the minute the aide arrives. I go shopping, run errands or visit friends. A couple of times I took my bills and mail to the library just to be out of the house. It's really an important break in the day for me. **❞**
—GRACE D.

While you can hire nurses independently, they typically work for home-care agencies and can work in your parent's home only under a doctor's orders. While they cost an average of $90 a visit—ranging from half an hour up to two hours—Medicare and Medicaid will cover the cost if it is deemed "medically necessary."

## THERAPISTS AND NUTRITIONISTS

As part of your parent's home care, the doctor may recommend that he be visited by some sort of therapist on a regular basis. Occupational therapists train people with rigid fingers, stiff hips, dim vision or other disabilities to perform daily tasks by working on muscular control and coordination, teaching them new ways to do things, setting them up with special equipment and making adjustments to the home. Speech therapists help people who have trouble speaking or understanding speech because of a stroke or another illness to communicate again. Physical therapists work the muscles and joints to improve mobility, flexibility and strength, usually after an injury, surgery or an illness (such as a stroke). Nutritionists will get your parent on a diet that is healthful, manageable and compatible with her medications and any illness that might be affecting her. Social workers often work as part of the home-care team, counseling clients and their families and referring them to appropriate community services.

All of these professionals make house calls, usually through a hospital or home-care agency. Prices vary, but they average around $80 per visit, lasting one or two hours. The cost is covered by insurance if it is part of a hospital discharge plan of care.

## A NOTE ON FINANCES

Home care is expensive, but almost any type of care your parent receives now will be costly, and in most cases, home care is the least expensive option. Look at the other options available, such as assisted-living homes and nursing homes. Compare prices, find out about any possible insurance coverage, and consider how much care your parent needs, how long she is likely to need such care and her own personal preferences. If your parent needs only a little help or short-term help, and good services are available, home care probably makes the most sense. But if she is chronically ill and needs extensive care, home care may be impractical in the long run.

Whatever you do, consider the nursing home option early. You need time to review the choices and you may want to get your parent's name on waiting lists. Also, if your parent's savings are running low, it may be better to apply while she still has enough to pay for six months to a year of nursing home care. Once she has little money left or is on Medicaid, she will have fewer choices.

# Geriatric Care Managers

If you are far away, busy with other responsibilities, or just need some guidance and support, a geriatric care manager (also known as a case manager) can assess your parent's situation, connect her to appropriate services and then oversee every aspect of her care on an ongoing basis.

Care managers, who are usually social workers or nurses with training in geriatrics or gerontology, can handle almost any facet of your parent's care, either short- or long-term. You can retain a manager simply to introduce you to community services, or to oversee a particular issue, say, housekeeping or nursing care, or to fill in, supervising home care while you take a break.

Often, care managers step in briefly when a situation gets tricky—your parent refuses to accept outside help, she is at risk of an injury and you don't know how much to intervene, or family members can't work together and need counseling. Or a manager can take over the whole kit and caboodle—hire, coordinate and monitor all home-care workers, make medical appointments and arrange for your parent to be escorted to those appointments, pick up the mail, respond to emergencies and, an invaluable bonus, offer a sympathetic ear and some reassuring support to you, the frazzled child. In most cases, you can take it a day at a time and expand, reduce or cancel the service at any time.

Typically, a geriatric care manager will first meet with family members, your parent and perhaps a doctor or others involved in your parent's care to discuss the needs and the urgency of the situation. He or she will watch your parent go about her daily tasks, note and address any limitations or obstacles she faces during the day, and take whatever steps are necessary to make her home safe and navigable. Then the manager will draft a detailed plan of action, outlining what services will be provided, when, by whom and at what cost, specifying the manager's role and fees. Once the services are in place, the manager will keep you posted on your parent's care and well-being. You should request a written monthly report, a weekly phone call or some other kind of routine communication.

A first assessment typically costs about $200 to $350, and once the service is in place, you can expect to spend at least $200 a month, or more than $1,000 a month if your parent needs a lot of attention. (Insurance rarely covers the cost of care managers.) The care manager's fee doesn't include the cost of the services themselves—home health aides, nurses, medical supplies or whatever else your parent requires.

Sometimes a local organization, like the area agency on aging or a senior center, will offer free or subsidized care management for a brief period. But typically you'll have to hire a care manager privately.

When you hire a geriatric care manager, find out how long she has been in the community—newcomers won't be as familiar with local services and also might lack rapport with important personnel—and how many clients she is currently serving. The fewer clients on a person's plate, the more time and attention she can give to your parent. A care manager with more than forty clients will spend, on average, less than an hour a week considering and monitoring your parent's situation. Is that enough time?

## TO FIND A CARE MANAGER

The National Association of Professional Geriatric Care Managers (602-881-8008) offers referrals from its list of members. The National Association of Social Workers (202-408-8600) can also help in locating someone to oversee caregiving services, but be sure to specify your needs.

# The Hiring Process

When a member of the local church or synagogue volunteers to call on your mother, you can go on instinct alone. But if you are contracting with a home-care agency, and especially if you are hiring a freelance worker, be sure to do some homework. Ask a lot of questions and get an agreement in writing. While you're at it, you might call the area agency on aging to see if the state has a home-care hotline or a senior advocacy organization that monitors services and agencies and receives complaints. Here are some questions to ask when looking for a home-care agency:

◆ What services do you provide? Who is on the home-care team—physicians, nurses, therapists, dietitians, social workers, home health aides, homemakers, companions, volunteers?

◆ What is the cost for these services? Is there a minimum of how much care my parent receives? Are there extra charges that might arise unexpectedly? (Ask to have all agreements, including services to be provided and financial arrangements, put in writing.)

◆ Is the agency certified to receive Medicare and Medicaid reimbursement?

◆ Can you subsidize care for people who cannot pay for themselves? (Government and voluntary agencies, such as a Visiting Nurse Association, often have public or private money to cover some care.)

◆ How do you determine what services my parent needs? Will a nurse evaluate her? Will he or she consult with my parent's doctor and my family? (Ask to have a plan of care drawn up and updated as your parent's condition changes.)

◆ How will her care be coordi-

> **"** *While I'm at work I have two companions who come in shifts to watch Mother. One is excellent and I love her dearly, but Mother is really awful to her. Frances, the companion, is an articulate, intelligent, retired professional who is doing this work just to keep active. She is very thoughtful, kind and sympathetic. Mother was a nurse and I think she feels resentful and threatened by having this capable person take care of her. She is rude, uncooperative and mean to her.*
>
> *The other aide is young and sweet, but, you know, nobody's home. Every day is a new day for her. I have to tell her everything all over again. Mother gets along just fine with her—perhaps because she is so simple.*
>
> *I spend a lot of time apologizing to Frances and a lot of time explaining things to Susie. I guess there's no perfect solution. Anytime you have someone caring for your parent, there's bound to be some problem.* **"**
> —JENNY Z.

nated? Who oversees workers? Will a supervisor visit regularly? How do I reach a supervisor if there is a problem?

◆ Is someone available 24 hours-a-day in case of emergency? Are backups provided when workers cancel or don't show up? (Again, get this in writing.)

◆ Will my parent be cared for by the same person consistently or will the guards change regularly (which is less desirable, but often unavoidable). If my parent doesn't get along with a particular worker, can someone else be assigned to her?

◆ Is the agency licensed by the state and in compliance with all state regulations? (Agencies that provide nursing and therapeutic care must be licensed, but those providing home-makers and health aides do not.)

◆ Is the agency accredited by a trade association, such as the National League for Nursing, which sets standards for the industry? (Accreditation means that an agency has met certain requirements with regard to staffing, training and supervision, but not all agencies choose to take part even if they meet the requirements, so don't rule out an agency simply because it is not accredited.)

◆ Is the agency bonded (which means that any court settlement will be paid from the bond)? Does it provide worker's compensation so you are not liable if an employee is injured while caring for your parent?

◆ Can I get references? Be specific when you ask for references, so you don't talk to the only three people who were happy with the service. For example, get the names of two clients who live within five miles of your parent, or two clients with dementia. Then ask these references specific questions—Did the agency respond quickly to the client's changing needs? Did the health aide arrive for work on time?

◆ When hiring someone on your own, instinct is your best friend. Is this person respectful, courteous and well-groomed? Could you get along with her, and more important, will your parent be happy with her? Ask about qualifications, training and experience. Is the home health aide certified? Does this person have experience working with the particular problems that affect your parent, such as dementia, incontinence, stroke? Is she physically capable of meeting your parent's needs—can the companion support your parent so he can move from a bed to a chair, for example? Exactly what chores and services will this person perform?

# Managing the Troops

If your parent needs constant home care and you are overseeing that care, it may seem as though you have taken a full-time job as staff manager. You have to ensure that workers show up on time, do what needs to be done responsibly, get along with your parent and don't leave until they're relieved by the next shift. And when they are good and you want to keep them, you have to be sure that they're content.

Even if you're used to managing people, this can be an uncomfortable and trying job. Home-care workers perform personal tasks in the most intimate surroundings. Seemingly small mistakes can cause enormous anguish and frustration. *She's always late. . .forgets to remind*

*Dad to take his afternoon pills...smokes in the house...argues with Mom....* It is a delicate situation, but open communication and a willingness to compromise will help you—and your parent—immensely.

**Lower your expectations.** No one is going to care for your mother in exactly the way you think she should be cared for. No one is going to give her the attention, devotion and individual care that you would give her, or that she deserves. And no one is going to treat her home the way you or she would. No one. Which means that you have to accept a standard that is considerably less than perfect and learn to ignore a few minor errors or irritating habits.

Try several people if necessary, but be ready to compromise, or you will be hiring and firing in rapid succession. The aide may be watching television when you think she should be tending to your parent, but if your parent likes her and she is doing a reasonably good job, hang on to her.

**Keep workers happy.** A worker who is treated with respect and kindness is more apt to treat your parent with respect and kindness. During these tough times, it may be hard for you to think about anyone else's needs, but do what you can. Welcome any worker into your parent's home, make sure she has a place for her belongings, acceptable food to eat and some privacy occasionally. Be sensitive to her needs and the pressure she faces, both on the job and away from it.

When there is a problem, don't assume it is the fault of the employee. And when things are done well, show your appreciation. Just saying "thank you" will mean a great deal, but if a worker is exceptional, write a note to her supervisor, give her a bonus or buy an occasional gift. (People working for agencies don't get paid as much as you might think; the agency takes a hefty portion of the fee.)

**Foster this relationship.** Remember that ideally you are the silent partner in this relationship. In most cases, it is less important that you get along with a home-care worker than that your parent and she get along with each other.

Encourage this budding friendship from the start. Tell the worker about your parent—what makes her tick, what she used to be like, what will win her over and what will infuriate her. And tell your parent about the worker—who she is, what

❝My mother is now on Medicaid, but I supplement the pay of the two women who take care of her. They earn so little and they work so hard. They are incredible with her. Vicky will wash Mom's hair, not because it needs it, but because Mom enjoys it so much. Kathy will stop at the store on her way to the house in the morning to pick up anything Mom needs. They really are wonderful. They are almost like family. And because of them I can stay in my own apartment and continue working. So I do everything I can to keep them happy.❞                —JACQUI L.

## WHEN THERE IS TROUBLE

Serious problems are rare, but they happen. A worker mistreats your parent, steals from him or gets drunk on the job. The best protection here is common sense. Don't leave money or jewelry in sight, no matter how much you trust a worker. Lock the liquor cabinet, if necessary. And don't ever give a worker access to your parent's bank account or wallet.

Be alert to any sign of possible physical abuse, such as unexplained bruises or wounds, and to indications of emotional abuse, such as a parent's unusual fear or nightmares. If your parent is confused, she may make accusations that are false because she is paranoid or anxious. Try to confirm her complaints, and then reassure her if you determine that she is inventing problems. If her accusations continue, even if they are untrue, you may have to find another worker with whom she is more comfortable.

When you suspect trouble and have reason to think that your suspicions are valid, act immediately. Dismiss the worker and call the area agency on aging to find out how to report abuse or exploitation. You may need to contact an elder abuse hotline, the Better Business Bureau, the local consumers' affairs office or a licensing agency. Notify the bank of your concerns if the problem has to do with your parent's accounts.

she does and why she does it. Then, step back and let them get to know each other.

If your parent is the one with lofty expectations—if she is never pleased with any worker, resents the fact that she has to be cared for, and takes it out on the aide, talk to her. Understand that she may be behaving this way because of her own painful emotions. Let her air her fears and then help her to see that while this situation may not be ideal, it has to be acceptable. Remind her that you are not abandoning her, that you will continue to see her and care for her. Talk with the worker, as well. Encourage her to be flexible and to have a sense of humor about your parent's criticism, and beg her to put up with some occasional wrath. Tell her to call you if she needs to let off some steam, and be sympathetic when she does.

**Communicate clearly.** Be direct and open from the start. Tell potential workers about your expectations and your parent's needs. Write out a detailed description of the worker's duties and a daily schedule so there are no misunderstandings about what is involved in this job. And make any house rules

❝ *We hired what was essentially a baby-sitter to stay with my father. Kim was about sixteen or seventeen at the time, trying to earn some money over her summer vacation.*

*One afternoon I arrived when she was leaving—we had a sort of changing of the guards each day—and I realized that she had been crying. I followed her out on the porch and we had a long talk about how my father reminded her of her grandfather, who had died a few years earlier. Apparently, she had been really close to her grandfather and she was reliving his death every day. It was very sad, but also very sweet. I had thought of her as a sitter, but after we talked I saw her as someone who was really sharing this pain with me, someone who really cared about my father.* ❞
—GRACE D.

clear—smoking, noise levels, food consumption, alcohol consumption or anything else that concerns you or your parent. Do it diplomatically, as a list of reminders, not orders.

Let any worker give you her house rules as well—what tasks she will do, what she won't do, when she likes to take breaks, how she likes to handle problems. Even if she doesn't express any needs, your asking shows that you respect her.

If there comes a time when your parent or you want things done differently, raise the subject right then, because the longer you wait, the more difficult it will be to institute change. Make a constructive suggestion or frame the problem as an oversight on your part. "I probably forgot to explain that it's easier to bathe my mother in the morning when she's calmer than in the afternoon when she's tired." Likewise, ask that workers be candid with you about their problems or frustrations.

**Monitor the service.** If your parent is able and alert, then she can supervise her own care. But if she isn't, it's important to make unannounced visits, or to have someone drop in occasionally for you. Be sure that workers arrive on time, are tidy and clean, meet your parent's needs and treat him respectfully and kindly.

If you are using a care manager, you still need to stay apprised of how things are going. In theory, a care manager oversees everything for you, but it's important that you have a hand on the reigns as well. Monitor the care to see if it meets the goals of the plan the manager has drafted. If you are far away, ask a neighbor or friend to check in now and then to see how things are going.

# Respite Care

Anyone with hands-on responsibility for a frail parent needs a break occasionally, if not regularly. Start using respite care as soon as possible. You will need it before you think you do. You also need to get your parent accustomed to other caregivers before he is deeply established in a routine that includes only you.

Respite is a broad term that may

mean having someone come over one evening a week so you can go out for dinner, but it typically means moving your parent temporarily to a nursing home or hiring round-the-clock workers for a week or two while you go on vacation, deal with a family emergency or simply escape the day-to-day rigors of caregiving.

You might believe that you are the only one who can care for your parent. You may be afraid that your father will hate you for "deserting" him. You may worry that if you move him temporarily or have someone replace you for a few days, he will fall to pieces. You may worry, and he may not like it, but you still need to do it.

Ask the area agency on aging about respite programs or call nursing homes, which sometimes provide respite care. Veterans hospitals may also provide respite as part of your parent's regular medical care.

Medicare covers respite when it is part of hospice care, but not in most cases. If the kind of care your parent needs is too costly—and it can be quite expensive—talk to family, friends and neighbors. People are often willing to help out for a brief time. Between community programs and family ties, you should be able to put together a schedule so you can take a break.

## When Using Respite

◆ Leave detailed, written instructions for anyone staying with your parent concerning medications, meals and habits, even if you have discussed each item thoroughly with them. Post a list of all emergency-

*"I have decided to take a week off by myself. I am going to a little cottage near a lake. I haven't told Mum yet, but I feel no guilt at all.*

*At first it felt like a ruthless decision. I thought I should keep being here for her. Or, if I took some time off, I thought I should visit friends or do something with my grandchildren. But the pressure has been intense. I feel so time-bound, so scheduled, as if my life is just about the needs of other people.*

*I really want a week to myself, for me, not for anyone else. Just to look at the water and clear my head. That's my gift to myself."*
—BETTY H.

phone numbers (fire, police, ambulance, doctor's office, your number and a neighbor's number). And show the respite helper where to find any emergency medical supplies.

◆ If you are an integral part of your parent's day, try a brief trial— a day or weekend away—before heading off for any extended trip.

◆ Have a backup plan. Companions and aides can cancel just when you are about to drive away. Talk to other family members who might step in if you are deserted, and make sure a home-care agency guarantees that your parent will be covered during your absence.

◆ Don't be talked out of this break, even if your parent says or hints that you are being selfish. She will survive your absence.

# Chapter Ten

# HOME AWAY FROM HOME

*When It's Time to Move • Sharing Your Home
With Your Parent • Senior Apartments, Group Homes,
Life Care Centers and Other Options*

........................................

H OME CERTAINLY IS WHERE THE HEART IS, BUT AT SOME
point it may not be feasible or desirable for your father
to stay in his own home—there may be no way for him
to manage the stairs, the upkeep may be too difficult or his care
may be too much for you and other family members to handle.
Whatever the reasons, when your parent can no longer stay in
his home, it's a major turning point for everyone involved.

For your parent, it may mean leaving a cherished place of his
past, and losing his independence and privacy. For you, it's a
time of doubt and worry. *Will Dad be all right? Is this really the
best thing to do?* You may find yourself sparring with siblings and
even with your father if he sees you as the force behind a move
he doesn't want to make. But once the dust settles, a move often
proves to be a good decision, as a new living arrangement can
provide friendship and stimulation, as well as the care he needs.

But where should he live? Fortunately, your home or a nursing
home are not the only alternatives. There is an expanding array
of options, ranging from shared housing and assisted-living
homes to full-service life care centers. Talk with your parent
about his needs and preferences and learn about the options

available in his community as soon as possible. Knowing the alternatives will help both of you to navigate this difficult terrain and make the best choice.

# Launching the Discussion

If you aren't in one already, don't wait until a crisis arises to consider housing, because then you will be left with few choices and little time to research options. As hard as it may be to discuss these issues in advance, find out what your parent wants in her living arrangement. What qualities are most important to her—privacy, activities, a garden to roam in, a place near family or in the country, plenty of companionship? What will her finances allow? If she were to need a lot of supervision, where would she want to be? How important is it to her that she not move a second time?

Unfortunately, most people have more trouble talking about changing residences than about living wills, perhaps because they find it easier to imagine a time when they will be disconnected from a respirator than a time when they will be disconnected from their homes. But urge your parent to talk about this. You might broach the subject by discussing the housing choices a friend is facing.

Remember, your parent's home, no matter how modest, means the world to her. It is where she built her life, raised a family and welcomed her friends. It holds her

*"My mother made the decision herself, without discussing it with anyone. She moved out of New York and into an elderly housing complex near me. I was upset because, you know, this is a thing that you dread. I thought she would be miserable. But she seemed happy there, and looking back I remembered that she had talked about going into an old-age home once with my father before he died. She said, 'Wouldn't it be nice to be in a place where they do everything for us?'"* —BARBARA F.

memories and is molded to fit her needs—or was before illness or disability changed them. More than anything, her home represents her independence and her privacy. Leaving it, especially to go anywhere that is earmarked for the elderly, may be unthinkable to her.

If your parent avoids this subject, delays a decision and, in general, clutches defiantly at the status quo—frustrating you to no end—she may have valid reasons. What you perceive as stubbornness may be a perfectly normal desire to stay in her own home, and a deep-rooted fear of what lies ahead.

Try to be sympathetic to these underlying feelings and get her to share her grief about this move or her fears about the future.

# Is It Time to Move?

You may be able to renovate your parent's house and hire home aides, but is that really the best option? Is it affordable or practical? Is it best for your parent or manageable for you? If time is on your side, weigh all the reasons for moving and for staying, visit a few residences, and then let the idea sit for a month or two before making a decision. While your parent's personal wishes are the top priority, there are other issues to consider:

**Her safety.** Your parent may need more medical care and supervision than visiting nurses and aides can reasonably provide at home. If so, and if her confusion or disability makes living at home dangerous, then staying where she is may not be an option. Your family needs to weigh the risks along with her right to decide. (See page 16 on when to intervene.)

**Your limits.** Your ability to help your parent will play a major role in determining when it's time for him to move. You and other family members may not have the time or the stamina to tend to his needs, juggle schedules, coordinate and oversee home-care services and fill in when workers cancel. Accept your own limits and recognize that they are important—just as important as your parent's needs.

**Costs.** Paying property taxes or a mortgage, keeping up with home

## PROMISES MADE . . .

Even though you may believe that you will never put your parent in a nursing home, you simply don't know what the future holds, either for your parent or for you. Your parent may become so ill or so perilously unaware that you cannot continue to manage her care. Your own life may change in such a way that you cannot give your parent the attention that you assumed you could. Given such possibilities, don't put yourself in the position of having to break a promise; don't make it in the first place.

If your parent asks you to promise that you will never put her in a nursing home, you don't have to be direct in your response. Tell her that you will do whatever you can to avoid it, that you will never abandon her and that you always will do whatever you can to protect her privacy, safety and dignity.

maintenance and hiring homemakers may all be too much for your parent's purse, especially if she is still living in a large family home. If finances are the only problem, look into homeowner loans that are paid off only when your parent dies, sells the house or moves. (See page

*"Dad wasn't all that frail, but he was lonely. He would come up with a hundred reasons to ask one of us to come over. A light bulb was out or a gutter was full or he couldn't get the television to work. There was always something, and I was always running over there or worrying about him and feeling bad that I wasn't with him. I turned to my sister one day and said, 'This has got to stop.' I have three kids at home and a job and I couldn't keep doing it. I couldn't handle the work and I couldn't handle the worry. That's when we started looking into other housing possibilities."* —SKIP R.

268.) Ask the local tax assessor's office or the area agency on aging about programs that help older homeowners save on property taxes through exemptions, limits, deferrals, credits and deductions. The local utility company may also offer subsidies or programs to help elderly people make their homes more energy-efficient. And, before your parent moves, consider innovative options, like taking in renters or adding an apartment to your parent's house (See page 202.)

**Location.** If your mother lives in the boondocks and cannot drive because of poor eyesight, she may need to move closer to public transportation. If winters in New England are too hard on your father's ailing heart, he may have to head south or find a housing situation that doesn't require scraping ice off windshields or plodding through snow drifts.

**Loneliness.** Loneliness is no small issue. Your parent may love his home, but it may be a little too hollow and too quiet, especially if a spouse has recently died or a beloved neighbor has moved. Companions and community visitors may fill the

## USER-FRIENDLY LIVING

If your mother remains in her home, it can be renovated to accommodate almost any disability. The American Association for Retired Persons (800-424-3410) issues a booklet that describes how to make a home user-friendly for people with disabilities, and another that offers more technical design information for builders.

The National Rehabilitation Information Center (800-346-2742) can supply further information on disabilities, rehabilitation, home modification and rehabilitation equipment. (See Appendix B, page 396 for a list of organizations that provide information on home modification and accessibility.)

void for a time, but he may yearn for more reliable and meaningful friendships. He might have someone move in with him, or he might move into an apartment building or a group living situation.

**Future care.** A diagnosis of Parkinson's, Alzheimer's or another debilitating disease means it's time to prepare for a future when your parent may not be able to live at home. She might rather move while she can still make her own decisions and can adjust more easily to the change.

# Should Mom Move Closer?

When your mother needs to move, you may be tempted to lure her to your own neighborhood. That way, you could spend more time with her, keep an eye on her, help her with shopping, cooking and other chores and arrange local services for her. She could see more of her grandchildren and you would save a lot of time and money on travel.

But consider this very carefully. Do you want her to move because it will truly make her life better, or because it will allow you to sleep at night? What will she do in this new place, without her own friends and community? Once she is nearby, will you really be able to do all that you think you will? And, in truth, do you really want her to be so close?

Before suggesting this move, be sure it is really best for both of you,

because once she moves, having her return to her own community will be painful and disruptive.

# Should Dad Move In?

When a parent suddenly becomes ill or handicapped and can't live at home any longer, you may have an instinctive response to take him in. It's a generous thought, certainly, but it's not always the best option, and sometimes it can be an enormous mistake. Having your parent move in with you is a serious commitment, so think it over carefully before extending the invitation. When in doubt, test the waters for a time. Ask your parent to live with you for a few months or a few weeks, being clear about the trial nature of the arrangement, and see how it goes.

If you decide against family living, stick to your convictions—no matter what Aunt Sally thinks. There are not many people who can live compatibly with a parent at this time of life. Nothing is wrong with deciding against doing so. It is simply honest. Trying such an arrangement when you know it can't work may be worse than not trying it at all, because it disrupts your parent's life and then makes everyone feel as though they have failed.

Some things to consider as you ponder the possibility of long-term togetherness:

**Can you get along?** It's not worth trying this if your blood pressure rises at the mere thought. Think about your relationship with your parent. What was your most recent visit like? Did you enjoy a pleasant afternoon together, or did you watch the clock until you could leave? Is your parent capable of respecting your privacy, your lifestyle and your authority in your own home? Can he respect your relationship with your spouse or other mate? Can you respect his privacy, lifestyle and decisions? While you might develop a closer relationship, it's likely that old problems and annoyances will be more pronounced when you are under one roof.

**What about the rest of the family?** How do your spouse and children feel about having your mother move in? Do others in the house get along with her? Call a family meeting or talk with each person individually and listen to their views. Don't alienate your spouse or displace your children because of a responsibility you feel toward your parent.

**Do you have the space?** This seems like an obvious question, but it's one that many people fail to consider fully. Communal living is far more successful in larger homes or those with separate living spaces (a bedroom, bathroom and sitting area with a separate entrance, for example). Tight quarters will exacerbate the unavoidable everyday problems and strip everyone of their privacy.

If you have the space, are you willing to give it up? How will it change your life to lose a study or a guestroom, or to move two children into the same room? If you are

*"My mother moved in with us at age ninety-five. I bought a reclining chair for our guestroom and a television set and flowers, and I bought her a beautiful nightgown and robe so that she looked lovely all the time. She started to accept herself again and her spirits came back.*

*It was very draining, though, because I was getting up during the night to change my mother's colostomy bag. And from the very beginning my husband and I missed our privacy.*

*I was glad to see Mother so happy, but I couldn't keep it up, so I brainstormed with my sisters, and we decided to split up the care. Now Mother goes to one sister's in May and June and to another sister's in July and August. The moving around is a little tough on Mother, but other than that it works pretty well.*
—MARGARET F.

adamant about this move, you may want to consider renovating the basement, building an attached apartment or buying a prefab unit for the backyard.

**Is your house equipped for this?** Ample space won't do you any good if the extra room is upstairs and your father can't get to it. Take a good look at your house in light of your parent's needs and disabilities. Are the hallways and doorways wide enough for his wheelchair? Can you make needed changes, such as installing handrails or ramps?

**How much attention does your parent need?** Consider his daily needs—help getting dressed, meal preparation, transportation. Can you meet all these needs, or are there adequate community services to support them? If your father needs home care, can you coordinate and oversee workers? What about entertainment? Will he be sitting in the living room every day with nothing to do, waiting for you to play a game or chat with him?

**Do your lifestyles meld?** Do you sleep late, but your parent gets up with the sun? Does your teenager listen to loud music in the afternoon when your parent likes to read quietly? Will you have to make meat-and-potato meals even though everyone else in the family is a vegetarian? Is your parent a chainsmoker, while your spouse is allergic to smoke? If your lifestyles clash, is there any way of living together in peace?

**What are the advantages?** If you have a reasonable relationship with your parent, you stand to gain from giving to her during the last years of her life. And your children may benefit from time spent with their grandparent.

There may also be tangible advantages to this arrangement. If your parent is still in relatively good health, she may be able to help around the house, do some shopping or stay with the children when you're out. Or perhaps she can help with some household expenses.

## RULES FOR LIVING TOGETHER

When an adult child lives with a frail parent, whether by choice or by default, there may be warmth and humor, but the stage is also set for trouble. You are giving up privacy and space not to just any boarder, but to a boarder whose opinions matter deeply to you, who may be able to electrify your nerves with a simple comment or a casual look, and to whom you may feel indebted. Your parent is not only losing independence, but losing it to his child, the one person who has depended on and looked up to him. He may feel embarrassed by this living situation and his own inabilities. As a result, the gratitude he feels may be mixed with resentment. So as you try to please him, he may be fighting to retain his autonomy. He may criticize you and yell at you.

## CLOSE, BUT NOT TOO CLOSE

If you want proximity but not total immersion, then accessory apartments and ECHO housing, described on page 202, allow you and your parent to retain your privacy and your own space but spend time together as well. If your house can be easily renovated to add a separate apartment, such arrangements are also less expensive than most other housing options.

And if he does, you are surely going to yell back at times.

Understanding the reasons for the antagonism, or simply the inevitability of some problems, should ease them—a bit. Starting off on a good footing with clear house rules will also help.

Establish these rules and routines right away. Work out the guidelines together, if possible, giving weight to your parent's needs as well as those of the rest of the family. Unfortunately, if your parent has dementia or is otherwise confused, guidelines may not help because she is likely to forget them. You may have to learn other ways of coping. (See Chapter Sixteen.)

**Remember your limits.** Your parent took care of you, so why can't you take care of him? Remember, you cannot ever repay what your parent has done for you. You need to accept the limits to what you can do for your parent, and you need to make room for your own needs as well as his.

**Recognize the head of the household.** Your parent used to rule the roost, but it is your turn now. If this may be a problem, make your roles clear from the start. You will probably want to run a democratic household, but in many cases, you and your spouse will cast the tie-breaking vote. If you have children, you may need to assert your role as a parent. Your parent should not usurp your job or undermine your authority. You and your spouse are the ones who decide how your children will be raised and your parent has to follow your lead.

> "My father has always been a big drinker and sometimes he likes to smoke a cigar after dinner. That was fine in his own home. But Mary and I don't like it.
>
> When we invited him to move here, I told him right away that the drinking and smoking would have to stop, or least be cut back. I was amazed at how well he took it. I'm not sure I've ever stood up to him like that. I think it caught him off guard. But he listened and, so far, he's respected our wishes."
>
> —BEN W.

**Set down rules, assign tasks.** If you are concerned about a specific issue—noise levels, smoking, telephone bills—or worried that you will end up serving as butler, cook and maid, make a list of rules and tasks on Day One, so there are no questions or misunderstandings. Give your parent certain chores to do, even if they are menial. He might make the morning juice, set the table or weed the garden. He'll be happier if he feels useful and knows what is expected of him, and you will feel less resentful.

**Protect everyone's privacy.** Devise a way to give everyone in the household a bit of privacy. Be sure your parent has a space where he can shut the door and be alone without being disturbed. Likewise, let him know which rooms are off-limits, and when. If possible, arrange things so each person can entertain guests without interference from others. If you plan on going out for dinners or away on vacations without your parent, make that clear from the start. Clarity will not only preserve some of your privacy, it will also allow your parent to enjoy your time together without worrying that he is intruding.

**Choose your battles.** When things don't work out exactly right, consider what you can live with and what is genuinely unbearable. Everyone will have to make compromises now. Decide which battles are worth fighting. If your parent is on the telephone too much, get another line. If she falls asleep with the television on each night, buy yourself some earplugs or program the TV to turn off at a certain time.

**Establish a forum for complaints.** Problems should be aired before frustrations build to a breaking point. Decide in advance how complaints will be handled. For example, hold a meeting once a month to allow all members of the household to express and work out their problems.

**Give it time.** The beginning may be turbulent, but in a few months you should all settle into a routine. Don't pack your parent's bags before you've allowed some time for adjustment.

**Know when to quit.** Once you've given this arrangement a reasonable chance, listen to your instincts. Any number of issues can bring family togetherness to a painful, grinding halt. There is no single moment, no simple indicator, just a realization that this living

*"I spent the better part of an afternoon trying to convince my mother that I was her daughter, not a servant, and when I went to bed that night I thought, 'We have to make another arrangement.' And that was it. The next morning I started making phone calls, and we found her an assisted-living home within a few weeks."* —JANE D.

arrangement is not working. You can try to ignore it, and it may last a few more weeks or months, but eventually you will have to speak up and make a change.

It's better not to wait until you are physically and emotionally depleted and your relationship with your parent or your spouse is strained or irreparably damaged. Start looking into alternatives as soon as you realize that a change must be made. Talk with your parent about the move and begin preparing for it. The transition will be smoother for everyone if it is done before you've become too resentful or resigned.

# Housing Options

Fortunately, the range of housing options available to the elderly is growing rapidly. Traditional nursing homes now represent only one end of the spectrum and they are a last resort. In the widening middle ground between home and nursing home are a variety of living arrangements. To find out about specific housing options in your parent's community, start by calling the area agency on aging and the local long-term care ombudsman. (See Appendix A, page 377.)

## ACCESSORY APARTMENTS

Also called mother-in-law apartments, accessory dwellings, mother-daughter homes and granny apartments, these are separate apartments within or attached to a home. An accessory apartment usually consists of a bedroom, a bathroom, a kitchen, a living area and a separate entrance. They can be created by renovating a basement or garage, or by attaching a wing to a house.

Accessory apartments often work well for parents who want to live near their children, but they also can be used for people who are not related. Your parent could move into an accessory apartment attached to someone else's house, allowing her to stay in her community in a smaller and less expensive dwelling. Or she might add an accessory apartment to her own house, live in either the apartment or the house, and rent the other section to a tenant. Some owners will make special arrangements, such as keeping the rent low in exchange for help with household chores or other assistance. (Be sure your parent understands that taking in renters requires some work on her part and that there can be problems if, say, a renter fails to pay the rent.)

Before building an accessory apartment, you need to:

*Twenty years ago my husband was transferred. My mother was all alone so we told her to sell her house and come live with us.*

*She is pretty easy to live with, except that she complains a lot. As the kids got older, the complaining got worse. It caused a lot of conflict. 'You should do this with the kids. You shouldn't do that.' You know, that sort of thing. I said, 'I'm the mother here. You're not their mother.' But it didn't work. So we sold our house and bought one with an in-law apartment. I see her in the afternoon, drop off her meals and drive her around, but we also have our own, separate lives. It's much better this way.* —LUCILLE L.

♦ Call the local zoning board or building department. Accessory apartments are not allowed in some communities zoned for single-family residences, and if they are permitted, certain restrictions and regulations may apply. If you are told that accessory apartments are not allowed, ask about getting a variance or a special-use permit, as some communities will make exceptions.

♦ Call the local housing authority and area agency on aging. Some communities offer low-interest construction loans, tax deductions and other financial assistance to help people build accessory apartments for the elderly.

♦ Consult a financial planner or accountant. If your parent builds an accessory apartment and rents out

## THE NEXT MOVE: HOUSING OPTIONS AT A GLANCE

| | Description | Costs |
|---|---|---|
| **Accessory Apartments** | An apartment within or attached to a house, or an outbuilding on the property of a single-family house. | Renovations for an accessory apartment vary. |
| **Shared and Congregate Housing** | Anything from a roommate situation between friends to group housing arranged by an outside agency. | From $200 to $500 a month, depending upon location and services provided. |
| **Senior Apartments** | Apartments set up specifically for elderly residents, sometimes by a private business, often through the government's Section 202 program. | Section 202 housing accepts only low-income residents. Others range from $500 to $1,000 a month. |
| **Assisted Living** | Group housing or large complexes (from 20 to 100 residents) that provide a range of services for the elderly who need supervision and help getting through the day. | Anywhere from $300 to $3,000 a month, depending on the location and the level of care provided. |
| **Continuing Care Retirement Communities** | Large complexes that offer the full spectrum of care, from apartments to assisted-living units to nursing home care. | Usually, one large entrance fee, which can be $75,000 or more, plus monthly rents of $1,000 and up. |

| Advantages | Disadvantages |
|---|---|
| Offers proximity while preserving privacy, if your parent moves in with you. Or your parent can take in renters to help financially or to do household chores. | These are not allowed in some towns. They can be costly to set up. And they may not provide your parent with enough help if she is infirm. |
| Companionship, shared expenses and, in some cases, services such as meals, transportation and housekeeping. | Less privacy than independent living. Older people who have lived alone for years may have no interest in group living. |
| Provides privacy and independence, and requires little home maintenance. Most offer some limited services, such as meals, housekeeping, laundry and transportation. | Typically there are long waiting lists for subsidized apartments, and they are sometimes poorly maintained. |
| Help and support—meals, housekeeping, supervision, activities and, often, custodial care—while maintaining independence and privacy. | Usually not appropriate for someone who needs a lot of care because of dementia or incontinence. |
| The peace of mind that all future care is covered and no more decisions will be necessary. Activities, independence and a mix of healthy and ill elderly residents. | The high cost makes this an option only for middle- and upper-income people. Residents usually must sign up while they are still relatively healthy, so it requires advance planning. |

one unit, the incoming rent will change his income level, which may affect his eligibility for Medicaid or Supplementary Security Income. He may have higher property taxes because of the larger house, but he will be able to claim deductions for some maintenance costs and the depreciation of the rental property.

◆ Talk with a real estate agent if you need someone to find renters and draw up lease agreements. (You can find generic lease agreements in most stationery stores.)

### *ECHO* HOUSING

Elder Cottage Housing Opportunity (ECHO) homes are modular homes that are temporarily placed on the property of a single-family house, usually in the backyard. They are about the size of a large garage, and include one or two bedrooms, a bathroom, a living room, a kitchen and an eating area. Designed specifically for older people, they are single-level, wheelchair-accessible, energy-efficient and well-lighted.

An ECHO home does not have to look like Mom drove up in a mobile home, although some do. Most can be designed to match an existing house, with the same windows, siding, roofing and roof pitch, or can be adapted to appear like a guest house on the property.

The area agency on aging or housing department should be able to give you information about local manufacturers of ECHO homes. A typical ECHO home is about 500 square feet and costs about $25,000.

Most can be removed when they are no longer needed.

Again, check with the local zoning board to see if ECHO homes are allowed in the neighborhood. You also need to find out whether local regulations require a minimum of yard space, the requirements for access and parking, if utility hookups are possible and how such a structure will affect the property taxes, if at all.

### SHARED HOUSING

Shared housing has become popular among the elderly in recent years, and understandably so. It saves money, provides companionship—and sometimes meals, housekeeping and other services—and allows residents to keep their autonomy, a precious asset.

By definition, shared housing is a situation in which two or more unrelated people live together as a family. The specific arrangements, however, vary from house to house, and apartment to apartment. Your parent can move into someone else's house and pay rent and a share of the household expenses. Or he might find a person to move in with him and have that person do chores instead of paying rent. Sometimes friends get together, find a house and share tasks and expenses.

When your parent (or you) interviews potential roommates, ask about pets, smoking, noise levels, visitors, laundry, sleep habits and arrangements for shared meals and chores, as well as checking personal and financial references.

## WANTED: HOUSEMATES

Some communities have services that link people with potential roommates or find group housing for them. Most provide this service free, although some charge a fee. To find out if such a program exists in your parent's community and to get more information about shared housing (including a list of interview questions for prospective roommates and a model lease agreement), contact the National Shared Housing Resource Center in Maryland (410-235-4454).

Once a match is made, prepare a detailed list of the house rules and each person's responsibilities. If a roommate has agreed to help around the house instead of paying rent, be specific about the chores and how often they need to be done. Be clear about how rent, utilities, groceries, repairs and other bills will be paid—how the costs will be split and when payments are due. Housemates should also agree in advance how bills and responsibilities will be handled if one person becomes ill.

Be aware that two or three people sharing a house usually goes unnoticed, but once four or more unrelated people share the same residence, local zoning officials may be alerted. Depending on local ordinances, the situation may be considered "group or multi-family housing," which may be prohibited. So check the local zoning codes.

## CONGREGATE HOUSING

Although in some areas the terms "congregate" and "shared" housing are used interchangeably, congregate housing typically includes more people, and offers a number of services such as meals, housekeeping, recreation and transportation. Residents may have bedrooms within a large house or a multi-family home, or they may have separate apartments within a building, often supervised by a house manager. All or most meals are shared in a central dining room, and residents sometimes share a living area.

Congregate housing is better than less formal shared housing for people who need more care and services, but it is likely to cost considerably more.

Many communities are leery of congregate housing because of the challenges it has posed to local zoning ordinances, but resistance is fading. Government, nonprofit, for-profit, religious and community groups have all gotten into the act, building, organizing and sponsoring such homes. The local housing department, senior center, or area agency on aging should be able to give you information about any congregate housing opportunities in your parent's neighborhood.

## SENIOR APARTMENTS

Some apartment buildings specialize in the needs of the elderly.

Not only are all of the tenants older, but the buildings are constructed for seniors—no stairs, ample pathways for wheelchairs, sturdy and stable furniture, good lighting, tight security. From small buildings with a few units to massive high-rises, these apartments are usually situated near shops or public transportation, and they often provide meals, activities and other services. Many are government-subsidized, but these often have waiting lists of up to four years, and they are available only to people with low incomes.

If your parent is frail and contemplating a move into a senior apartment, find out exactly what services are provided, including whether there are emergency provisions—an emergency call button in the bedroom and round-the-clock staff who can respond to emergencies. Also, find out in advance if your parent would have to move should he become ill or immobile. Some senior apartments evict residents who become infirm, even if they can afford to hire personal health aides or companions.

## FOSTER HOMES

Some families will take in an older person for a fee (anywhere from $500 to $3,000 a month). Most elderly people who live in foster homes have some limitations and need help with daily tasks. The foster family cooks meals, does laundry, provides transportation, and generally helps the person through the day.

Foster care can be a good option, especially if the foster family embraces and nurtures your parent. You may feel considerable relief, and you may even develop your own close relationship with the foster family. However, foster care can also elicit unexpected reactions. You may worry about whether a foster fam-

## COMMUNAL? NO WAY!

Group living arrangements like home-sharing and congregate housing are not for everyone. They are economical and provide companionship, stimulation and sometimes other support. However, if your father has been a loner all his life, he's not likely to adapt well now to communal living.

Is your parent ready to share a living space, or does he need a good deal of privacy? Can he get along with others and enjoy their company or does he find most people to be a nuisance? Can he compromise, adjust his schedule and habits, and be sensitive to other people's needs? If he doubts his capacity to be flexible in these areas, he may want to have a trial run before signing any long-term lease agreements.

> "*One day when she called and sounded particularly low I said, 'Oh Mum, I think I really missed the boat. I should have helped get you into a retirement home where you could have been with other people, because you love people so much.'*
>
> *I made it sound like a compliment. And I left it so that if she was interested, she could bring the subject up later, as though it were her own idea, not something that I was pushing on her. It takes some time for this sort of thing to settle in her mind. She needs to mull it over, without any pressure from me. If I had suggested straight out that she move, she would have gotten all indignant and resistant.*" —BETTY H.

ily is treating your parent well, whether they are neglecting or even abusing him (so far, few such problems have been reported, but the field is still new). You may also be visited in the late hours of the night by your old companion, Guilt, who tells you that strangers are doing what you should be doing. Or you may grow jealous of the relationship that is developing between your parent and his foster family. *Mom wants to spend the holidays with them instead of us. I can't believe it.*

In the clear light of morning, the fact that your parent has found a good home should outweigh such anxieties and concerns. Your best assurance is to visit frequently and establish a rapport with the foster family, letting them know how much you value and respect your parent.

States have their own rules on foster care, specifying how many adults can live in one foster home, regulating costs and defining eligibility requirements to become a foster family. The area agency on aging should know about any adult foster-care programs in your parent's state. Usually the cost is shouldered by the older person or his family, although some states are now allowing partial Medicaid coverage for foster care.

## ASSISTED LIVING

They exist under a variety of names—board-and-care homes, personal-care homes, sheltered care, adult homes, enriched housing, residential care—but whatever they are called, these residences are ideal for people who need help getting through the day, but don't require the intensive supervision and medical services of a nursing home. Because residents are usually encouraged to do as much as possible on their own, they tend to remain more active and healthier than people who enter nursing homes prematurely.

Assisted-living spaces range from large houses to giant hotel-like complexes. In some places, residents share bedrooms, in others they have private apartments. Whatever the size and style, most offer three meals a day in a common dining room, transportation, recreation, housekeeping and laundry services, help with bathing, dressing, toileting and other personal tasks, and round-the-clock emergency services.

## A QUALITY CHECK

When you research housing options, be sure to ask the local area agency on aging or the long-term care ombudsman about licensing or any quality assurance program within the state. Also, check with the Department of Consumer Affairs or the Better Business Bureau to see if any complaints have been filed against a particular residence. Most important, talk with people who reside in the facilities you are considering.

The services, staffing and philosophy of assisted-living arrangements can vary enormously, so find out exactly what is offered in each home. Above all, look for a place that respects the privacy and autonomy of its residents and really urges them to be active. Then get a detailed list of services offered. All meals or just some? Full laundry services or only sheets and towels? Housekeeping in your parent's room or only in the common areas? Is there custodial care (bathing, dressing, grooming, toileting)? Transportation? Group activities? Any nursing care? The more services that are offered, the more expensive this will be. But some services, particularly custodial and nursing care, also mean that as your parent grows more frail, she may not have to move to another facility to receive a higher level of care.

You might also consider the mix of residents in the facility. Are they at a comparable level of functioning? Are they active and interesting? Do they like to do some of the things that your parent likes to do? And if people share rooms, how are roommates matched? What happens if your parent does not get along with her roommate? (For a list of other issues to consider, see Appendix F, page 417.)

Although a few assisted-living residences welcome people with special problems, many refuse those with dementia, incontinence or other problems that require a good deal of attention.

Assisted living can cost anywhere from $300 to $3,000 a month. The costs are not covered by Medicare or private insurance, but certain states provide some rent subsidies or limited Medicaid coverage, and some residences offer financial assistance.

## CONTINUING CARE RETIREMENT COMMUNITIES

Continuing care retirement communities, also known as life care centers, are the *prix fixe* meal on the menu of housing options. They offer it all—from independent living to nursing home care—usually for one fairly hefty, fixed price.

Most such communities accept only people who can get around and live independently. Once a resident has been admitted, however, he receives whatever care is necessary for the duration of his life.

The centers usually include apartments or houses for those who

## CONTINUING CARE INFORMATION

The American Association of Homes and Services for the Aging (202-783-2242) issues the *Consumers' Directory of Continuing Care Retirement Communities*, which contains information about hundreds of these communities. The most recent directory can be found in public libraries or can be purchased through the Association.

The Association also sponsors the Continuing Care Accreditation Commission (202-783-7286), which inspects and accredits these communities. The Commission can send your parent a list of accredited CCRCs that meet certain criteria with regard to finances, medical care, resident life and management. (Accreditation is a helpful, but far from perfect, yardstick. Application is voluntary and the CCRCs pay a fee to be evaluated. Those that are not accredited may still have high standards.)

are living independently and offer a variety of activities such as golf, swimming, bowling and lectures. They also have an assisted-living complex which provides more care and services, and a nursing-home unit for residents who become frail or chronically ill. Consequently, there is a mix of residents, many of them healthy and active, so the atmosphere is less dreary than in a typical nursing home environment.

While they are expensive, these communities offer enormous peace of mind. Your parent doesn't have to worry about if or when he will need nursing-home care, where he will go and how he will pay for it. Everything he will ever need is paid for (depending upon the type of contract signed), and he will never need to move again.

Entrance fees vary greatly, ranging anywhere from $20,000 to more than $300,000. Part of the entrance fee is sometimes returned to the resident's estate upon the death of the resident. There are also monthly fees, ranging from $500 to more than $3,000. Residents are usually asked to choose from among several arrangements:

◆ Extended, or all-inclusive, contracts are the traditional life-care contracts. The entry fee and monthly fees cover any and all services needed, including unlimited nursing care.

◆ Modified contracts cover only a limited number of days of nursing care each year. After that, the resident pays a fee that is usually about 80 percent of the full rate.

◆ Fee-for-service contracts provide residents with independent-living and assisted-living services, but

**"***About three years ago, my parents
and another couple moved into a
life-care center in the neighboring
town. My sisters and I were shocked.
They were all basically healthy and
active. It seemed to us as if they were
giving up. We couldn't understand
why they moved.*

*Now I am grateful. They love
being there. They don't have the
responsibility of caring for a house,
they do what they want to do and
they have each other. It's not gloomy
or depressing. In fact, it's really
nice—much more like a country club
than an old folks' home. Best of all,
we don't worry about the future. It's
all taken care of. It's really a
blessing.***"**        —ELIZABETH J.

require that they pay the full cost of
any nursing care needed.

Because this is a long-term
commitment and an enormous investment, your parent should have
a lawyer experienced in such matters examine the contract. Be sure
to check the financial stability of the
community, the refund policy, any
additional fees, health insurance requirements, possible increases in
fees, and the availability of nursing
home beds. You should also find out
how decisions are made to move residents from one level of care to the
next.

Keep in mind that if your parent is moving into a life-care center, long-term care insurance may be
redundant. (See page 255 for more
on long-term care insurance.)

# Chapter Eleven

# A GOOD NURSING HOME

*What to Look for in a Home • Getting In*
*• Moving Day and Beyond • Your New Roles—as Visitor*
*and Advocate • Getting Adjusted*

Y OU HOPED IT WOULD NEVER HAPPEN. MAYBE YOU EVEN
promised yourself or your parent it would never happen.
But at some point—perhaps after great effort to avoid it,
disputes with siblings and agonizing days of sadness and
indecision—it becomes clear that moving your parent into a
nursing home is the only practical thing to do.

Although it may not seem so at the time, this move is often
the best choice. If your parent suffers from dementia or
incontinence, is immobile or has another chronic ailment that
demands an enormous amount of attention, a nursing home can
provide him with a level of medical care, supervision and welcome
activity that he cannot possibly receive at home. More than 40
percent of people over the age of 65 are expected to spend at least
some time in a nursing home during their lives.

Your involvement—and the involvement of other family
members—is vital to the success of this move. Your parent needs

your support and encouragement, and he needs someone to
monitor his care and to act on his behalf when things aren't right.
Sorrow may be unavoidable now, but try to shake off any guilt you
may be feeling. You are doing your best, you will continue to do
your best and your best truly is good enough.

# The Decision

The mere thought of a nursing
home may conjure up images
of muttering old people warehoused
in stench and isolation, of hostile orderlies, indifferent nurses and helpless patients strapped to their chairs.

It happens, but it happens far
less than it used to. Public lobbying, consumer advocacy, litigation
and federal reforms have all forced
nursing homes to rethink their mission and responsibilities. As a result, many have cut back extensively
on the use of physical restraints and
sedative medications, eased rigid
schedules, renovated rooms and
lounges and developed a range of
activities to keep able residents en-
tertained and stimulated.

Certainly, inspections continue
to turn up instances of substandard
care, but there are more and more
examples of success—nursing homes
where residents make friends, become involved and receive good
medical and personal care. If you do
some legwork and get your parent
into the best nursing home you can
find, then visit her regularly and act
as her advocate, her move to a nursing home is likely to be a good one.

Nursing homes are invaluable if
your parent needs more medical care

*"I know my limitations as a per-
son. I knew what I could do for her
and what I couldn't. My mother
lived with us for almost five years,
and at the beginning we were able
to manage. But she became too sick,
too demanding. Moving her into a
nursing home was the only choice. It
was time. I don't have any guilt
about it."* —NANCY S.

than is practical or possible at
home; when family members cannot handle the physical and emotional aspects of caring for an
infirm person at home; and when
living in any other type of residence
is not an option because of your
parent's particular disabilities or behavior—for example, dangerous
wandering, limited mobility, incontinence or abusive or otherwise
harmful behavior.

Most nursing homes offer
round-the-clock nursing supervision
and on-call physicians in addition
to meals, laundry services, personal
care, counseling, recreation, nutritional guidance, social services, rehabilitative programs and pharmacy
and laboratory services. Some now
also offer "subacute medical care"—
special wings or floors that provide
hospital-level care.

## TEN COMMON REACTIONS TO HAVING A PARENT IN A NURSING HOME

❖ Guilt that you are not doing enough for your parent
❖ Anxiety that the nursing staff won't do enough for him
❖ Guilt because you promised you would never put him in a home
❖ Anxiety about whether you will end up in a nursing home
❖ Guilt that your parent isn't in a nicer, more expensive home
❖ Anxiety over the high cost of the nursing home he is in
❖ Guilt that you don't visit him more often
❖ Anxiety about having to visit so often
❖ Guilt for feeling relief that your parent is in a nursing home
❖ Anxiety that it won't work and you'll have to devise another plan

While they are typically needed for long-term care, nursing homes are also used for brief periods while a person recuperates from an injury or illness, or to give a family a break from the rigors of home care. Homes are usually privately owned, publicly supported or run by a nonprofit religious or civic group.

## WHO PAYS?

What shocks most families is not just the high cost of nursing homes, but the fact that Medicare and private insurance almost never cover it. The average nursing home charges about $40,000 a year, but many charge two or three times that amount. Private long-term care insurance will pick up much of the tab, but few elderly people today have it because it's a relatively new option. Medicare will pay for a few months of nursing home care, but only in very specific situations. As a result, most elderly people pay out-of-pocket until their pockets are empty, at which point they apply for Medicaid.

If your family acts right away, your parent may still be able to protect some of his assets before going on Medicaid (see page 263). But bear in mind that he should keep some of his assets liquid—at least enough to cover up to a year in a nursing home, if possible—so that he is a good candidate for admission to a relatively good one. And be sure that any facility you consider is certified to accept Medicaid patients so that if your parent enters as a paying resident and runs out of funds, he cannot be evicted. If your parent is a military veteran, call the local veterans affairs office to find out if he is eligible for free or low-cost nursing home care.

## CHECKING THE COST

When comparing nursing home prices, use caution. Nursing homes charge a range of fees based on the level of care provided. But one home's "enriched care" may not be the same as another home's "enhanced care." The Health Care Financing Administration has identified 44 different names for the various levels of care provided by nursing homes.

You should also know that any price quoted is apt to be only a base rate. Every extra service can be added on to the base price, and in some homes, doing laundry, monitoring catheters and preventing bedsores are considered "extras." A survey by *Consumer Reports* found that nursing homes sometimes charge up to $1,000 a month for such extras.

## The Search

Ideally, to find a good nursing home you need time to tour a number of facilities, revisit some and ask a lot of questions. But quite often, time is not on your side and the search is hurried or even frantic.

If your parent is in the hospital, the discharge planner can lead the way, which has its advantages and disadvantages. Discharge planners may know quite a bit about local nursing homes, and they often have relationships with administrators, so they may be able to expedite your parent's admission. Also, nursing home administrators often give priority to a hospital patient whose care will be covered, at least in the beginning, by Medicare. Keep in mind, however, that a discharge planner's main objective is to get your parent out of the hospital, so she may pressure your family to make a hasty decision.

This decision is too important to hurry if you don't absolutely have to. Research nursing homes that the planner may not have suggested, and use your own judgment—or your parent's judgment—as you inspect and review the options. Find the best home for your parent, even if this means fighting for additional Medicare coverage for the extra hospital days, paying for those days privately or even taking your parent home temporarily while you find a suitable facility. If you "try out" a nursing home with the thought of moving your parent to a better one later, you will disrupt her life twice, create more work for yourself, and possibly hurt her chances of getting into another residence, as her placement will then seem less urgent.

Start your research—whether or not your parent is in the hospital—by putting together a list of nursing homes in the area. Talk with friends and acquaintances, and call the state long-term care ombudsman (see Appendix A, page 377 for the telephone number). Each state has an ombudsman—and some

**"***I refused to put my mother in a nursing home. I wouldn't have it. My sister and brothers kept telling me that we had to do it, that she was too difficult to manage, but I wouldn't listen. I cut back my hours at work and used up pretty much all of her savings to pay for aides and nurses at home. I stuck to my resolve.***

*Then a friend of mine told me that I had created a home for my mother that was worse than any nursing home. And she was right. My mother didn't do anything or see anyone. She never got out or had any stimulation. And, in the meantime, I was ruining my own life.*

*I finally gave in, but I was mortified any time I had to tell people where she lived. The staff at the nursing home was reassuring and I gradually felt better, but it took time. I regret being so stubborn, but I was only doing what I thought she would want.***"** —ALEX B.

counties have a local ombudsman—who acts as an advocate for nursing home residents and their families, helping them find good residences and resolving problems once they are in a facility. These ombudsmen visit nursing homes routinely, so they know a great deal about what each offers and the quality of care available.

Be aware, however, that while ombudsmen are an excellent source of information, they are government employees and don't like to make waves. An ombudsman may not come right out and say that a nursing home is unacceptable; he or she

may try to redirect you more subtly. *Why would you select Serene Acres? I think you should look at Barton's Landing. Are you sure Cedar Hollow is right for your parent?* Listen carefully for those cues.

You might also call geriatric care managers, local senior centers, the area agency on aging or members of the clergy who visit people in nursing homes and may have some recommendations. As you gather your initial list, don't pass over nursing homes sponsored by religious organizations even if your parent is not affiliated with that religion. While your parent should be in a place where she feels comfortable and won't be isolated because of her religious beliefs, a good home, no matter who runs it, is certainly worth considering.

Once you have the names of several nursing homes, call and find out about the location, size, costs and services available. Ask about Medicare certification and how many beds are set aside for Medicaid patients. (About 80 percent of homes are certified to receive Medicare and Medicaid.) Also find out whether your parent is eligible for admission.

## THE TOUR:
### WHAT TO LOOK FOR

Once you eliminate those facilities that don't seem promising, begin your on-site research by dropping by briefly as a visitor during regular visiting hours. Don't be blinded by fancy interior decorating or lush gardens—walk the corridors and observe how the residents

## KEEP YOUR PARENT AT THE HELM
*(even if you are charting the course)*

No matter what your parent's physical and mental limitations—even if she doesn't seem to be fully aware of what is happening around her—try to keep her involved in all stages of this decision, talking about the options, touring homes, choosing one and signing up. The more involved she is and the more you talk about what is happening, the easier the transition will be.

If your parent can't tour nursing homes herself, collect brochures, menus and activity schedules for her, and describe what you saw. If she can't be involved at all, keep in mind what makes her happy.

A common mistake adult children make when helping a parent relocate is selecting a place that is convenient for them but far from his friends and others who might visit. Or they pick a place that is attractive and pleasant to visit, but not so great to live in. A beautifully-renovated building may reassure you, but your parent may feel more at home in a smaller, less fancy facility with a warm and caring staff.

---

are cared for, because that's what really matters. If you like what you see, make an appointment for a formal tour. (If you live far away and are doing this investigating on your own, you may have to do more calling and less touring.)

When you go on a formal tour, be sure to see more than the public rooms—the lounges, library, gym, dining room, game room, etc. Ask to look at a typical bedroom and bathroom, the kitchen, the infirmary and the dementia wing or any other special unit. Meet the director or manager of the residence, the heads of nursing and admissions, and staff members in charge of various aspects of residential life—the social worker, activity director, nutritionist, cook, medical director.

You need to see whether the institution is clean and well-maintained, and whether the residents are well cared for. See Appendix F, page 417, for a detailed checklist of questions to ask on a tour and A Resident's Bill of Rights. Here are some general issues to consider:

◆ **The homeyness factor.** Would this be a comfortable place to live? Are the lounges cozy and the rooms adequate? Is there some privacy for residents while also a sense of community? Are there gardens or grounds where residents are free to roam?

◆ **Well-scrubbed and safe.** That first waft is a good indicator of cleanliness. A facility shouldn't smell musty or rancid, but it also shouldn't be filled with perfumes or heavy ammonia. Also, are the building and furnishings in good repair or is there plaster cracking off the walls? Is the residence safe—are the pathways cleared to prevent falls or is there construction going on in a hallway that residents use?

♦ **A caring staff.** Is the staff pleasant and helpful, or do they seem overworked and on edge? Do they welcome your questions? Do they seem to have warm relationships with the residents? Do they like working here? Is there a high rate of turnover?

♦ **The folks that live there.** The single most important part of your tour will be the residents themselves. Are they well-groomed and well-dressed? Are they involved in activities or bored? Does it seem that they have developed friendships within the facility? Try to talk with them out of earshot of staff so they can be candid. Are they content? Do they find they have enough to do? Do they like the staff? Are they treated with respect and dignity? What are their biggest complaints?

♦ **What's in a day?** Is independence encouraged and stimulation provided? Look at the activities schedule. Is there a wide range of choices? Is there anything on the schedule that would interest your parent? Do some of the activities entail taking residents out of the facility and into the community? Is the activities director willing to offer new classes or organize new events based on a resident's interests? How many people actually participate in a given activity? Are residents who are physically able encouraged to leave the grounds and to do things on their own?

♦ **Medical care.** Are nurses available around-the-clock? Is the

*"I visited two homes with wonderful reputations and found that while the grounds and buildings were absolutely beautiful, the staff was nasty to the residents and clearly unhappy in their work. Four others I visited were better—not as attractive, but without that icy atmosphere—but I still wasn't satisfied. I stayed on the phone night after night, calling friends and friends of friends, trying to get more leads. Then a friend's mother mentioned a place that I had never heard of. She said it had been a wonderful nursing home many years ago, but now was in a bad neighborhood.*

*I went out to see it anyway, and while it didn't compare aesthetically with the other places I'd seen, it was immaculately clean and the staff was actually cheerful. They were extremely professional, but there was also a sweetness about them. They seemed truly fond of the residents, and never seemed to be exasperated, even when patients were difficult.*

*My mother was very frail and confused, but she seemed content there and I felt good about it. The neighborhood was poor, but not dangerous, and it was only a half-hour ride from my office."* —SARA B.

facility close to a hospital? Are residents unnecessarily restrained, either physically or with medications?

◆ **The chow.** When you go on your tour, arrange to have a meal in the dining room so you can sample the daily fare. Is it tasty? Nutritious? Fresh? Does the daily menu offer several alternatives and does it change often?

◆ **The head honchos.** While you certainly need to discuss finances, services and eligibility with administrators, try also to get a feel for the philosophy of the institution. An administration that is genuinely concerned about patients—and not just dollars—will see to it that your parent gets good, continuous care. If, for example, he has financial trouble or develops an ailment that requires more care than the

## A FRIENDLY TAG-A-LONG

If you are touring without your parent or a sibling, ask a friend to come with you, preferably someone who has been through this experience. It's not easy looking at nursing homes and imagining your parent living in one of them, and it's physically tiring to do so much walking and interviewing. A friend can help you think more clearly and less emotionally, and give you the moral support you need on such a difficult trip.

home can provide, administrators who are devoted to patients will find a way to keep him at that residence or make sure that he moves to an equally good facility.

If a residence seems promising after a formal tour, try to return in the evening or on a weekend, when staffing may be lean. Keep a low profile. Stroll the halls and talk with residents and then find a perch where you can sit unnoticed for a while—perhaps reading a magazine in the corner of an activities room—and watch how staff members interact with residents. This will tell you far more about the home than you will learn in any guided tour.

## ASK FOR THE INSPECTION REPORT

Be sure to look at the nursing home's most recent inspection report, which will give you invaluable insight into the kind of care provided at the residence. Nursing homes that receive Medicare or Medicaid funding are examined every year by inspectors from the Health Care Financing Administration. Their reports will reveal any violations, from the temperature of the tap water to cases of outright physical abuse.

Your request may ruffle some feathers, as many nursing homes would rather keep these reports private, but don't be intimidated. Inspection reports—also known as surveys—must, by law, be made available to the public. If the nursing home makes this difficult, ask the state long-term care ombudsman or the state office that licenses nursing homes for a copy of the report.

When you review the inspection report don't seek perfection, because it doesn't exist. Instead, look for repeated violations and the kinds of violations that directly affect a patient's well-being, such as failure to follow a "plan of care" or overuse of restraints.

Ask about any violations that concern you. The way the staff answers your questions—whether they are direct and apologetic, or indifferent—will tell you a great deal about how they regard their mission.

# Getting In

Unless your parent has plenty of money—in which case she should be able to get into almost any nursing home she chooses—finding a good nursing home is only half the battle. The second half is getting your parent accepted there. Popular nursing homes will have plenty of candidates vying for admission, and administrators pick and choose freely when accepting residents. The person with the most money or the best Medicare coverage will be given priority.

When you meet with an administrator, be discreet in what you say about your parent's angry outbursts or demanding personality. Focus on the side of her that is calm and easygoing. And while you shouldn't hesitate to ask questions, be tactful. A family perceived as unreasonably demanding may be turned away in favor of one who un-

**"**Getting my father into a good nursing home was like getting someone with very poor grades into college. He was on Medicaid because we'd spent all of my parents' money during my mother's illness. He had advanced dementia and he had become angry and disruptive. A social worker said that nursing homes in the area would not consider taking such a patient and suggested that we get him admitted to a hospital and let the hospital staff pull some strings.

We represented my father as being cooperative and agreeable, as he had been before the dementia set in, and finally found a nursing home that we liked that was willing to admit him. We whizzed through the application process because we were afraid they would refuse him once they understood how difficult he could be. They took him, thank goodness, but it was quite an experience.**"** —SARA B.

derstands the pressures of nursing home work.

You can't hide your parent's financial problems because the nursing home will look through his records. Homes prefer patients who qualify for Medicare coverage and self-paying residents—the longer someone can foot the bills privately, the better. Because of this, in some cases it is best to get your parent admitted to a hospital first so that she can qualify for Medicare coverage and skilled nursing care.

## SPECIAL CARE FOR DEMENTIA

If a nursing home claims to have special programs and services for people with dementia, find out exactly what that means. An "Alzheimer's wing" may be a few rooms with a locked door, or it may be a carefully designed unit with a highly-trained staff. The only way to know what's really offered is to see for yourself.

A good unit for people with dementia—and it doesn't have to be solely for people with dementia; many of the best facilities mingle residents —should be quiet and calm, but also provide physical and mental stimulation. Residents should be encouraged to do simple exercises, engage in easy and entertaining projects, and receive lots of encouragement to do all that they can for themselves. The floor plan should allow them to find their way around easily and to wander safely. The staff-to-patient ratio should be high, with one staff person to every four or five patients. Schedules should be flexible to meet the diverse needs of residents, including those who are awake during the night. The number of patients on sedatives or other psychotropic (mind-altering) medications should be low, perhaps less than 20 percent, and the use of physical restraints, such as straps or body vests, should be virtually nonexistent.

---

The majority of nursing homes accept Medicaid, but because the reimbursement rate is relatively low, many of them limit the number of Medicaid residents they will house at any given time. A nursing home with 150 beds, for example, may have only 10 or 15 beds earmarked for people on Medicaid. This means your parent will have fewer choices of facilities and is likely to face lengthy waiting lists.

If he has trouble being admitted, talk to the long-term care ombudsman, a local consumer's coalition and if possible a savvy eldercare attorney. States have varying rules about Medicaid, and sometimes a person's needs will determine the coverage, and in turn, their chances of getting in. Build a rapport with the nursing home's administration, and if your parent is put on a waiting list, call often and be persistent about making sure that he gets the first bed available.

### THE CONTRACT

The admissions process can be lengthy and exhausting, and requires that you submit a variety of your parent's personal, financial and legal records. The nursing home's financial officer will tell you what is needed.

Any nursing home contract should include detailed information about costs, payment schedules, services to be provided, penalties for failure to pay, the facility's refund policy and bed-holding policy should your parent be hospitalized or temporarily absent for some other reason, the rules of the house, and the responsibilities and rights of residents. Read the contract carefully or have an experienced lawyer read it. Ask the nursing home's director or the state's long-term care ombudsman to clarify any provision that concerns you or your parent. Beware of clauses in the contract that free an institution from liability for injury or lost possessions.

### THE PLAN OF CARE

As soon as your parent is admitted to a nursing home, the staff will do a full assessment of his physical, functional, social, mental and emotional condition. They will then put together a "plan of care" that outlines his medical treatments; describes the therapy and nursing care he will receive; recommends activities he should or shouldn't engage in; and specifies his diet, exercise regime and daily schedule. The plan should be devised in a way that keeps your parent as active and independent as possible.

Your parent and your family should be integrally involved in designing the plan of care, so try to attend the initial conference. If he has dementia, be sure the staff understands what gives him pleasure, what upsets him, what calms him

down, what times and tasks are most confusing for him, and anything else that might help them.

Get a written copy of the plan, and be sure it is updated every three months, or at any time there is a change in your parent's physical or mental health. When you visit, check to see that the plan of care is being followed.

# Moving Day

Moving day can be wrenching for everyone. You may feel anxious or guilt-ridden. Your parent may be nervous, depressed or frightened. Try to put your own worries aside for the moment so you can empathize with her and reassure her. And if you have advance notice before the move, here are some other ways you can make the transition easier for her:

♦ In the weeks before the move, try to bring your parent to visit her new home. This time she will see it through the eyes of a future resident, which will give her a different perspective. Introduce her to other residents and staff and tell them when she will be arriving so they can greet her.

♦ Ask friends and family to offer her encouragement and support.

♦ Hold a party for your parent a few days before the move. (Have it around her hospital bed, if necessary.) Guests should bring gifts for her new life—framed photos, silk flowers, a knitting bag, bathrobe, slippers, easy-to-wear clothing, a

*"I was prepared to be uncomfortable, to hate this place. But I was surprised. It was attractive and, more than that, many of the people living there were much healthier than I expected. One older gentleman even flirted with my mother in the elevator. I think we both liked the home more than we expected, and that came as a great relief."*
—FRAN M.

scarf, scents and powders, a calendar with visit dates already written in, some potpourri, a new bed quilt, a child's drawing for the wall.

◆ Before loading up the car, find out exactly what your parent is permitted to bring, and what is not allowed, so you don't arrive only to be sent home with half of her belongings. Leave valuables behind unless they are absolutely necessary (things get lost and stolen in any institution), but include objects of comfort, such as a special chair, a favorite afghan or family photos. Put name labels on all your parent's clothes and belongings.

◆ If your parent has fixed habits and routines, ask the staff if they can be accommodated. After years of doing something a certain way—having a cup of coffee first thing in the morning, staying up every evening to watch *The Late Show*—it's hard to change the pattern. Being able to keep some of his old routines will make this move easier.

◆ Get others to lend a hand. They might help you arrange your

parent's room and then stay and have a meal with her.

◆ If you go as a group, be sure to space your departures so that your parent doesn't have to deal with one enormous good-bye. The group might continue on to your house to give you some support and comfort at the end of what is bound to be an emotionally draining day.

# Your Role as a Visitor

Visiting can be stressful and time-consuming for you, but remember, even if a visit is brief, your parent complains the whole time or she forgets that you came at all, your presence is invaluable. It lets her know that you still care and that she is not alone, and it helps you keep tabs on how she is doing.

Visit as often as you can manage (but not more often than that). And when you do visit, make it count. Take note of your parent's well-being, consult with staff members about how she is faring and offer her lots of reassurance. Help her to see the positives—the care she is receiving, the friendships she may be forming and the entertainment that she didn't have before. A few more visiting tips:

◆ While nurses and aides can be helpful in letting you know when your parent needs a visit, don't routinely schedule your trips via the staff. By dropping in unexpectedly now and then, you will be better able to monitor her care.

♦ Try to plan your visits around your parent's schedule. For example, don't interrupt her nap time or her favorite class.

♦ If your visits are tense or awkward, do something new. Play a game of cards, take your parent out to lunch, read her mail or a newspaper aloud to her or take her for a drive. If your parent has dementia, tour the home together (it will always be fairly new to her), let her reminisce or look through a photo album with her. You might also diffuse tension by talking to other residents. That will help your parent make friends and allow her to show you off as well.

♦ Pamper her. If you are used to having a hand in your parent's physical care, don't hesitate to continue in that role. Fix her hair, help her put on makeup, rub her back or give her a foot massage.

♦ Bring the children, unless your parent or a child specifically asks you not to. Children radiate joy, spirit and energy—which is appreciated by most elderly people.

♦ Don't say you will visit at a certain time unless you are sure you can do so. If your parent is mentally alert, visits can trigger a lot of excitement, and a canceled visit can be a huge let-down.

♦ Keep your parent up-to-date on what is happening with friends and family. Don't hide bad news, as tempting as that is. It's best to be open and let your parent grieve when a friend or relative dies, and to react to other unhappy news.

♦ Take a few minutes during a visit to review your parent's wardrobe. Does she need new clothing or shoes? Ask an aide who regularly cares for her if you can get something that might make her more comfortable—such as sneakers, slippers, a new robe or elastic-waisted pants.

♦ Use your visits to establish a rapport with the staff. Get to know them and let them know how much you appreciate their efforts.

## WHEN YOU ARE FAR AWAY

If you cannot visit your parent, try to get someone else to. Talk with relatives and friends, and find out about local volunteer visitors—a nursing-home social worker, the state long-term care ombudsman or a local consumer advocacy group should be able to tell you about groups that visit the facility. If you cannot find volunteers, look into hiring a companion or even a geriatric care manager (see page 182).

Ask a nurse supervisor how to best stay in touch with the staff and when you should call to get regular updates on your parent's care and condition. Also, contact the nursing home's family/resident council, an advocacy group which represents the needs and concerns of patients and their families. It will keep you abreast of what's happening in the home and make others aware of your parent's situation.

And when you can't be there, use the telephone. Lots of calls, even short ones, can fend off the loneliness your parent may be feeling

*"When my mother stopped recognizing me, I stopped visiting her as much, not because I thought she didn't know the difference, but because it was so hard for me. To have her turn and look blankly at me, to have her ask, 'Who is this woman in my room?' was very painful. I used to shout at her, 'Mom, it's Nancy!' and then be depressed for days after the visit.*

*I still don't go quite as often as I used to, but I've learned something that helps. When I visit, we look through this old album together. It is filled with pictures of her and her brothers when they were little. We look at the same pictures every time. She doesn't have any idea who I am, but she knows who they are, and I see how it comforts her to tell me about them. For that one hour, she is a child again, living in a brown house in Richmond, Indiana, with a great, big slide and two fun-loving brothers. And for that hour, I think she is happy."* —Nancy S.

now. Or send her a video or cassette tape of you and others in the family. (If there is no video cassette player at the home, you might want to buy one for your parent.)

## WHEN CONFUSION TAKES HOLD

A failing memory is a cruel foe—your parent doesn't remember that you visited and then insists that you never come to see him. But you can give his ailing mind a boost. Mark a large calendar with your name written in large, bright red letters on the days that you will visit. If you live far away, send a note and a picture of yourself, telling your parent who you are and that you are coming to see him. Ask the staff to remind him that you are coming. Then send notes between visits reminding him of what took place during your last visit and when you will visit next.

If none of this helps, don't keep pushing your parent to remember something that he truly can't. What difference does it make, really, if he knows when he last saw you? Live in the present with him. And definitely ignore any urge to visit less. It is more important than ever that you keep tabs on his care, now that he cannot fend for himself. And even if he doesn't remember a visit, your presence is still reassuring to him. He can still hear your familiar voice or feel your warm touch. On some level, he knows that you were there and will be more at ease because of it.

# Your Role as an Advocate

When you visit or call, consult with those staff members who care for your parent most. You need to be your parent's advocate, especially if he cannot or will not speak up for himself. If his roommate keeps him up at night, if you notice a change in his moods, if he can't eat the food from the dining room, urge him to speak up or speak up for him. Know his rights (see A Resident's Bill of Rights in Appendix F, page 421) and then protect them.

In particular, stay abreast of those less dire ailments that are often overlooked or not adequately treated by nursing home staffs. These include vision and hearing problems, bedsores, incontinence, poor eating habits, insomnia, depression and overmedication. If you can't be there in person, ask the staff about these issues, and ask to be notified if your parent falls, becomes ill or is given more than her routine medications.

Also, be sure that your parent is treated with respect and that he has some privacy, as these are so important to self-esteem and so often lacking in communal living situations. Perhaps there is a time each day when his roommate can let your father have the room to himself, or maybe there is a corner of a lounge or a card room where he won't be disturbed. If your mother is uncomfortable about having strangers help her dress or bathe, see if the job might be limited to one or two regular attendants.

If your mother has a particular interest, say in gardening, talk with the activities director about how she might become engaged in some relevant task. If your father says his days are meaningless, ask if he can visit people in the infirmary, read to residents who have trouble with their vision, help in the gift shop, or deliver flowers or mail to others. It's amazing how a little giving can lift the spirits.

## TWO GOLDEN RULES

When you act on your parent's behalf, keep two points in mind:

♦ Strike a balance between advocating for your parent and supporting those who are responsible for his care—the supervising staff, nurses, aides, social workers, orderlies, cleaning crew, etc. They will often show your parent the same kindness and respect that you show them. Develop a rapport with them, ask them about their own families and lives, and show that you understand the pressures they face.

When someone makes a special effort or is especially kind, be sure to thank him or her. If you want to go a step further, give the person a gift or send a letter of praise to a supervisor. Tips are almost always appreciated. Ask a floor supervisor or the family council how to proceed. If tips are not allowed, the family council might pool contributions for a staff gift or party.

*There were a couple of very bad months at first. I spoke to the social worker at the home and she asked me if I could hire a part-time aide to help my father adjust. Because he was on Medicaid, this wasn't really above board—he would have been cut off if they knew we were paying for private care—but we did it anyway. And it succeeded beyond our expectations. The place became a home for him. He joked with the aides and nurses and they treated him with affection.* —LILIAN R.

When you have a concern, work together with the staff to find solutions or resolve problems. Staff members can often make adjustments once they are made aware of a problem, but they will do so more readily, and care about your parent and your family more genuinely, if you show a sense of humor about any mishaps and express appreciation for their work.

◆ Choose one person from your family to act as a spokesperson. You don't want a phone call from your brother to jeopardize an understanding you have carefully developed with the staff, or a visit from your sister to discontinue a special menu you have worked out with the dietitian. Having one spokesperson is easier for the doctor and nurses and reduces the possibility of mix-ups. (See more on dealing with siblings in Chapter Twelve, page 229.)

# When Trouble Brews

When you notice a problem in your parent's care, bring it to the attention of the staff as soon as possible. The longer you wait, the more difficult it will be for you to discuss the situation, and the harder it may be for the staff to correct it. First, talk with the person directly involved—the orderly who has repeatedly left your parent sitting unattended, the housekeeper who fails to change his wet sheets—and be specific about your concerns. If the problem is not resolved, talk to an immediate supervisor, and move on up the ladder until you get some results. Be calm and kind when you deal with each person, but remain firm in your resolve.

If there is still no resolution, find out about the facility's grievance procedure and file a formal complaint. By law, all nursing homes are required to have such a procedure. The resident or family council, if there is one, should be able to advise you or may even step in on your parent's behalf.

> **"**One of the aides, whom my mother loved, had heard a rumor that I had complained about her. I hadn't, but it took over a year to break down this barrier. I said to one of the home's social workers, 'Look, if she wants to be angry with me, fine. I can take it. I just don't want her to be angry with my mother.' I tried very hard to mend the fences because I knew that much of the quality of my mother's care depended on what they thought of me.**"**   —BARBARA F.

Being rude or difficult might adversely affect your parent's care, but reasonable complaints that are respectfully registered should not. In fact, once the staff realizes that you are going to stay involved, your parent may receive better attention.

## NEGLECT, ABUSE AND EXPLOITATION

Despite improvements in nursing home care, residents are still

## RESTRAINING RESTRAINTS

Nursing homes have been ordered by Congress to cut back on the use of restraints—both physical and chemical means of controlling patients—but some facilities have been more successful than others at curtailing this practice. Know what to look for and how to keep your parent as free from restraint as possible.

Physical restraints include everything from full body vests to innocuous-looking wheelchair trays. Chemical restraints include tranquilizers, antianxiety drugs, antidepressants, sedatives and hypnotics. Any restraint is dehumanizing and potentially dangerous. The drugs can cause side effects—from confusion, agitation and insomnia, to changes in blood pressure and appetite. Physical restraints can lead to loss of appetite and cause bedsores. They can also choke or severely injure a person who, in a state of panic, tries to escape, or who simply tries to get up in the middle of the night.

Recent studies show that restraints are rarely necessary and do not necessarily prevent serious injuries. For example, if your parent is agitated, letting him walk around may calm his troubled mind. And with a little ingenuity, risks can be reduced so falls don't happen or, when they do, they are not harmful. They can be prevented through exercise (which improves balance and strength), the use of supportive shoes, lower beds and chairs, better lighting, clear pathways, handrails and walkers. A wedge of foam tucked into a chair can prevent a person from sliding out, and sensors can be attached to a bed to alert the staff when a confused person is trying to get up.

Anytime your parent is restrained, find out why. Restraints can be used only under a doctor's order. Mind-altering medications are more difficult to monitor, but if your parent is unusually groggy or inattentive, find out what drugs she is being given and why. If a drug is necessary to treat an ailment, perhaps she can take a lower dose or be treated with a nonsedative or short-acting alternative.

When falls or other problems cannot be avoided without restraints, weigh the risks and benefits of the situation. Often it's better to risk a minor fall than to have your parent tied down. In any case, studies suggest that restraints do not reduce the number of injuries. If used, they should be a temporary answer. Talk with the doctor, social worker or nurses about other solutions.

mistreated at times. Physical and emotional abuse and neglect, financial exploitation and theft do occur, especially when residents are too sick to fend for themselves. Be alert to signs of trouble. Drop in unexpectedly now and then. Ask about any unusual marks or bruises on your parent. (If he has fallen or otherwise been injured, you should have been notified immediately.) If your parent has dementia, learn to distinguish between his routine accusations about those who care for him and what may be a valid complaint. Check to see that his possessions and bank accounts are safe.

And don't ignore subtle warning signs; if something doesn't seem right to you, follow up on it. A person doesn't have to touch your parent to be abusive. Saying things that make him feel threatened, demeaned or afraid constitutes abuse. Isolating a person, ignoring his emotional needs, or failing to keep him clean and toileted all constitute neglect.

As soon as you notice something troubling, alert the staff supervisor, the director of the home and the doctor. If there is any question at all of danger, get your parent out of the situation right away or ask that the person or people responsible—if you are sure you know who they are—be removed from your parent's care immediately.

## GETTING OUTSIDE HELP

If you get no help from within the nursing home or if a problem is severe, go outside for help.

◆ Long-term care ombudsmen have no power of enforcement, but they have both the legal authority and the experience to work with a nursing home to resolve problems. They are required by law to investigate all complaints and can refer serious ones to other agencies. Some states permit ombudsmen to file lawsuits on behalf of residents.

◆ The agency or agencies that have licensed, accredited or certified the nursing home should investigate any serious complaint immediately. If the problem is not urgent, inspectors should look into it during the next inspection. The ombudsman should be able to tell you how to reach the appropriate inspectors and licensing agency.

◆ If you believe the nursing home is exploiting your parent financially, notify his bank and ask that his account be monitored.

◆ Contact the National Citizens' Coalition for Nursing Home Reform (202-332-2275), a very helpful organization that can guide you through trouble or refer you to a local consumer advocacy group.

◆ The area agency on aging can direct you to other state offices you need to notify (the Medicaid office, a local protection and advocacy agency, the attorney general's office) and should also be able to refer you to available legal services if necessary.

If you file a formal complaint—within the nursing home or with an outside agency—build a record by following up all phone calls with letters, and requesting a written response. This assures that any agreement is clear, and gives you backing in case the problem is repeated or becomes more serious.

# Is This Move Working?

Your mother's belongings are in place, her room is relatively comfortable, the staff is supportive and you have both settled into a new routine. But she seems unhappy. Her health has deteriorated. She is more confused than before and she complains endlessly. Was this the best thing to do?

Give it time. Elderly people usually need at least six months, and often longer, to adjust to a new environment, a new routine and new relationships. There are often setbacks early on, but your parent probably will adapt with time.

Monitor her care closely and be sure that her plan of care is being followed. If she has become incontinent, is she being helped to the toilet regularly? If she is weak, is she getting exercise? If her mind is in a fog, talk with the doctor about her medications and other health problems that might be making her confused.

If your parent's complaints are vague, help him to be specific. Is there something he needs or wants, or does he simply need to air his fears and worries? Once you've discussed his complaints and tried to address any problems, ask him to think of three things he likes about his new home. Redirecting his attention to the positive changes in

his life will take his mind off the less desirable aspects of it, at least temporarily.

If you believe that your parent's care is good, keep these realities in mind:

♦ Nursing home residents sometimes complain bitterly and ap-

*"At first my father didn't want to stay and he kept trying to leave. The staff was kind and understanding about it, but we were really afraid that they would decide that he couldn't stay. He was angry and demanding a lot of time, he was notoriously picky about what he ate, and he complained about everything. The staff told me not to worry, that he would adjust, but I couldn't believe it. I was sure he would wear them out and then what would we do? I also felt like a monster for leaving him there because he seemed so miserable.*

*About two months after his move, I went to see him and arrived to find him all smiling and happy. I have never been so grateful to anyone in my life as I was to the nurses who were so patient and good to him. They never suggested medicating him to make him less rambunctious, or made me feel that he was in any way a burden. It's odd. You love these people, these strangers, who care so tenderly for your parent, who do what you wish you could do. They become your friends and you want to do good things for them."*

—BRENDA S.

pear depressed when visitors are around and then, as soon as the guests are gone, they return to activities, their friends and a more pleasant mood. If there is a staff member who has a good rapport with your parent, ask how your parent's mood changes with your visits. If your father simply needs to complain and you are an easy target, let him. Just be aware that you are getting all the bad news and none of the good, and take his complaints with a grain of salt.

◆ If your mother appears worse each time you visit, it may not be that her condition is rapidly deteriorating, but simply that you are more aware of her decline. When you see someone every day, it's difficult to notice subtle changes in health or mental abilities. When you visit every couple of weeks, the changes become more apparent.

◆ Adult children often project their own emotions onto parents

they have placed in nursing homes. Who is really unhappy, your parent or you? You may not like seeing her in a nursing home, but she may be doing just fine.

## FOR MORE HELP

**National Citizens' Coalition for Nursing Home Reform 202-332-2275**

For information about residents' rights and the laws governing nursing homes.

**American Association of Retired Persons 800-424-3410**

For brochures on finding a nursing home and protecting your parents' rights once she is in one.

# Chapter Twelve

# THE INNER CIRCLE

*Working with Siblings • The Family Meeting • Spouse and Children • Balancing a Career and Caregiving*

...................................

A CRISIS IN YOUR PARENT'S HEALTH OR WELL-BEING CAN strengthen some relationships—you may find a new appreciation for your husband or develop a closer bond with your sister—but it can drive a sharp wedge into others. Unfortunately, the people we are closest to, the ones we have known the longest and the most intimately, are also the ones who can most infuriate and hurt us. Perhaps we expect too much or give too little. Whatever the reasons for it, at no time is this dynamic more apparent than during times of stress, when we need more from each other yet have less to offer.

Your involvement in your parent's care is likely to affect all your relationships. Siblings, who may have been at the fringe of your life, are now smack in the center. A mate or children, who may not be able to fully understand what you are going through, may feel neglected. At work, bosses and colleagues offer a valuable diversion from your parent's care, but they create yet another layer of stress as you struggle to balance the demands of the job with the demands at home.

To some extent, you have to accept that things are going to be a little rocky for now. These other people in your life will survive without your undivided attention for a while. (Remember you are not responsible for everyone's happiness.) The most important thing you can do right now for any relationship is to keep the lines of communication open and your priorities intact.

# Working with Siblings

Your mother has been hospitalized with acute emphysema and needs to move into a nursing home. Your sister flies in, one brother drives up for the weekend. Your other brother decides not to make the trip, but asks you to keep him posted. Over the weekend, the three of you make repeated visits to the hospital, meet with a discharge planner and nursing home administrators, and then gather in the evening, exhausted and distraught. You hug, cry and do your best to help each other through the storm.

And then, just when life calms down—your mother settles into the nursing home and your siblings return to their homes—new troubles begin to brew. Your sister thinks the family should hang on to Mom's house, as she may get better. The absentee brother has heard of a tax loophole and suggests that you talk to a lawyer about putting the house in all of your names. You resent him for ordering you around. Your younger brother, who thinks the house should be sold, bows out because he feels that no one is listening to him. And your otherwise supportive sister is a bit testy because she is jealous of the time you are spending with your mother.

## THE ONLY CHILD

An only child does not have siblings to argue with, but he also has no siblings to share the worries, decisions and responsibilities of this stressful period. If you are caring for a parent on your own, talk with a counselor or join a support group. You need some outlet where you can express your concerns and learn the ropes from others.

Sound familiar? When a parent becomes ill, sibling relationships are tested and even friendly alliances can become volatile. Discussions are heated and opinions strong because the matters at hand—a parent's health, living situation and finances —are ones that everyone cares about. Reunited, perhaps at a family home, siblings may revert to childhood roles and behaviors, competing, once again, for Mom's affection or Dad's praise. Who is the closest? Who does the most work? Who is being selfish?

If your parent's needs are pressing, don't try to resolve old conflicts. You can't possibly come up with the emotional reserve needed for it, nor should you divert so much of your attention to something that can wait.

However, you should acknowledge any tensions and find ways to work around problems that are getting in the way of your parent's care.

## ADAPTING TO NEW ROLES: THE PRIMARY CAREGIVER

Typically, when a parent grows frail, one sibling gravitates toward the role of primary caregiver and takes on the majority of the work. This person may be closest to your parent geographically or emotionally. She may be the one who always takes charge, the one with the most time to give or the one who typically takes care of others. However the role is established, it can make everyone in the family uncomfortable. The primary caregiver may feel she is doing too much, and the others may feel shut out.

If you are the primary caregiver, get your siblings involved right away (perhaps by holding a family meeting). Early on, you may believe that you can handle your parent's care and that no one else can do it as well. But those reigns can become very heavy, very quickly. If you don't share them now, you may find yourself stuck with them later. In addition to the sheer work involved, this can be a lonely undertaking. You need siblings to share the decisions, the worries and the stress.

Siblings usually want to help, but they may not jump in eagerly because they feel that they would be interfering with your role, because they don't want to take directions from you or because they don't agree with the way you are handling things.

If you hold a family meeting, discuss the specifics of your role. You might even draft a detailed job description of what you've been doing and let your siblings revise it. This not only helps them to see all that you are doing and how they might contribute, but it gives you the go-ahead to do certain tasks.

Over time, if you maintain the role of primary caregiver listen to your siblings' concerns, keep them informed about what is happening and let them help. Whether or not

*"My brother refused to believe that my mother had dementia. I would tell him specific things that she did and how impossible things were becoming but he always came up with an excuse for her. And then he would tell me that I was the one with the problem, that I was being overprotective.*

*I brought Mom to his house one Saturday. I knew that the only way he would realize what was happening was if he saw it for himself, if he spent some real time with her. When we arrived I told him that I had to go out of town and left Mom with him for the night. I didn't give him an out.*

*When I came back for her the next day, he took one look at me and for the first time in my life I saw my brother cry. It was very sad, and I felt sorry for him. I understood—he really hadn't wanted to see it. But I had to do it. I needed his help and his support. I couldn't handle it alone any longer.* **"** —TERRY B.

## WHEN RELATIONSHIPS GET ROCKY

When you just can't get along, you and your siblings need to find a way to care for your parent without stepping on each other's toes. You may have to schedule visits so you don't run into each other, for example. Or you may need to hire a geriatric care manager to divide the duties or cast the deciding vote when you can't agree on the best course of action. However you handle the specifics, you need to accept that each of you has a unique relationship with your parent, and then make room for each of those relationships to work in its own particular way. And lastly, make a concerted effort to let go of certain issues. If a brother absolutely refuses to help in your parent's care, stop wasting your breath trying to get him to do more. Move on to more productive tasks.

they're able to express it, your siblings care tremendously and need to be kept up-to-date.

If you are not the primary caregiver, maintain your own relationship with your parent by visiting, calling or writing regularly. Offer whatever help you can, and then try to support the primary caregiver. Even if you don't always agree with her, acknowledge the work she is doing, let her blow off steam and give her a break from her duties whenever you can.

When there is a problem, when you feel shut out or ignored, talk to your sibling. Explain what you are feeling, but be sympathetic to her situation. You may think you see things more clearly from a distance—and perhaps you do—but she is the one living with your parent's care day in, day out, so she has a certain right to make decisions. And she has little energy to worry about your feelings or needs now.

### A FAMILY MEETING

No matter how you feel about your siblings, get together with them—either informally after a holiday meal or at a more structured meeting, with an agenda and perhaps a family counselor. Such a gathering will enable all of you to take a hard look at Dad's situation, plan for the future and, if necessary, take responsibility for specific duties. It also provides a forum where each person can air his or her views, learn what others are feeling, share much-needed emotional support, and devise a way to work as a team— if not in harmony, then at least with some sort of temporary truce.

The first meeting may be a little rough. The room may be filled with concern, discomfort and fear, as well as love and a desire to help. You may all have your own agendas and may not yet be able to listen to others. Don't give up. This is the beginning of a process. Just getting together and acknowledging that you need to work together is in itself an accomplishment.

◆ **Who comes.** Although it's important to keep your parent centrally involved in any discussion about her care and her future, you may want to hold one or two meetings without her to talk about subjects that might upset her needlessly, or so that you can talk more freely.

It's best to limit participants to siblings in most cases. You might include someone who is deeply concerned or involved in your parent's care (a parent's sibling or an adult grandchild) or a relative who can offer some expertise (a sister-in-law who's a lawyer or a cousin who's a nurse). But keep the number small and manageable.

Family members who cannot attend can participate by conference call. Those who say they do not want to get involved or that they have nothing to offer should nevertheless be urged to come. They should know what is happening, may have some valuable suggestions, and might be persuaded to help.

◆ **A moderator.** When emotions are high, or the issues particularly complex, find a moderator who can guide the discussion, make sure everyone has a chance to talk and encourage members to listen to each others' perspectives. This should be a neutral party, someone who is not related to the family and who is good at mediating disputes— a family friend, a member of the clergy, a hospice counselor, a social worker or a geriatric care manager.

◆ **An agenda.** Though it may seem very formal, having an agenda will make it clear why you are meeting and help keep the conversation on course. Sometime before the meeting, each sibling should write down three or four topics that he or she wants to discuss. A moderator or a sibling who's been chosen in advance to organize the meeting should incorporate these suggestions into a manageable agenda. Don't try to settle everything in one or two meetings, or you will become tired and cranky and the discussion will rapidly deteriorate.

◆ **Some guidelines.** To make sure everyone is heard and the meeting accomplishes what you want it to, agree upon some rules in advance. Ask others for suggestions or adapt the following guidelines to suit your family:

One, no one is allowed to dominate the meeting. If you don't have a moderator to direct and focus the discussion, agree that each person will talk for no more than, say, ten minutes at a time—and use a timer, if necessary.

Two, when someone is speaking others must listen without interrupting. Listening, and really digesting what others have to say, is an essential goal of these meetings. If you get nothing else accomplished, be sure that you all hear each others' views. If people have trouble absorbing what others are saying, ask each to briefly repeat the last speaker's message before taking his turn.

Three, each person should use sentences that begin with "I"—

"*My mother lives with us, and my two sisters got very resentful because I was telling them when they could visit her. I didn't want them just dropping in whenever they were in town. It's invasive and I'm not the greatest housekeeper in the world. Besides, I hoped they would plan their visits when I couldn't be home so Mom wouldn't be alone. I would say, 'I have a class on Tuesday and Thursday and it would be helpful if you could visit then.' But they got indignant and accused me of trying to keep them away from her. It got so that we were hardly speaking to each other.*

*When Mom needed more help, I spoke to a social worker at the hospital, and she asked everyone to meet with her. When we started to explain how we were feeling without yelling at each other, everything seemed so simple and sort of childish. I think we were all worried about Mom, and taking it out on each other. We have a lot more understanding of each other now. There are still sparks sometimes, but we've really pulled together as a family.*"
—CAROL G.

speaking only about his own opinions, feelings and actions—and avoid finger-pointing statements that begin with "you."

Four, since your parent's care is the reason for this meeting, all discussions should relate to this subject. Steer away from old arguments and debates that are not relevant.

◆ **What to discuss.** First, everyone needs to be clear about the facts and the issues. What is your parent's diagnosis and prognosis? If there is confusion about your parent's health, get his doctor or a nurse to briefly outline the situation in a note to the family before the meeting. What are the biggest concerns right now and for the future—health care, housing, day-to-day functioning, finances?

Then determine what needs to be done. (Be sure to let your parent voice *his* concerns and opinions first.) Make a detailed list of all jobs—researching available community services, touring nursing homes, meeting with lawyers, contacting a geriatric care manager, doing housework, transporting your parent to the doctor, paying bills and filling out insurance forms, finding and organizing important documents.

Include in your list of duties the job of spokesperson—someone who will represent the family if your parent is unable to confer with professionals herself. This person will not control any aspect of your parent's care, merely serve as the family's voice. She should, for example, talk with your parent's doctor, asking any questions that siblings might have, and then relay information to the others. (If your family is large, create a telephone chain so the spokesperson doesn't have to make all the calls.) Communicating with one spokesperson is far easier for professionals, and it reduces the risk of misinformation and misunderstandings. The spokesperson may or may not be the same person for each issue—one may be the medical liaison while another deals with lawyers.

♦ **Divide up the duties.** Once you have a list of tasks, divide up the duties. Start by letting people volunteer for jobs, and be leery of excuses. *I live too far away. I'm too busy with the children. I'm not good at this.* Everyone can do something. Siblings who live far away can handle bills, make regular phone calls to a parent, research local agencies by phone, handle some paperwork, and offer the primary caregiver support and respite. Those with children can cook meals occasionally for your parent (they have to cook for the children anyway), bring the children for a visit, get prescriptions filled, pick up books at the library and pay bills.

It's almost inevitable that one person will shoulder a disproportionate share of a parent's care, but one of the main goals of this meeting is to even things out as much as possible. Make it a priority because an unfair workload can create lasting resentment. Anyone already carrying a heavier load has to let go of some of it, and others have to pick up the slack.

Once you agree upon some relatively fair division of labor, make a clear and detailed schedule of who will do what, when and where. Make sure everyone involved has a copy. Then, give your plan a trial run. Within three months or so, you should reconvene to discuss how things are working, to reassess your parent's needs, and to make any necessary adjustments to your plan.

# Significant Others

If you have a strong and supportive relationship with a spouse, it will be an enormous help to you now. A spouse who listens, empathizes and takes on some additional household responsibilities is a godsend and deserves huge thanks. But whatever problems exist in the relationship will be exacerbated. A parent's care often causes marital rifts, some of them quite deep.

If your parent needs you for the short term, your spouse will have to make do without you for a time. You may not be with him physically or you may be absent mentally. Either way, your parent's care is a priority and you both have to make compromises, at least for now. However, if her care becomes a long-term

❝*I live with my mother and needed help. At our first family meeting, everyone agreed to pitch in, but to be honest, it didn't work. So finally, when I couldn't deal with it anymore, I left home.*

*It's hard to admit that I did that, but it got results. I told them, 'I'm not going back home until there's a written schedule and it's adhered to.' Once they realized exactly what was going on, once they lived it and saw what I was dealing with, they were willing to help. We made out a schedule and most of the time it works.*❞ —LINDA K.

*"Last time I visited my mother, Richie came with me. I got a sinus infection while we were there and spent a lot of time in bed, so he was in charge. Each day, when he went off to read the paper, Mom would come down and say, 'Now don't let me disturb you, dear. Keep on reading.' But then she would talk and talk and talk at him for hours.*

*I wouldn't have wished this on him, but in retrospect I'm relieved that he had that experience. Now he can understand why I come home from these visits feeling so exhausted."* —CARLA P.

and all-consuming undertaking, if you are absorbed by her needs for more than a few months, do not jeopardize your marriage. It is too important. Your parent will have to do with less of you because your mate, even if he doesn't say so, needs a little more of you. Here are some approaches that should help during this time:

♦ **Clarify who's responsible.** Is each of you solely responsible for your own parents, and not at all responsible for your spouse's parents? Is the woman responsible for both sets of parents? (Of course not, but this assumption is made with frightening regularity.) Should a spouse be expected to give up his weekends, vacations and evenings to join you when you visit your parent? Or should a spouse give up the pleasure of your company because you believe you should be at your parent's side whenever you're not working?

These perceptions will vary enormously from couple to couple, and you need to talk about them. Don't make assumptions or hang on to hidden expectations. Come up with an agreement.

In general, your parent is your responsibility and you can't expect your spouse to take on your family duties. But you can reasonably expect him to support you through this period, to offer a shoulder to cry on and a sympathetic ear, and to pick up some of the household duties—housework, childcare—that you can no longer manage.

♦ **Be clear about how your spouse can help.** Your spouse may want to help, but may not know how. He may offer advice, only to find that it triggers an argument. Unable to "fix things" for you, he feels inadequate and resentful.

Don't expect your spouse to read your mind or assume he knows how you feel. Tell him what you are feeling and what you need from him, whether it is emotional support and understanding or more tangible assistance. "I need to stop by Mom's house two nights a week. It would be great if you could shop and make dinner on those days."

Even if the help you receive is minimal, remember to thank your spouse for it. He will be more apt to help in the future.

♦ **Consider his feelings.** Your spouse will certainly be affected by the stress you are under and the changes in the household. Not only is he getting less of your attention, but if he has been your confidant in the past, he may feel shut out be-

❝*When my mother-in-law became sick, I started visiting her, fixing her meals, making sure that she was all right. I guess it's my nature to take care of people. But then I became resentful. I don't really like her—she is very critical—and I had my own parents to take care of. I couldn't hide my resentment, and it caused regular spats between Steve and me.*

*Finally I told him that I was glad to help, but that I would not be responsible for her care. I was firm about it. I explained what I would and would not do.*

*He was incredibly understanding. He didn't realize that I had been feeling any of this. Through our conversation, he began to realize that he'd been denying the whole thing about his mother, and dumping it on my shoulders.*

*I still visit her, but not nearly as much, and always with lots of support from him, which is all I really wanted in the first place.* ❞

—ALICIA B.

cause he can't share your grief. He may be afraid that if he voices his own needs or opinions, he will appear selfish or unsympathetic. And no matter what is happening with you, he will have his own grief to deal with. He may be forced to think about his parents' future, or may be painfully reminded of his own aging process.

With all that you are dealing with, it's hard to think about someone else's sadness or anxiety, but try.

Your distraction may be mistaken for a sign that you don't care, and small misunderstandings can expand into large ones if not attended to. Encourage your spouse to talk about his feelings. And give him the time and the space to vent them.

◆ **Make time for your mate.** When a parent's care is chronic, don't forget to take time out for a dinner with your spouse, quiet walks together or brief getaways. Make time not simply for heavy talks, but for play, shopping, relaxing and simply staying in touch. These dates may not seem like a priority at the moment, but they are vital not only to your marriage, but to your own mental health.

# The Sandwich Generation

Your parents are elderly, your children are still children, and you are being pulled by both ends of the age spectrum. Each day you face a dilemma: Do you take Dad to his doctor's appointment or get your son to school on time? Do you visit your mother or watch your daughter's soccer game? When the day is done, there is practically no "you" left, just the echoes of all the people who need you.

This dual demand of child and aging parent is now so common that it has its own names—"the sandwich generation," "women caught in the middle," "the caregiver crunch." The situation has potential benefits—a child might pitch in and

## KEEPING SANE AT HOME

If your parent's care consumes a great deal of your time and emotions, call a meeting of your own immediate family—your spouse and children. Holding a meeting to discuss an issue, rather than talking about it here and there, over the laundry or TV, tends to lead to more productive conversations.

Follow the guidelines outlined for family meetings earlier in this chapter. Let each person talk about what he or she feels, and then discuss how everyone can work together and support each other, assigning specific chores and duties if necessary. When the issues are knotty, a family counselor, found through a mental health center or a family doctor, can be helpful.

help, and a grandparent might enjoy a child's company—but it can also leave you feeling torn, guilt-ridden and irritable.

Don't let your child get lost in the commotion, slipping down your ladder of priorities until he is hardly on it anymore. Address his needs and concerns, and be sure that your parent's crisis does not compromise the quality of your relationship with him.

◆ **Be honest.** Children, even very young children, can understand much more than we give them credit for. Tell your children what is happening, what you are feeling, why you are sad, and why you don't have as much time for them. Encourage them to ask questions, and then answer their questions directly. If a parent is dying, talk about that as openly as you can, too. (For more on children and death, see page 373.)

◆ **Take time to listen.** Don't assume that you understand a child's concerns. Let her tell you about them. Children respond to illness in unexpected ways and worry about issues that adults may not even consider. For example, a child may be wondering if she is going to have to give up her bedroom if Grandpa moves in, she may be worrying more about your health than about a grandparent's health or she may be concerned that Grandma's ailment is contagious.

Your child may not open up on your schedule, so be ready. When you sense that a child wants to talk, stop what you are doing. Get off the phone, stop cooking dinner. A child might not "save" his emotions for later, when you are free.

When he does open up, no matter what he says, be careful not to make him feel that his emotions are wrong, trivial or silly. And let him know you've really heard him.

◆ **Set aside time for him.** In your bulging schedule, planning a trip to the zoo may seem like a joke, but it's not. Spend some time, just the two of you, doing something unrelated to caring for Grandma. If you can't go to the zoo, take a slight detour on the way to the grocery store and go to the park or a toy store, even briefly. Have a private lunch together. Or if you have to make a long car trip, take your child with you and turn it into a special occasion.

♦ **Let him help.** If your child shows any interest in helping with your parent's care, give him a job to do. Just keep your requests reasonable. Even a toddler can stroke Grandma, carry her blanket to her or draw a picture for her. Children want to be included in family situations and will be proud of what they can do to help.

♦ **Let her refuse to help too.** Younger children may be eager to help but older children, especially adolescents, may want to keep a distance. They may be uncomfortable with their grief or sadness, or feel "grossed out" by aspects of your parent's care. Or they may be preoccupied with what they consider to be more important aspects of their lives—friends, parties, music or sports. While these priorities may seem skewed to you, they are a normal and a necessary part of teenage development. Urge teenagers to understand the importance of family and responsibility, but allow them to be children, too, even if it means distancing themselves some from you and your parent's situation.

♦ **Get at the cause of bad behavior.** Children have an uncanny ability to pick up on stress. Your stress makes them feel stressed, and young children often don't know what to do with it except to cry and whine and run in circles.

They also misbehave to express their own pain, jealousy and confusion. Sometimes, if the only way a child can get your attention is by doing something bad, then that is what he is going to do. For him, an angry reaction from you is better than no reaction at all.

*"My father has been quite frail for three years and I feel angry sometimes that my children aren't seeing the man I knew. I tell them what he used to be like, but they just see this very weak person who needs a lot of peace and quiet.*

*Last time we were there, the kids were playing in the garden, and he said, 'When the hell are you going to leave? This noise is too much.'*

*I don't know whether to bring them up next summer when I go. It's hard on him and hard on them."*
—JANE C.

Remember that you are the adult here. Your child is far less able than you are to deal with all these emotions. Spending time with him and talking openly should fend off some problems. But when there are outbursts, remain calm and try to understand the root of the problem. Don't condone his behavior, but allow some of it. Everyone needs a little forgiveness right now. If things become unmanageable or worrisome, talk with a family counselor or a child psychologist.

◆ **Show your child your younger parent.** If your parent is very sick, confused or grumpy, pull out some old photos or, better yet, some home movies. Show your children what Grandpa used to be like in his younger and stronger days. You might tell them stories of things you used to do together. Help them to understand who this man is and what he means to you. Help them to separate the sickness from the person.

# In the Workplace

You are sitting in your office and the phone rings. It's your father. His speech is garbled and he seems confused. You're worried, but you have a meeting with your boss in twenty minutes. What do you do?

Your mother goes to adult day care until five o'clock each day, but you don't get home until six. What do you do?

When a parent needs help, some caregivers cut back their work hours, some end up quitting their jobs, some change jobs. Most continue on, but many jeopardize their futures with the company. Before you veer off your career track, think long and hard about your options.

◆ **Organize your day.** Make a schedule of your day, and look for ways that you might be more efficient. Are there errands that can be skipped, or done in the morning or during breaks at work? Are there certain chores that others in your household might be able to take over? Are there routine commitments that you can drop or cut down on?

◆ **Reduce stress.** Enroll in a stress management class, or take 10 minutes out each day for yoga or meditation, or even just a quiet moment alone. Find the time because it will allow you to be more productive and to have greater stamina for your responsibilities.

◆ **Set down rules.** If you are called at work frequently by your parent, health aides, care managers and others involved in your parent's care, set down some firm rules about when you can be interrupted and under what circumstances. It sounds heartless, but it's better to be clear than to be annoyed with home-care workers (or your parent), or to be reprimanded by your supervisor.

## DISCRETION AROUND THE WATER COOLER

At work, be careful what you say to whom. If necessary, talk to your boss directly—*before* gossip about your long-distance phone calls or exhaustion at work gets back to him, and the situation becomes distorted.

## THE FAMILY AND MEDICAL LEAVE ACT

Under the 1993 Family and Medical Leave Act, employees must be offered at least 12 weeks of unpaid leave to care for an ill family member—a parent, spouse or child (but not a grandparent or the parent of a spouse). The Act applies to all businesses with 50 or more employees (at sites within 75 miles of one another). An employee must have been with the company for at least one year and must have logged at least 1,250 hours in the previous 12 months (about 24 hours a week) to be eligible for leave. The Act mandates that:

- If possible, employees must give 30 days notice that they are taking a leave.

- Employees (except for those in the 10 percent of highest-paid positions) are entitled to get their old job back, or a post with equivalent duties, benefits and pay.

- Employees are entitled to their full health benefits while on leave. However, an employer can demand to be paid back for insurance premiums if the employee quits the job at the end of the leave.

- Leave can be taken in bits and pieces—a few days or even a few hours at a time—if the employer and employee both agree on the arrangement.

- An employer can require that vacation or sick days be used at the beginning of the leave.

◆ **Enlist help.** Talk to relatives, family friends and neighbors, or find a volunteer visitor who can check on your parent when a minor crisis strikes during work hours. Be sure to have more than one name and number in case the first person on your list is not available.

◆ **Contact the office of human resources.** Most large companies have personnel who can provide information about eldercare and community services. Some businesses also provide national referrals and free counseling to employees, and some sponsor support groups, seminars and information fairs on eldercare. They can also tell you about work flexibility rules.

◆ **Plan ahead.** If you know that your parent is going to need you in the near future—if she is very ill and the doctor says she could have another stroke any day, for example—talk with your boss and take responsibility for making provisions to get your job done if you are called away.

## NEGOTIATING
## WITH YOUR BOSS

Bosses want employees to be happy, sure, but their number one concern is getting the job done. So when you talk to a boss about changing hours, taking time off or other work arrangements, couch it in terms a boss can appreciate.

Rather than telling a sob story and asking your boss to help you, come up with a solution and then pitch your plan to the boss. Work out all the details in advance and then explain why your plan will be at least as good as the current way of operating. (You might want to provide a written proposal, outlining the plan, before you meet.)

As you sell your idea, be sure to keep the focus on your professional goals and the goals of the company, rather than on your personal needs. And let the boss know that you are committed to this job.

Then propose a trial period, which gives both you and your boss a chance to test this arrangement before buying it.

## A Company Plan

If your workplace has a large pool of employees who are caring for an elderly relative, talk with company executives about flexible hours, a shorter work week or job-sharing. More and more companies are allowing such arrangements, as employees increasingly find themselves caring for an elderly parent or a young child. Some companies have contracts with eldercare services which provide referrals nationwide along with counseling and caregiving tips. Making such an arrangement is good business, in terms of worker productivity. Some of the larger referral services include Work/Family Directions at 800-635-0606, Child and Eldercare Insights at 216-356-2900, Partnership Group at 215-643-8383 and Dependent Care Connection at 800-873-4636. Or contact the American Association of Retired Persons at 800-424-3410 to request a package on how companies can develop eldercare services for employees.

Use statistics and studies to back up your proposal. Nationwide, 10 to 20 percent of the work force has some responsibility for an elderly person, and many workers have significant duties, spending 20 to 40 hours a week caring for an elderly relative. Studies show that with company support (referral services, flexible hours, etc.) employees are less apt to use their business phones for personal calls, arrive late or leave early, call in sick, use drugs and alcohol or have financial problems. (Don't lay it on too heavy, though, or your boss may start screening job applicants and hire orphans only.)

Find out what other companies in your area or in the same industry are doing and use them as role models. Employers often respond to competition.

# Chapter Thirteen

# PAYING THE WAY

*What Medicare and Medicaid Really Cover
• Medigap and Long-Term Care Insurance
• Financial Planning • Homes as Collateral •Tax Tips
• Financial and Legal Counsel*

O F ALL THE ISSUES INVOLVED IN PARENTCARE, THE financial ones are often the most daunting, especially those having to do with health care and nursing homes. How do you pay for those whopping medical bills? How much insurance is enough? When, if ever, do you dig into your own savings? And how do you sort through the Byzantine rules governing Medicare and Medicaid, taxes and estates, which are full of exceptions, constantly changing and, in most cases, different from state to state?

No family is exempt from financial headaches. If you are not concerned about your father's day-to-day survival, you may be worried about his future security or a dwindling inheritance. If you are not dealing with a mother who is unwilling to spend a dime, you may be trying to contain one who doesn't realize how little money she actually has. Then there are the siblings who may bicker about what is being spent, saved or given away.

Finances are a private and often touchy subject, but if you can, help your parent to look at the full picture and plan for what may come. This chapter and the next lay out the groundwork. But whatever financial problems you face, the best solutions require advance planning, so don't delay.

# Talking About Money

Tread gently when you raise the subject of money with your parent. Older people in particular perceive money as deeply connected to issues of personal independence, control and dignity. Your mother may not want to divulge her financial situation. Your father may not want your advice. You walk a thin line between respecting such wishes and trying to ensure your parent's financial security—security that is important to both his care and his self-esteem.

Consider the issue from your parent's perspective. Not only did he grow up in an era when money wasn't discussed, but much of his identity may be invested in his role as a provider. He may feel that talking about his finances with you will strip him of that role. Furthermore, your parent's view of saving and spending may be quite different from yours. He lived through the Depression, watched prices rise astronomically throughout his lifetime, and now faces an unknown future, perhaps on a fixed income. As a result, he may be fiercely protective of every penny. He may not be willing to spend now in order to save later, to hire a lawyer, to buy adequate insurance or to pay for necessary home health care.

First ask your parent if he wants your help. Then listen to his views about his situation—his sense of what his problems are, his priorities and his solutions—before offering your own opinions. If he doesn't want to reveal financial details, you can discuss or describe basic financial tools and options without prying into the specifics of his situation. And let him make choices whenever possible. It's not easy, especially when you feel you know what's best, but remember, it's not just his money at stake, but his pride and self-worth.

If your parent would be more comfortable talking with someone outside of the family, give him the name of a good financial planner or lawyer. (See page 273.) If that doesn't work, consider the gravity

*“I have a joint checking account with my mother, but I still pay for a number of things out of my own pocket. She examines the statements carefully and would have a fit if she knew what some things cost. I've hired extra help and paid for a few minor repairs on the house. I also paid some of her lawyer bills because otherwise she would never have hired a lawyer. Anytime I do this, I keep receipts, so I can show my brother what I've spent. He's not apt to challenge things like that, but you can never be sure how people are going to react.”* —RHODA B.

of the situation. If your parent is facing a serious and immediate matter, spell out the consequences. Tell him calmly and clearly that if he doesn't get a loan he will have to move out of his house, or that if he doesn't pay his health aides enough, he will be left to manage on his own. If you still come up against a brick wall, back off. The landlord may evict him and the government may get your inheritance, but unless you have the right to control his bank account, there is nothing you can do but live with his decision. This is, after all, his money and his life. (If you believe he is making irrational decisions because of incompetence, you may need to obtain guardianship over him. See page 286.)

Whatever you do, unless you are very wealthy, don't dig into your own pockets. Don't spend your child's college savings or your retirement account on your parent's care. Buy him new clothes, nice meals and other gifts if you so desire. Cover some minor expenses if you feel it is necessary. But stop there. It may seem callous not to help, but you have set aside money for your own retirement, your children, your old age and your future pleasure, and you will need it. Give your parent your love, your time, your assistance, but not your savings—a recommendation that bears repeating because it is often so difficult to accept.

If you do dip into your own savings for some reason, treat it as a

## WHOSE MONEY IS IT?

You may find that as much as you want the best for your parent, you are also eyeing her assets with some thought to yourself. How much is there? How much might be passed along? How can your parent's money be protected?

To some extent, these are healthy thoughts—conscientious, not greedy. Your parent should protect whatever she can. Certainly, it is better that her money go to her heirs than to the government.

But be careful not to overstep the boundaries of helpful financial planning. This money belongs to your parent, not to you. It should be used, first and foremost, for her comfort and care, even if that means spending every dime on private nurses and medical equipment.

If your parent's money is disappearing because of decisions she is making which you believe to be foolish and there is nothing you can do to change her ways, resign yourself to the situation and accept the fact that you will never inherit any of her savings. You will save yourself from aggravation now and from disappointment when everything is gone.

business deal between two strangers. You might give your mother a loan that will be paid off at her death, or buy a share of her house and let her remain in it as a renter. Write up a contract that clearly defines the terms and the penalties, and have it signed by both parties.

If you find yourself paying for a substantial amount of your parent's expenses—and they do add up—keep a record of them, because you might be reimbursed from your parent's estate after her death. But alert your siblings to the expenses you are paying and make sure they agree to any reimbursement plan. Then send them regular financial reports and keep meticulous records, including all receipts, bills and cancelled checks. You are not betraying any assumptions of goodwill by being businesslike about these matters. Even the closest family relationships can be torn apart by financial issues. (See Chapter Twelve for more about sibling relationships.)

# Paying for Health Care

If medical and nursing-care bills are not pouring in now, the prospect that they will lies ominously ahead. The numbers can be staggering—$27,000 for a two-week stay in the hospital, $1,700 a year for routine medications, $8,500 for a month of rehabilitation, $30,000 a year for various home-care services, and $50,000 a year for nursing home care. Who can afford it? Where will all that money come from?

Ideally, public and private insurance programs combine to pay for this health care, but in reality they only cover a portion of it, often leaving families financially devastated. Your parent's insurance and finances must be in good order if he is to get the best possible coverage. If he hasn't already done so, it is imperative that he or you evaluate his health insurance immediately. Too little health insurance leaves him exposed to enormous financial risk, while too much means unnecessary payments for premiums, and delays if the plans overlap and insurance companies disagree on who should pay. Act now because your parent may become ineligible for certain types of insurance as he grows older, or if he is diagnosed with a serious illness.

Your family's greatest concern is probably long-term care—that is, extended care in a nursing home or at home. Hospital stays and doctor bills are largely covered by Medicare and individual health insurance policies, but long-term care is not, and

## FINANCIAL ALERT

Planning ahead for any necessary long-term care is an urgent matter. Your parent's choices will be increasingly narrowed the longer she waits. Consider long-term care insurance, life-care centers and other options now. This is a decision that should not be put off.

these costs can be exorbitant. Your parent should consider long-term care insurance if he is still relatively healthy, or talk with a lawyer about planning for Medicaid if he is nearing eligibility. (See page 260.)

## MEDICARE

Medicare (www.medicare.gov) is federal health insurance for people over 65 and certain disabled people under 65. The program is run by the Health Care Financing Administration, with the help of the Social Security Administration. Most people over 65 who have been employed or who are married to or widowed from someone who was employed are eligible for Medicare. Others may be able to enter the program by paying a small premium or by meeting certain income limits.

Everyone who receives social security payments automatically gets a Medicare card at age 65. If your parent doesn't receive social security, he should apply for Medicare three months before his 65th birthday. (The "enrollment period" begins three months before this birthday and ends four months after it, but get the paperwork done early. Failing to enroll during this time will mean delays in payment and possible penalties.)

Medicare is divided into two parts: Part A, hospital insurance, and Part B, medical insurance. The hospital insurance covers most hospital bills and a very limited amount of nursing home care. Recipients are responsible for certain deductibles and co-payments. Part B covers medical bills, including most doc-

---

### MEDICARE REQUIREMENTS

❖ Services must be provided by a Medicare-approved hospital, agency or institution, except in emergencies.

❖ Services must be "medically necessary"—that is, ordered by a physician in order to diagnose or treat an acute or chronic illness.

❖ Services must be provided within the United States or, in some circumstances, Canada or Mexico.

---

tor's fees, medical equipment, diagnostic tests, outpatient care and some medications. A monthly premium is required ($42.50 a month in 1996), and can be deducted automatically from social security payments. The annual deductible ($100 a year in 1996) must be met before payments begin, and a co-payment of 20 percent is required in most cases.

Although Part B (medical insurance) is optional, everyone is automatically enrolled when they become entitled to Part A. Most people subscribe to Part B—and your parent should as well—but if for some reason he doesn't want it (he is adequately covered by another policy), he should contact the local social security office to cancel the coverage. He should enroll in Part A in any case because if he waits to apply once he is hospital-

# MEDICARE PART A: HOSPITAL INSURANCE*

|  | COVERED | NOT COVERED |
|---|---|---|
| **Hospital stays** | ❖ Once the annual deductible ($768) is met, Medicare covers bills for the first 60 days of hospitalization; it requires a co-payment ($192 a day) for the next 30 days. This coverage begins anew with each "benefit period."** Any time a person is hospitalized for more than 90 days, the co-payment is quite high ($384 a day) and only 60 of these extra days will be covered in a lifetime. | ❖ Private-duty nurses<br>❖ The extra cost of private rooms unless privacy is judged "medically necessary"<br>❖ Personal services within the hospital, such as television and telephone |
| **Nursing home care** | ❖ The first 20 days in a benefit period are covered fully; a co-payment ($96 a day) is required for the next 80 days. No coverage is provided after 100 days.<br>❖ "Skilled care" (nurses and occupational, speech and physical therapists)<br>❖ Medications, meals | ❖ Care must come within 30 days of a three-day or longer hospital stay and must be related to the hospital stay; otherwise care is not covered.<br>❖ Any care on days beyond the 100 days allowed in a benefit period<br>❖ Custodial care (help with bathing, dressing, grooming, etc.)<br>❖ Extra charges for a private room |
| **In-home health care** | ❖ Part-time or intermittent home health care (nurses, therapists and home health aides) when prescribed by a doctor for treatment and/or rehabilitation, and when the patient is homebound<br>❖ 80 percent of approved fees for medical equipment | ❖ Full-time nursing care<br>❖ Homemakers, companions, health aides, meal-delivery and other services unrelated to prescribed treatment and/or rehabilitation<br>❖ Medications |
| **Hospice care** | ❖ All medical and nursing care, medical supplies, short-term hospitalization, home care and counseling<br>❖ Some of the cost of drugs and inpatient respite care | ❖ A portion of the charge for drugs and inpatient respite care |
| **Psychiatric care** | ❖ 190 days, over a lifetime, in a free-standing psychiatric hospital (as opposed to a wing of a general medical center, which would then count as general hospitalization) | ❖ Any care that exceeds 190 days |
| **Blood** | ❖ Unlimited coverage after the first three pints | ❖ The first three pints in each calendar year |

* Dollar amounts are 1999 figures.
** A "benefit period" begins after at least 60 days free of hospitalization or skilled nursing care.

## MEDICARE PART B: MEDICAL INSURANCE*

| | COVERED<br>(at 80 percent, after a $100 deductible is paid each year) | NOT COVERED |
|---|---|---|
| **Doctor's fees** | ❖ Most doctor's bills, including second opinions and some care from Medicare-approved special practitioners, such as nurses, social workers and physician assistants | ❖ Charges in excess of approved fees<br>❖ Routine physical exams<br>❖ Routine dental care, some chiropractic care and foot care |
| **Outpatient hospital care** | ❖ Medical services and supplies, including emergency-room visits, one-day surgery and some rehabilitation | ❖ Mental health services require a 50 percent co-payment |
| **Therapy** | ❖ Limited outpatient physical, occupational and speech therapy | ❖ Anything beyond $900 for such therapy |
| **Laboratory services** | ❖ Blood and urine tests, X rays, scans, biopsies, etc. | |
| **Medical equipment and supplies** | ❖ "Medically necessary" equipment, including wheelchairs, oxygen equipment, walkers, etc. | ❖ Eyeglasses, hearing aids, dentures |
| **Ambulance service** | ❖ Cost of ambulance transport | |
| **Preventive care** | ❖ Mammograms and pap smears, pneumococcal vaccine, hepatitis B vaccine | ❖ All other preventive care, including routine screenings, vision and hearing exams |
| **Drugs** | ❖ Drugs administered by a doctor or nurse | ❖ Most prescription and nonprescription drugs |

\* As of 1999

ized, he will be faced with a mountain of paperwork and bureaucratic delays at an already difficult time.

## Accepting Assignment

Medicare tries to keep costs under control by determining in advance what it will pay for each medical procedure. When a doctor accepts this assigned fee as full payment for a given service—called "accepting assignment"—your parent pays only the yearly premium, the deductible and the 20 percent co-payment. More than 70 percent of doctors are "participating physicians," which means that they accept assignment on *all* Medicare claims.

If a doctor does not accept assignment—for example, if a doctor charges your parent $220 for a test when the approved Medicare fee is only $200—then your parent pays the 20 percent co-payment *plus* the $20 difference between the doctor's fee and Medicare's approved fee.

There is a limit to how much a doctor can charge, however. In 1995, doctors were permitted to add no more than 15 percent to Medicare's approved fees. This means that when Medicare's approved fee for a service is $100, the most a doctor can charge is $115. (Of course, a doctor may charge any price he chooses for services that Medicare does not cover, like routine physicals.)

If your parent is happy with his doctor, he may choose to pay the extra charge. Otherwise, he can find a doctor who accepts assignment either by calling doctors' offices or by looking in the *Medicare Participating Physician/Supplier Directory*, which can be found in public libraries, social security offices and senior citizen centers.

## Medicare Extended

If your parent has little in the way of income and assets, he may be able to get under the Medicare umbrella at a discount—no premiums, deductibles or co-payments.

*The Qualified Medicare Benefi-*

## HELP WITH INSURANCE FORMS

Doctors' offices file Medicare claim forms (and they have 12 months to do so, so you may need to prod a bit if your parent is waiting to be reimbursed), but your parent is responsible for other insurance forms and any Medicare appeals, as well as questions about billing. It's easy to postpone these tedious tasks, particularly when you have a lot of other things on your mind. In fact, many people fail to get money owed to them from insurance programs because they put off filing forms and appeals indefinitely.

If the bills, papers and forms are too much for your parent or you to handle, call the area agency on aging or the local legal aid office. Some states offer help, at least with Medicare claims and appeals, if not with other insurance paperwork, free of charge or for a nominal fee.

You can also hire an insurance claims agent (aka a medical billing agent, public health adjuster, medical insurance consultant) to handle this job. These agents usually will meet with you for one free consultation, and then either charge 10 to 15 percent of the amount reimbursed, set an hourly fee of $25 to $55, or bill a flat amount for each claim.

The field is new and unregulated, so be sure to get references before you hire an agent. For referrals or information about the field, contact the National Association of Claims Assistance Professionals (708-963-3500).

ciary Program (QMB), also known as the Medicare Buy-In Program, is for people with incomes at or below the national poverty level, and with limited assets. The state pays Medicare premiums, deductibles and most co-payments.

The Specified Low-Income Medicare Beneficiary Program (SLMB) is for people whose incomes are up to 10 percent above the national poverty level. Under this program, the state pays just the Medicare Part B premium.

To learn more about either of these programs (requirements vary from state to state), contact the state or local Medicaid, welfare or social services office.

## Appealing a Medicare Decision

Don't think for a minute that it's not worth challenging the bureaucracy of Medicare. It is. According to the Health Care Financing Administration, which manages Medicare, about 70 percent of all appeals are successful to some extent. If you disagree with a Medicare decision—if coverage has been refused or is inadequate, or if there is some other problem—request a review of the claim. Tackling all that red tape may fill you with dread, but your chances of winning your case are quite good.

If an institution, an individual or another health-care provider tells your parent that Medicare won't cover a performed service or procedure, ask the provider to send in a claim anyway, so you can get an official determination from Medicare. Then, to challenge that decision, follow

*"The hospital was going to discharge my mother because Medicare allowed only so many hospital days for her procedure and then they wouldn't pay anymore. But I knew she wasn't well enough to be discharged, so I told the discharge planner that I was leaving her there and contesting the decision.*

*It was a battle, but in the end Medicare paid the additional hospital bill, which was about $5,000. It was definitely worth the trouble. You can't let these guys get the best of you. You have to fight for what's right."* —LUCILLE L.

the instructions on the back of the notice. For more information on how to appeal decisions, contact the local social security office, the Medicare intermediary or carrier (private insurance companies contracted by the government to oversee Medicare claims) or the state Peer Review Organization, a physician watchdog group contracted by the federal government to monitor the hospital care of Medicare recipients.

The local social security office or area agency on aging can tell you how to contact these organizations in your parent's state.

## MEDIGAP

Medigap is the colloquial term used to describe private insurance that fills some, but not all, of the holes in Medicare coverage. Typically this supplemental insurance

## THE TEN STANDARD MEDIGAP PLANS

|  | PLAN A | PLAN B | PLAN C | PLAN D | PLAN E | PLAN F | PLAN G | PLAN H | PLAN I | PLAN J |
|---|---|---|---|---|---|---|---|---|---|---|
| Basic benefits* | yes | yes | yes | yes | yes | yes | yes | yes | yes | yes |
| Hospital (Part A) deductible |  | yes | yes | yes | yes | yes | yes | yes | yes | yes |
| Nursing care coinsurance |  |  | yes | yes | yes | yes | yes | yes | yes | yes |
| Foreign travel emergency ($250 deductible, 80% coverage) |  |  | yes | yes | yes | yes | yes | yes | yes | yes |
| Part B deductible |  |  | yes |  | yes |  |  |  |  | yes |
| Part B excess doctor fees |  |  |  |  |  | yes 100% | yes 80% |  | yes 100% | yes 100% |
| Personal care at home** |  |  |  | yes |  |  | yes |  | yes | yes |
| Prescription drugs ($250 deductible, 50% coinsurance) |  |  |  |  |  |  |  | yes up to $1,250 | yes up to $1,250 | yes up to $3,000 |
| Preventive medicine ($120 a year) |  |  |  |  | yes |  |  |  |  | yes |

*co-payments for hospitalization and, after Medicare benefits are used up, full coverage for 365 days (over a lifetime); coinsurance on other expenses under Part B of Medicare; three pints of blood each year

**only when a person is also receiving skilled home care covered by Medicare

pays the cost of premiums, co-payments, deductibles and physician bills that exceed Medicare's approved charges. It does not cover much, if anything, outside of Medicare's realm, including long-term care.

Medigap insurance is highly recommended for most people, to protect them against ongoing medical expenses. But it isn't for everyone. For example, it may not be a good choice for anyone who is nearing the financial eligibility limits for Medicaid, or for someone who is enrolled in an HMO or other managed-care plan or group-health plan that provides ample coverage.

If Medigap insurance is necessary for your parent, he should, if possible, buy a policy within six months of enrolling in Medicare Part B. During this window of opportunity, he cannot be denied coverage because of existing medical problems. But after this six-month enrollment period is over, insurance companies can increase the price of the policy, refuse to cover your parent or attach an array of conditions to the policy.

## Ten Medigap Plans

To make shopping easier, states limit Medigap to ten standard plans—ranging from plan A, the core plan which is available in all states, through plan J, the most comprehensive and expensive plan. By law these plans cannot vary from company to company or state to state. And to further simplify life, the language and format used in all of the plans are also standardized.

But—yes, there is always a but—there are a few exceptions to all this standardization. Some states do not offer all of the plans, so your mother in Kentucky may not be able to buy the same plan that Aunt Marjorie bought in Illinois. Some states offer special "Medicare SELECT" policies, which work like managed-care plans—patients are required to use a designated group of doctors, clinics and hospitals. And finally, insurers are allowed to add benefits to a standard plan, thus making it no longer standard.

So despite standardization, you or your parent should read any policy carefully to understand exactly what is covered and what, if any, exclusions or restrictions exist. Ask the company for a clearly-worded summary—something insurance companies are required to provide. By and large, your parent will be comparing apples with apples, so she should be able to decide with relative ease which type of plan she wants, and then to shop around for the best price and service and the most stable and reliable company.

## Medigap Shopping Tips

The National Association of Insurance Commissioners and the Health Care Financing Administration recommend these guidelines for people buying a Medigap policy (if you have any problems with an insurance company or agent, contact the state insurance department or call the Medicare Hotline at 800-638-6833):

◆ **Don't buy more policies than you need.** Duplicate coverage is expensive and unnecessary. It's also generally prohibited.

◆ **Be careful when replacing an existing policy.** Your parent must be given credit for the time spent under the old policy in determining if any restrictions on preexisting conditions apply under a new policy. And while he must sign a statement saying that he plans to terminate the old policy, he shouldn't cancel until he's sure he wants new one.

◆ **Don't be pressured.** Take time to pick the best policy. Your parent shouldn't be forced or frightened into buying a policy. (Pressuring prospective buyers is against the law, so report it.)

◆ **Know the company you're dealing with.** Check with the state insurance department to make sure a company or agent is licensed. Beware of any claims that a policy is sponsored by a state agency or that an insurance agent is working for the government—neither is true.

◆ **Check the right to renew.** States now require that Medigap policies be guaranteed renewable.

This means that the company can refuse to renew your policy only if you do not pay the premiums or you made material misrepresentations on the application. Beware of older policies that let the company refuse to renew on an individual basis. These policies provide the least permanent coverage.

◆ **Check for preexisting-condition exclusions.** Don't be misled by the phrase "no medical examination required." If your parent has had a health problem recently, the insurer might not cover treatments related to that problem until the policy has been in effect for six months.

◆ **Complete the application carefully.** Do not believe an insurance agent who says that the medical history on an application is not important. If you leave out any of the medical information requested, coverage could be refused for a period of time for any medical condition you neglected to mention. The company could also deny a claim for treatment of an undisclosed condition or cancel your policy.

◆ **Use the "free-look" provision.** Insurance companies must provide at least 30 days to review a Medigap policy. If your parent doesn't want the policy, he can send it back within 30 days and get a refund of all premiums paid.

## MANAGED-CARE PLANS

As a Medicare beneficiary, your parent has the choice of using the traditional fee-for-service coverage and buying a Medigap policy to cover what Medicare doesn't, or he can sign up with a managed-care plan that has a contract with Medicare. Managed-care plans, also known as coordinated-care plans, are what most people refer to when they talk about health maintenance organizations (HMOs), but in fact they include both HMOs and another type of plan, competitive medical plans (or CMPs).

Don't let the alphabet soup confuse you. Managed-care plans are simply health insurance and health care wrapped into one. They provide comprehensive coverage, usually at lower rates, but they also dictate who provides the health care and where it is delivered. Members must get their medical care from a network of physicians, nurses, therapists and other professionals within the plan, and usually they must use only specific hospitals, nursing homes and other institutions. These practitioners may be perfectly good at what they do, but the choice is limited and the list may not include your parent's doctor or the best medical specialists in the area.

Still, if your parent likes the doctors and the affiliated institutions in the network, these plans can provide an attractive package. Managed-care companies that have contracts with Medicare receive premiums directly from the government—your parent pays no premiums—and the plans cover all the services normally covered under Medicare as well as many services not covered by Medicare, such as dental care, preventive care, hearing aids, eyeglasses and prescription drugs. Because this coverage is so extensive, Medigap insurance is unnecessary.

Be aware, however, that if your parent joins a managed-care plan and later decides to cancel her policy and return to the traditional fee-for-service coverage, her age or her physical condition may limit her choice of Medigap policies.

## LONG-TERM CARE INSURANCE

The missing piece in all these policies is coverage for long-term care—and it's a very large piece indeed. Nursing home care, which can cost $50,000 a year or more can quickly devour a family's savings. In-home care often costs less, but it's still expensive, and the time and effort required to supervise and coordinate it take such an enormous toll on families that many end up sending a parent to a nursing home.

So who pays for all of this? Medicare has so many restrictions that it pays for only about two percent of all nursing home costs nationally. Private insurance currently

---

**FOR VETERANS ONLY**

If your parent is a veteran, he may be eligible for free or low-cost medical and nursing home care, and he may not need much in the way of supplementary health insurance. Call the local Veterans Affairs Office for more information on services and coverage.

---

picks up only about one percent of the tab. The rest is paid privately by individuals and, when they run out of money, by Medicaid, the government's insurance program for people who are poor.

Until recently, private long-term care insurance was prohibitively expensive and fraught with restrictions. Now the premiums are more reasonable and the coverage is more extensive. Nevertheless, it's still somewhat of a luxury.

Because these changes are relatively recent, your parent may not have long-term care insurance. And if she is already quite old or ill, she may not be eligible for it now. Often it's not an option after age 80, or if a person has been diagnosed with a debilitating illness. But if your parent is eligible, and if he has substantial assets to protect, long-term care insurance is worth investigating.

Prices for the policies vary, depending upon the type of plan and the age of the buyer. A 65-year-old person in good health can expect to pay around $3,000 a year for a pol-

---

**❝**I'm looking at long-term care insurance for myself, because it's too late for my parents. But when I think about the expense I wonder if it's really worth it. I'm only fifty-three—too young to think about nursing homes. But then, that's what always happens with these things. You don't think about them until you really need them, and then it's too late.**❞**                    —NELLY O.

## PAYING FOR LONG-TERM CARE WITH LIFE INSURANCE

If your parent already needs long-term care and doesn't have long-term care insurance, under certain circumstances he may be able to collect life insurance dollars to pay his bills. Hundreds of insurance companies now offer an arrangement known as living benefits (or advanced or accelerated benefits), in which policyholders collect benefits early—rather than passing them on to heirs—in order to pay for nursing homes, home care and other related expenses.

The specifics of each plan vary, though most require that the policyholder be expected to live for less than a year. Some life insurance companies pay only a fraction of the total benefit, while others pay almost all of it. Some pay the benefit in one large check, while others provide monthly payments. Some offer living benefits only on new policies, while others will add riders to existing ones.

Living benefits should not be confused with "viatical settlements," in which a third party pays an individual cash in return for becoming the owner and beneficiary of the policy. Under these agreements, a company or individual takes over a life insurance policy, pays the remaining premiums, and gives the owner a fraction of the value of the policy—often just 50 to 80 percent, depending upon life expectancy. These arrangements are often more flexible than living benefits, but they pay less and may affect taxes and other benefits, and they are often subject to abuse.

Before your parent cashes in his life insurance, he and you need to study any agreement carefully. Consider the reasons for cashing in, and find out if the income will be taxed, and if it will affect his Medicaid eligibility.

icy, but premiums can reach as much as $8,000 a year for an older person. Most policies then pay a fixed amount for each day of nursing home or in-home care, or they pay a percentage of the cost of services, up to a set maximum. Remember, your parent can't buy a long-term care policy once he is sick, so if he is thinking of buying one, he should do it soon.

### Who Should Buy Long-Term Care Insurance?

◆ **Those with ample assets.** The primary reason to buy long-term care insurance is to protect one's assets. Certainly your parent should not buy a policy if he would be eligible for Medicaid within, say, 12 to 18 months of entering a nursing home. As a rough guideline, to consider a long-term care policy he should have at least $50,000 in assets (not including his house and personal belongings). For a couple, the amount is higher, about $150,000 in assets. Those with $1 million or emore in liquid assets may not need the coverage because they can pay for care.

♦ **Those with adequate income.** Can your parent afford to pay another $300 to $500 a month? Some experts suggest that long-term care insurance should not cost more than 5 percent of a person's total income. If your parent fails to pay his premiums his policy will be cancelled. As you consider your parent's ability to pay, be sure to take into account how premiums will go up and how that will affect your parent's future budget, when it may be more limited than it is now.

If your parent is already spending too much on premiums, he should consider reducing a Medigap policy in order to buy long-term care insurance. After all, his biggest financial drain in the future is likely to be long-term care, not prescription drugs or co-payments.

♦ **Those who are likely to need long-term care.** No one can see the future, but based on the history of longevity and disease in the family, as well as your parent's current living situation, you can make an educated guess. If your father is at risk for heart disease he is less likely to need long-term care than a person who has a family history of Alzheimer's disease. If your mother lives with your sister who is

## MEDICAID PARTNERSHIP

A few states have established or are in the process of establishing innovative partnerships between Medicaid and the insurance industry, in which people who buy coverage for, say, three years of long-term care can go on Medicaid when their insurance coverage runs out and still protect all or some of their assets. Call the state insurance department or talk with an insurance broker to find out if such programs exist in your parent's state.

a retired nurse, she is less apt to need long-term care than a person who lives alone and far from family support. Also, is there a wealth of local volunteers and services on which your parent can rely, or does he live in a community with little in the way of social services?

### Selecting a Long-Term Care Policy

Your parent should compare several policies to find the one that best suits her needs. The state insurance department can tell her which companies sell long-term care insurance in her state. (She might also look into the possibility of adding a rider onto her current health insurance policy.)

When reviewing policies, be sure that any special features are worth the price paid in higher premiums. Any extras will add substantially to the cost. Your parent shouldn't simply decide what she wants and get a price; she should compare basic packages with more extensive policies, see what each item adds to the price of the policy, and then determine if it makes sense to pay the higher amount.

Some features to look for:

♦ **Broad coverage.** Be sure a long-term care policy covers in-home care and "custodial care"—supervision and help with dressing, eating, bathing and other daily tasks—in addition to nursing care. People often grow frail and need this custodial care, but only very limited nursing care.

If your parent is adamant about staying in her own home and willing to pay for the extra coverage, investigate policies that cover a range of home-care services, such as homemakers, companions and respite care.

♦ **Few restrictions.** A policy should not have prerequisites for coverage, such as specifying that nursing home care be preceded by hospitalization. Coverage should be based on need, not "medical necessity." Your parent should be covered as soon as he needs help with at least two personal tasks, such as bathing, dressing or eating.

If a policy denies coverage for preexisting medical conditions, the restriction should last for no more than six months.

♦ **Adequate reimbursement.** Most policies pay a fixed amount for each day of long-term care, and your parent pays the rest. Home care is usually covered at about half of the rate of nursing home care, so a policy might pay $100 a day for nursing home care and only $50 a day for home care. Of course, the higher the amount of daily coverage, the higher the premium.

To determine how much coverage your parent needs, calculate how much he can afford to spend on future long-term care—that is, how much is left over after he has paid his regular bills. And then find out the average per-day cost of nursing home care in his area. From there, it's simple subtraction. If nursing home care costs $120 a day and he has $40 a day in discretionary income, then he needs a policy that offers $80 a day in coverage.

*"My sisters think that my father should be in a nursing home because it would be cheaper, and they say he doesn't know or care where he is anymore. I think he should stay in his home with private nurses because I believe he does know the difference.*

*It's true, we're spending a tremendous amount of money for his care. All of his money is disappearing. I know what they're feeling because I'd planned on having some inheritance, too. But I think we have to make his life as comfortable as possible. I don't want the inheritance if it comes at such a price."*
—KATHERINE S.

♦ **Inflation protection.** If your parent buys $80-a-day coverage today, but doesn't need it for 15 years, the price of nursing home care may have gone up so much that his policy won't even cover meal service. For most people, a policy should allow for at least 5 percent inflation, compounded annually. Inflation protection is important for relatively young people (in their 60s or early 70s) though it may not be necessary for someone who is 75 or older, and therefore expected to need long-term care sooner. In this case, it might be worth buying a more generous policy with no inflation protection.

♦ **A reasonable waiting period.** The longer the waiting period before coverage kicks in, the cheaper the policy. Any waiting period less than 20 days will make the policy too expensive. However, a waiting period of more than 100 days reduces the chance significantly that your parent will ever put the policy to use.

♦ **A reasonable maximum.** Very few long-term care policies offer unlimited nursing home care, and those that do are expensive. Sometimes coverage is limited on a "per-stay" basis—a policy might cover 100 days and then as long as there's a break of at least 90 days in between, it will cover 100 days again. Other policies have lifetime limits—a given number of days or a specific dollar amount that will be covered over your parent's lifetime. Your parent should buy a policy with the highest maximum that she can comfortably afford. Be sure to check the limits on both nursing home and in-home care, as some policies set different maximums for each.

♦ **Waivers.** A policy should include a waiver that frees your parent from paying premiums while he is receiving long-term care.

♦ **Coverage for dementia.** Most policies today cover Alzheimer's and other "organic diseases of the brain" (as opposed to mental illness, alcoholism and drug addiction, which most policies do not cover). But check to be sure.

♦ **Guaranteed renewals.** Almost all long-term care policies are now guaranteed renewable, but be certain to check because this is imperative. A company should be allowed to cancel a policy *only* if the premiums are not paid, and under no other circumstances.

♦ **Fixed premiums.** Because your parent is likely to be living on a fixed income, he should find a policy that has fixed premiums. Otherwise he may find that just when he most needs this coverage, he can no longer afford to keep it. (Once a policy is purchased and the terms agreed upon, a company is permitted to raise premiums only if it does so for all its policyholders or a certain group of policyholders, not on your parent's policy alone.)

♦ **Nonforfeiture protection.** This provision can add 20 to 50 percent to the price of the policy, but is important for buyers who are relatively young (under 70). Nonforfeiture guarantees that the buyer will receive some value from the policy even if the policy is canceled.

The value—either some money back or partial long-term care coverage—is based on the premiums paid prior to cancellation. The longer the policy is held, the more value it accumulates.

◆ **A solid company.** Buying from a strong company is essential because the field is young, and companies have little history upon which to base their underwriting assumptions. A strong company will be better able to absorb errors. Check rating directories such as *The Insurance Rating Guide* published by Standard & Poor's (available in most public libraries) and be sure the company has one of the highest ratings.

Be leery if a company salesperson tells you that the state guarantees coverage if the company defaults. The premiums may be higher for such policies, and if the company fails, the coverage offered by the state won't be as generous as the terms of your parent's original policy.

## MEDICAID

Unless your parent is very comfortable financially, learn about Medicaid (Title XIX), the government health insurance program for low-income people. Many people who think they won't ever need it find that they do, because the cost of long-term care quickly drains a person's savings. Medicaid ends up paying for about half of all nursing home care nationally.

Learn the rules (or, better yet, confer with a lawyer) early on so that your parent doesn't scrape the bottom of his savings account need-

> **"**Our father told us years ago not to pay for expensive caretaking if he began to suffer from severe dementia the way his father did. He protected his assets so he would be eligible early for Medicaid. It all happened the way he'd imagined. I'm grateful he had such foresight.**"**   —FRED S.

lessly. He may qualify for Medicaid long before he thinks he will. He also may be able to protect some of his assets before going on Medicaid. (When older people use up their money to become eligible for Medicaid, the process is called "spending down.") See page 263 for more on protecting assets.

The Medicaid program covers almost all of a person's health-care costs, including nursing home care, but there is a price to pay. Many doctors and nursing homes won't take patients on Medicaid, or will accept only a limited number because the reimbursement rates are low. As a result, Medicaid patients sometimes seek health services in clinics where they wait and wait and wait, and then receive mediocre care. Or, quite often, unable to find a place in one of the better nursing homes, they settle for substandard care.

Despite these liabilities, Medicaid is a vital and welcome safety net. If your parent wants to protect his assets before going on Medicaid, get him to meet with a lawyer who specializes in Medicaid planning because the rules are complicated. If your parent cannot afford to hire a lawyer, contact the state legal services office or the state bar

## MEDICAID AND NURSING HOMES

There is a myth that any-one who is on Medicaid will automatically receive inade-quate, unacceptable nursing home care. It's true that the plushest nursing homes do not accept people on Medicaid. It's also true that most other homes limit the number of Medicaid patients they will accept. But plenty of attractive, well-man-aged nursing homes accept Medicaid patients—about one third of all nursing homes have at least some Medicaid patients.

Remember, an expensive nursing home isn't a guarantee that your parent will get loving, devoted care, just as a run-down exterior doesn't always mean shabby care. Appearance is an important clue to what kind of service is provided, but the qual-ity of care comes from the peo-ple who work in the facility— the philosophy of the adminis-trators and the devotion of the staff.

Many of the residences that accept Medicaid favor self-paying patients and admit only

a small number of Medicaid patients. A nursing home with 200 beds, for example, may admit only 15 or 20 Medicaid patients at any given time. Consequently, to get your par-ent into one of the better Med-icaid-certified homes, you need to get his name on waiting lists early or help him set aside enough money so that he can apply as a self-paying resident. If your parent has some sav-ings—enough to cover at least six months of nursing home care, and preferably more—he will have a far better chance of being accepted by the home of his choice. Once he is admit-ted, he cannot be discharged when he goes on Medicaid, even if those beds set aside for Medicaid patients are full.

Once your parent is in a home, you can see to it that he gets the best care possible by establishing a rapport with the staff and monitoring his care closely. (See Chapter Eleven for more information on nursing homes.)

association about legal aid to the el-derly, or call the organizations listed on pages 395 and 396 for counseling and information.

### What's Covered

Medicaid rules vary from state to state, but coverage must include:

- Inpatient and outpatient hospital services
- Physician services
- Periodic diagnostic tests and screenings
- Laboratory and X-ray services
- Rural health clinic services
- Nursing home care

• In-home health care for people eligible for nursing home care
• Medical transportation.

Beyond this list of "musts," many state Medicaid programs also cover dental, foot and eye care, prescription drugs, less intensive home health care, social workers, private-duty nurses, rehabilitative therapy (speech, occupational and physical), dentures, eyeglasses, case management, prosthetic devices and hospice care.

Medicaid usually covers the entire cost of an eligible patient's health care, although some states charge a small deductible or nominal co-payment for certain services.

## Who's Eligible

Broadly speaking, in order to qualify for Medicaid a single person is permitted to own no more than a home, personal belongings, a car and some small amount of savings (perhaps $2,000, plus some money set aside for burial and funeral expenses), and must have a meager income (a few hundred dollars a month or less in most cases). These standards vary, depending upon the individual's disability and medical needs, what other public assistance he receives, his life insurance, and other issues that a specific state deems important.

Because a spouse who remains at home continues to need financial support when a mate enters a nursing home, the rules for couples are more generous. Generally, a spouse can keep, in addition to a home, car and personal belongings, half of the couple's assets, but usually no more than $80,000 and no less than $16,000. Spouses can also keep their own income and usually some portion of their partner's income (usually no more than $2,000 a month), depending upon the well spouse's needs and the state's limits.

Beyond these broad federal guidelines, each state has its own unique and bewildering set of rules and exceptions. And workers in the department of social services are not in a position to advise potential applicants how to get on Medicaid early and protect their assets.

Here's an example of why it's important to know the rules: In some states the spouse who remains in the community is allowed to keep whatever assets are necessary to produce enough income to pay her regular bills. A person who receives $300 a month in social security but has $200,000 in the bank earning three percent—or $500 a month—might be allowed to keep the entire bank account so that she has enough income to live on. Most people are not aware of this provision and thus might wait until the $200,000 was virtually depleted before applying for Medicaid. In other states a spouse can refuse to contribute to nursing home bills and can keep all of her own income.

## How to Apply for Medicaid

The area agency on aging or, if your parent is in a hospital or nursing home, the facility's patient advocate, can tell you how to apply. In most states you need to contact the local department of social services or the human resources administration. Your parent will have to show proof of age and citizenship, a social security card, proof of current income from social security and retirement benefits, current bank statements, bank books and other financial statements, receipts from rent and utility bills and any other health insurance policies.

## Protecting Assets to Qualify for Medicaid

Your parent saved diligently so he could pass something on to his children. Maybe he wanted his parent's home or a piece of land to stay in the family. But faced with the prospect of hospital or nursing home bills, his savings, perhaps even the house or the land, are all in jeopardy. Your parent may be able to protect some of his assets and still become eligible for Medicaid, but to do so he has to plan well in advance. The sooner he acts, the more he will be able to protect.

For the time being, in most states your parent can protect his assets by giving them outright to others or by putting them in an irrevocable trust, one that he cannot touch or benefit from. (See page 291 for more on trusts.) But strict lim-

---

## A QUESTION OF MORALS AND MONEY

For some people, protecting assets and then going on Medicaid raises troubling moral questions. Medicaid and other public programs certainly are not intended to protect anyone's inheritance or extra spending money; they are meant for those who are truly needy. What your parent saves, taxpayers pay.

Your family has to be guided by its own moral and political code on this matter. Some people argue that whatever money an older person has should be spent on making his last years as comfortable as possible—it should not be protected for his children—and that receiving public assistance is demeaning. Others believe that using public monies when personal funds are available is criminal.

A third group contends that lifelong taxpayers who believed they were sufficiently covered by Medicare and were not offered adequate long-term care insurance (because until recently, it didn't exist) are justified in protecting whatever assets they can. Affluent people set up trusts to protect their estates from taxes, so why shouldn't people with smaller estates protect themselves from nursing home bills? The decision is up to your family. Familiarize yourself with the facts and do what's right for you.

**"**_When the lawyer talked to me about putting Dad's house in my name, I thought it was a great idea. Then I got home and I began to feel it was wrong. Dad believed in paying his own way. That was important to him. I didn't think he would want me to do this._

_The more I thought about it, the more confused I felt. I know he wanted us to have his house but I also know he wouldn't want to be on welfare or have us do anything dishonest. Here I was, choosing between these two horrible things, and he couldn't express his opinion because he was too sick._

_In the end, I didn't put the house in my name. I just felt it was wrong. We still have it now, but the lawyer tells me that the government will come after it eventually._**"**
—ANNE P.

itations and exceptions apply and they vary from state to state and change from year to year.

If your parent chooses to protect his assets in order to qualify for Medicaid early, don't let him be overly zealous about it. He needs money to live on. And remember, he would be well advised to keep enough money so that he can apply to a good nursing home as a self-paying resident. Also keep in mind that the opportunities to protect assets are becoming narrower and may eventually disappear. What is permitted today may not be permitted tomorrow.

To illustrate the nature of Med-

icaid planning, here are some examples of requirements and the practices used to comply with them.

♦ When a person applies for Medicaid, officials examine his financial records for the past 36 months to see what, if any, gifts or transfers have been made. Anyone who has given a substantial gift or otherwise transferred assets during this "look-back period" may not qualify for Medicaid until some time in the future. Usually the person must wait the number of months it would take for him to spend on nursing home care the amount that was given away or transferred.

For example, a person enters a nursing home and immediately gives his children $60,000. If the average cost of nursing home care in his area is $5,000 a month, then he would not be eligible to receive Medicaid for one year, the length of time it would take to spend $60,000 on his nursing home care.

One possible solution: Give only half of the assets away. If this same person gave only $30,000 to his children, he would have enough money to cover his nursing home bills during the penalty period, now only six months, but he would still have protected half of his funds.

♦ While individuals are allowed to keep a home as well as certain personal belongings, states will claim anything remaining in the estate after death to recoup what has been spent on nursing care.

A possible solution: Depending upon the state's rules, your parent may be able to protect his home by putting the deed in a child's name

**FOR MORE HELP**

**State counseling offices** that offer insurance advice can be found through the Medicare Hotline (listed below) or the area agency on aging.

**Local social security offices** have Medicare forms, *Your Medicare Handbook*, a directory of health-care professionals that accept Medicare as full coverage for most services and other information on Medicare.

**The local social services office** has information about Medicaid in your parent's state.

**The state insurance department** has brochures on state insurance rules, and Medigap and long-term care insurance. The department also handles complaints about insurance and can direct you to free or low-cost insurance counseling for the elderly.

**The Medicare Hotline** (800-638-6833) can answer general questions about Medicare, Medigap policies, insurance fraud and special Medicare beneficiary programs.

**Consumer Information Center** (Department 33, Pueblo, CO 81009—inquire by letter only) will send government publications such as the *Guide to Health Insurance for People with Medicare*, and other publications concerning Medicare.

**The National Insurance Consumer Helpline** (800-942-4242) is run by the insurance industry to answer questions about home and life insurance.

**The American Association of Retired Persons** (AARP) (800-424-3410) issues numerous helpful pamphlets on Medicare, Medigap, long-term care insurance, Medicaid and other insurance options. It also runs a Medicare/Medicaid Assistance Project.

**United Seniors Health Cooperative** (202-393-6222) is a nonprofit organization of older people who work to help other older people live healthy and independent lives. The group does much of its own research, publishes a newsletter and has a number of publications on insurance matters that are available to the public.

**Local senior organizations** usually have information on insurance policies and programs.

**The Internet has information** and answers to common questions. Try Health Care Financing Admininstration at www.hcfa.gov or search by topic.

(or that of another person). Even if your parent lives in the house during his lifetime, it would then be out of reach of state officials and other creditors.

# Financial Planning

If there is any question about your parent's financial state of affairs, she should do some planning. After reviewing her entire situation, she needs to create a current spending budget as well as a strategy for investments and insurance that will protect her in the future. If she has a large estate, she also needs to think about protecting her assets from taxes. (See page 289.)

You and your parent can do this together, you can do it for your parent if you have the authority to handle her finances, or she can hire a financial planner. If you are involved, remember to restrain any urge to take over—respect your parent's privacy, autonomy and her right to make her own choices, even foolish ones.

A comprehensive financial plan shouldn't take an inordinate amount of time and it is time well spent. It should protect your parent's future and give both of you some peace of mind today. The following guidelines will help you get started.

### Assess the Current Situation

Estimate your parent's financial worth by calculating the total value of all her assets (including savings, investments, real estate) and subtracting the amount of all debts (mortgages, loans, outstanding bills). This will give you an overall framework to consider as you review her finances.

Now calculate her current income, including pensions, social security and income from securities and retirement accounts. Then add up her monthly expenses, including mortgage or rent, food, utilities, home maintenance, insurance premiums, property taxes, clothing, transportation, medical bills, travel and entertainment. Re-

## AS EASY AS AUTOMATIC

Insurance premiums, mortgage payments and other routine bills can be paid automatically from a bank account so that policies don't lapse and credit is not jeopardized. This also frees your parent or you from one more monthly chore. Likewise, income such as social security and pension checks, can be deposited automatically so checks don't pile up or get thrown out accidentally. (If your parent doesn't want her bills paid automatically and you are concerned that she may forget to pay them, ask the creditor to notify you or another family member if bills become overdue.)

viewing past entries in a check-book may reveal some of her regular expenses.

If there is a net outflow, then how much of your parent's savings is being spent each month? How long can she continue this way? Are there expenses that can be trimmed or eliminated? Are there other sources of money (a home that can be used as collateral against a loan, a life insurance policy that can be cashed in, properties or other assets that can be sold)?

## Anticipate the Future

What will your parent's income and expenses be in three, five, ten years? What if he becomes ill, or more seriously ill? If the crystal ball portends trouble, how might your parent save for the future? Are there tax credits or deductions, or any free services which he might be eligible for now or in the future?

Also, is your parent's insurance adequate? Is the coverage redundant? Be sure that policies have not lapsed, or that he is not still paying for an old policy that is no longer necessary.

While looking at the future, your parent needs to consider ways to protect his assets. If they are substantial, he can protect some of them from estate and inheritance taxes, or if he is, say, $60,000 shy of Medicaid eligibility, he may be able to protect some of his money from nursing home and medical bills.

If both your parents are alive and you are helping them with their finances, explore how each of them would fare financially if the other became ill or died. Determine how each spouse's income and expenses

*"My parents have done nothing to prepare for their old age. They have simply spent whatever money they had without thinking of the future. They never listened to us when we told them to save. Now they are running out of money. Neither one of them is healthy and they are both growing helpless. I'm sure one of them, and probably both of them, will need nursing care at some point soon. And they won't be able to afford it.*

*My brothers and I are wondering who's going to pay for this. I probably have the most money of the three of us, but I also have four children. I can't afford to pay for nursing care nor do I think I should. I feel for them and I want to help, but I'm also angry at them for dumping this responsibility on us."* —DIANE P.

would change and how they might protect themselves now.

## Discuss Your Parent's Priorities

As you create a financial plan, talk about your parent's goals and priorities. What does he need money for and what is most important to him? Does he want to enjoy these years as much as possible, or is he committed to setting aside money for his children? Is he adamant that he pay all his bills without going on public assistance or borrowing? Encourage your parent to consider these issues so that he can arrange his assets to meet his goals.

## HOLDING ON TO THE PURSE STRINGS

While it is tempting to throw your hands up in the air and assign the whole financial mess to a professional, finances are too important a matter to relinquish to someone else's judgment. Financial advisors and lawyers should be used for just that—advising. Your parent, you or another family member should carefully oversee everything that a professional does. (If you don't understand something, keep asking until you do.) Under no circumstances should your parent give a financial planner, lawyer or other professional the legal authority to make financial decisions on her behalf without her (or your) approval.

### Develop—and Follow—a Plan

Once you know your parent's financial strengths and weaknesses, come up with a plan to meet her needs. This may include changing her spending habits, buying a Medigap policy, renting out a room in her house, setting up a trust, selling some assets or revising her investments to include more bonds and fewer stocks. (Again, you may need the help of a financial planner or lawyer. See page 273.)

Be sure your parent follows the course that's been laid out. It does no good to spend hours figuring out ways to save money if the cost-cutting measures are ignored. Give your parent encouragement and support about altering long-ingrained habits. And keep after her because, as you know, waiting is a dangerous game.

Review the plan in six months or a year, or any time there is a change in your parent's circumstances—a divorce, an accident, an illness or a financial windfall.

# Getting Cash Out of a Home

If your parent is cash-poor but home-rich, he should consider taking in renters, sharing his home or adding an accessory apartment. Or he can borrow money by using his home as collateral.

With a home equity conversion (HEC) plan, your parent may be able to get a lump of cash to renovate his house, receive a constant flow of cash to pay ongoing bills or obtain a line of credit to cover unpredictable expenses. Unlike home equity lines of credit, which require that the debt be repaid in monthly installments, HEC loans are usually not repaid until the home is sold or until your parent moves or dies. Eligibility requirements are typically based on age, income, assets, need, the value of the home and any outstanding debts and mortgages.

Borrowing is a complex business and a bad deal can get your parent into serious trouble. He should consult a lawyer to make sure that any arrangement he makes is a safe one. And he should be sure that any loan will actually cover his financial needs, now and in the future, because once he has used the equity in his home—and some of these loans have high interest rates—he may have little else to offer as collateral.

## REVERSE MORTGAGES

Reverse mortgages, the most common type of home equity conversion loans, are available in most states, usually from a bank or public agency. The various types include:

**Federally-insured loans.** Insured plans, also known as HECMs or Home Equity Conversion Mortgages, are the most popular and the most widely available reverse mortgage plans. While more expensive than some other reverse mortgages —lenders charge a closing cost and a premium—they are protected should the value of the loan exceed the value of the home. This guarantees that your parent will be allowed to stay in her home, and that the lender will not try to claim any other assets in addition to the home if the house depreciates. Also, payments to your parent are guaranteed in case the lender defaults on them—a reassuring advantage.

Ceilings exist, however, on the amount of equity that one can borrow against—about $150,000 in most states.

**Uninsured loans.** Loans that are not insured by the Federal Housing Authority are known as fixed-term loans, meaning that the loan must be paid back on a predetermined date, usually within three to ten years. Such loans are useful if your parent needs money for a specific period of time and expects to sell his home before or at the end of the term. Fixed-term loans are available only in a few states, and sometimes only in certain areas of a state.

**A reverse annuity mortgage.** In this arrangement, some of the money borrowed is used to purchase an annuity from a life insurance company, which in turn makes monthly payments to your parent for life. The loan has to be repaid when your parent moves, sells the house or dies, but the monthly payments continue, no matter where your parent lives, for the rest of his life (or until the last borrower dies, if a couple takes out a loan together).

It's a bit of a gamble though. If your parent lives a long time and receives years of payments, a RAM is a great investment. If he dies soon after the papers are signed, however, the cost is exorbitant (because the annuity purchased was expensive and little was paid from it). Borrowers are usually required to be more than 60 and sometimes older than 70.

## HOME REPAIR LOANS

Home repair loans, which are typically offered by government housing agencies or nonprofit organizations, provide a one-time lump sum for home repairs (fixing a roof, or repairing plumbing, weatherstripping and insulation) or renovations that make a house accessible for people with disabilities (installing ramps, grab-bars, a lift or lower cabinets). Home repair loans cannot be used for cosmetic work or additions judged to be unnecessary.

The loans are usually offered without interest, or at a very low interest rate, and the construction may increase the value of the home enough to cover the loan and possibly even leave some profit.

## PROPERTY-TAX DEFERRAL LOANS

In many states, elderly people who meet certain income limits can defer paying property taxes. The amount owed, plus interest (which is fixed by law, usually at around six to eight percent), is paid off when the person sells the house, moves or dies. For more information, call the local tax collector.

## SALE-LEASEBACK PLANS

Unlike other plans, which are offered by government agencies or private lenders, sale-leaseback deals are usually made between individuals. Your parent sells his home to another person, but remains in it indefinitely as a tenant with a guaranteed lifelong lease. While your parent gets cash and is no longer responsible for the expenses and responsibilities that come with being a homeowner, he also relinquishes full control over his home.

 **FOR MORE HELP**

**The American Association of Retired Persons (800-424-3410)**

AARP operates a Home Equity Information Center.

**The National Center for Home Equity Conversion 7373 147th St., Suite 115, Apple Valley, MN 55124**

Send a check for $1.00 and a self-addressed, stamped envelope to receive an updated list of local programs that offer these loans; for a book on the subject, send $24.95.

# Tax Tips

◆ Many older people are not required to file federal tax returns, so make sure of your parent's tax status before doing unnecessary work.

◆ People over 65 are entitled to a tax credit and a higher standard deduction.

◆ People over 55 have the option of taking a one-time capital gains tax exclusion on $125,000 from the sale of a home.

◆ Individual states offer various tax-relief programs for seniors. Call the local tax office about them.

◆ Elderly people are not required to pay taxes on most public assistance, such as mortgage assistance, home improvements paid for by the state to reduce home energy costs, nutrition programs and veterans benefits. They may be required to pay taxes on part of their social security income, however.

◆ Your parent can deduct medical payments that exceed 7.5 percent of his adjusted gross income. This includes all medical and hospital care not reimbursed by insurance, dental care, nursing home care, health insurance premiums and co-payments, prescription drugs, nursing services, medical aids such as eyeglasses and hearing aids and medical supplies.

Your parent can also treat as a medical expense the cost of any home improvements that have been made because of a disability or medical condition, such as installing railings or widening hallways and doorways to accommodate a wheelchair. If the change increases the value of the house (say your parent installs central air conditioning because of his asthma), then he can deduct the amount spent minus the amount the property increases in value (which has to be determined by an appraiser).

◆ If you are paying your parent's medical bills, you can add them to your deductions *if* you provided more than half of your parent's total support in that year (whether or not you claim him as a dependent on your tax return).

◆ Claiming your parent as a dependent, and taking all the related deductions and credits, is possible only under the following circum-stances: if your parent's annual income, not including social security, is less than a few thousand dollars, *and* you pay for more than half of his care and living expenses (if your parent does not live with you, then you have to pay half the cost of keeping up his home for that year), *and* no one else claims him as a dependent.

◆ If several siblings are sharing the costs of your parent's care, then one of you can claim a "personal dependency exemption" by filling out a Multiple Support Declaration.

◆ Tax credits are available for certain home services, adult day care and supervision. If, for example, you hire someone (and pay their social security contributions) to care for your parent while you work, you can take a credit of up to 30 percent of the cost of the care.

---

**"***After my father died, I had to file his tax return. My father was incredibly orderly. But I have never seen such a disorganized mess as his tax information, including masses of past tax forms and receipts. I hired an accountant to help me and we sorted through papers for months.***

***Dad always hated the IRS and taxes. He died on April 15th which has become a little joke in our family—maybe, lying in that hospital bed, he started thinking about his taxes and the IRS and it was just too much for him to bear. Taxes. It should be on his death certificate as cause of death.***"** —GLORIA C.

## GETTING TAX HELP

**Tax Counseling for the Elderly** is a program funded by the Internal Revenue Service that offers free tax help to older people. The counselors (all volunteers) are trained in issues pertinent to the elderly, such as social security benefits, tax credits and rebates. The volunteers set up shop each year in early February in public libraries, senior centers and banks (some will make house calls). The American Association of Retired Persons sponsors some of these volunteer tax counselors through its program, Tax Aide. Call a senior center, the local IRS office or the local chapter of AARP.

**Volunteer Income Tax Assistance** is also sponsored by the IRS. VITA workers provide free tax preparation to low-income seniors, non-English-speaking taxpayers and disabled people. The local IRS office should be able to refer your parent to VITA workers.

**The IRS.** For answers to tax questions, call your local IRS office or the IRS tax information number (800-829-1040). Tax forms and publications on specific tax issues (such as "Tax Information for Older Americans") can be ordered by calling 800-829-3676.

# Protection Against Fraud

Elderly people are popular prey for high-pressure salespeople and scam artists. Even if your parent is conscious about protecting herself from cons, discuss the following do's and don'ts with her:

◆ Trust your instincts. If someone doesn't seem honest, he probably isn't. If a claim sounds too good to be true, it probably is.

◆ Beware of lures of friendship, entertainment or promising investments. Loneliness, boredom and financial fears sometimes lead the elderly to sign up for products, memberships and investments that cost them dearly.

◆ Don't be pressured into buying anything. Be leery of any salesman who ignores your refusals or tries to force you to act immediately.

◆ When salespeople come to the door, do not invite them to come in. Ask for identification and then let them give their pitch from outside.

◆ Always get receipts, avoid dealing in cash and never send cash in the mail.

◆ Give donations only to established, reputable charities or to causes with which you're personally familiar.

◆ Never give a credit card number over the phone unless you have initiated the purchase.

◆ Steer clear of contests and sweepstakes. The odds of winning are ridiculously low, and you may end up buying something you don't want, or find your name on every junk-mail list.

◆ Be suspect if anyone who is repairing your house or car suddenly finds a number of things that need fixing. Get another opinion before having any additional work done.

◆ Never leave workers unattended in your home or give a stranger your key.

◆ For help or information concerning fraud, call the local consumer protection agency, police department, area agency on aging or the local Better Business Bureau. The National Consumers League has a toll-free consumer protection line (800-876-7060).

◆ Be wary of anyone offering investment advice, and of brokers who push you to buy and sell often. Call the Securities and Exchange Commission at 202-942-8088 to find out if a person is a registered broker, or at 202-942-7040 to file a complaint about an broker. The National Association of Securities Dealers (800-289-9999) can give you information about the registration of or disciplinary action against individual brokers or brokerage firms. Or call them at 301-590-6500 if you have a question about the legalities of certain actions taken by a broker or brokerage firm. .

# Financial and Legal Counsel

Friends, colleagues, doctors and social workers may all offer financial and legal suggestions about your parent's situation. Be leery. Even people who are trained in these matters have a hard time keeping up with the fine print and the ever-changing rules.

Seek the advice of a reputable and experienced financial planner, lawyer or other professional. While it is expensive, the price of the advice is usually more than covered by the savings it produces.

## WHO NEEDS PROFESSIONAL ADVICE?

Professional advice is helpful to anyone who:

• Is nearing Medicaid eligibility and may want to protect some assets and become eligible early

• Is drafting a will or a durable power of attorney

• Has, alone or with a spouse, assets of more than $600,000 (including the value of a home and any life insurance policy)

• Has legal questions about a housing contract, nursing home regulations, consumer rights, social security or other such matters

• Wants to make a financial plan, including a review of spending habits, investment holdings, insurance policies and other assets

• Carries a large amount of debt and needs help with creditors

• Has finances that are relatively complicated—because of, say, a vast array of assets or a jointly-owned business.

## HIRING A PROFESSIONAL

Get recommendations, preferably from other professionals—lawyers, financial planners, professors at law or business schools, business acquaintances, accountants. Or consult library directories (for example, the *Martindale-Hubbell Law Directory*.) For national organizations that provide referrals to financial planners see Appendix B, page 388.

Once you have the names of three or four people who sound promising, make an appointment to meet them. Some issues to discuss:

◆ **Training, experience, expertise.** What is your specialty—estate planning, investments, taxes, insurance, health care? What degrees, certification or special training do you have? How long have you been practicing? (With few exceptions, it should be at least three or four years.) What percentage of your clients are elderly, or the families of elderly people? Can you describe other cases or accounts you have handled that are similar to this one?

◆ **How much?** How do you charge—an hourly fee, a flat fee, a commission or a combination of these? (If the person receives a commission, consider whether he or she will be acting in the best interests of your parent or simply working to

sell a policy, an investment or another financial or legal tool.) What is your estimate of the total cost? What happens if the cost exceeds this estimate? (The professional should get written permission before exceeding the estimate.) Are your bills itemized? Is an advance payment required? How often do you bill?

Fees are almost always negotiable, so once you find someone you like, compare prices and ask if he or she can bring the price down. Then get a written agreement concerning

## TOO MANY COOKS

If your parent is dealing with more than one professional—an estate lawyer, a financial planner and a tax advisor, for example—be sure they are willing to work together. In the best of circumstances, such professionals should work as a team, with one person acting as a coordinator. Otherwise, a financial planner may be dedicating certain assets for future use while a lawyer is protecting them in an untouchable trust, and an insurance agent advises using the money to buy a new policy. Talk with each person involved and choose one to oversee all of your parent's dealings, though none should have the right to make important decisions without his approval.

bills, payments, penalties and services provided.

◆ **The time frame.** What needs to be accomplished and how long do you estimate it will take? When will the plan or the portfolio be updated, and how much will this cost?

◆ **Other helpers.** Who else in the office will work on this matter? If an assistant or associate, will his fees be lower and how much supervision will he receive?

◆ **References.** Get the names of two or three clients, preferably people in a similar situation, and then call and find out how long they have used this professional and how helpful, open and knowledgeable they have found him or her to be.

◆ **Compatibility.** As you talk, get a sense of the person's character and personality. Do you share a basic approach to or philosophy about this problem? Do you sense that this person will be honest and direct? Does he or she answer questions so that you and your parent can understand the situation clearly? Can this person assure you that he or she will return phone calls within one business day?

# Chapter Fourteen

# THE LEGAL ISSUES

*Wills • Power of Attorney • Advance Directives • Guardianship • Estate Planning • Probate • Dividing an Estate*

..........................................

Y OUR PARENTS HAVE $30,000, OR MAYBE $3 MILLION, tucked away in various accounts, a home and personal property. When they die that money, the house and their other assets will go to you and your siblings, right? Not necessarily. Unless they have a will, the state will decide how those assets are divided. And without proper financial planning, taxes can consume up to 70 percent of a large estate.

What if your mother becomes incapacitated? The doctor, the lawyer and the bank manager will turn to you and other family members for guidance and decisions, right? Maybe, but maybe not. If your mother hasn't signed a durable power of attorney and a health-care proxy form, you may have to go through arduous court proceedings to prove your parent's incompetence and to be named her legal guardian.

Regardless of your parent's health or wealth, she should sign four documents right away if she hasn't done so already: an up-to-date will, a durable power of attorney, a living will and a health-care proxy. It's not expensive to execute these papers, and they will guard your family against sometimes lengthy legal proceedings and potentially bitter arguments.

This chapter describes these essential documents along with

the strategies your parent needs to follow to protect his estate from taxes. The information here is meant to serve only as a guideline; your family should work with a lawyer who is knowledgeable about the laws in your parent's state and experienced in issues concerning the elderly.

# Wills

Lawyers will tell you that pretty much everyone of legal age should have a will. Of course, they have a vested interest in getting people to execute wills, but in this regard, they are right. Anyone with children or assets—a house, a savings account—should have a will. Most lawyers will draft a simple will for under $200.

A well-drafted will ensures that your parent's belongings will be divided according to her wishes. It can prevent, or at least diminish, family squabbles and reduce the time and cost of probate. And in some cases it can reduce the amount of taxes that are owed. If your parent dies without a will, the court will decide how the property is to be distributed, and appoint someone to oversee the closing of the estate—someone who may charge a fee that can be as much as five percent of the value of the estate. When your parent dies you will have a lot on your mind; a clearly-drafted will can make this period easier for everyone.

If both your parents are alive, they should each have a will, as a joint will can complicate matters. If your parent already has a will, be sure it is up-to-date. Wills should be reviewed every year or two and also whenever there is a major change—for example, a death in the family, a divorce, a move to another state, a change in assets or a change in heirs.

Typically, a will describes a person's assets, property and belongings and explains how they are to be doled out after the person dies. Most wills include a general bequest, giving all assets to a spouse or dividing them equally among the children, but they may contain specific instructions assigning certain items to individuals, and instructions for establishing a trust. A will also names an executor (or executrix, if it's a woman), who will pay taxes and debts out of the estate and be sure that the assets are distributed in accord with the will's instructions.

Legally, a will affects only that part of the estate that goes through probate. Anything in a trust, jointly owned, or given directly to a beneficiary named in a life insurance policy is not under the jurisdiction of a will.

Be sure you know where your parent keeps his will, codicils (amendments) to the will and any letter of instruction that accompanies the will. If he doesn't already have a safe spot for it, suggest that he keep it in a lawyer's office, a strongbox or with a state registry service. A safe-deposit box in your parent's name is not the best place to store a will because the box may be sealed by the court at the time of death.

## LETTER OF INSTRUCTION

Your parent's will explains in broad, legal terms how his estate is to be passed on, but does anyone know, for example, what is to be done with his beloved cat, Pester? Or who should get the family's photo albums? Or which of his col-

leagues should receive the books, files and computer equipment from his office?

Beyond the scope of a will, there are often a number of practical matters that need attention. Get your parent to write (or dictate, if he can no longer write) a letter of instruction, which is an informal, nonbinding document that explains any personal matters not mentioned in the will. The more comprehensive it is, the better, especially if your family is prone to disagreements or your parent has failed to talk with

## GENERIC LEGAL FORMS

Many of the forms that your parent needs—a will, power of attorney, even the papers to set up a trust—can be found as generic documents at stationery or legal supplies stores, public libraries and the county recorder's office. A variety of computer software products also enables individuals to draft wills and other legal documents. But is this a safe bet?

In some cases, these forms are fine. Generic advance directives, for example, are usually adequate, as long as they are specific to your parent's state and any special instructions are written in. And a computer-generated will may be sufficient as long as your parent's estate is small and uncomplicated.

These forms are not appro-

priate for many situations, however, and should always be used with caution. Some states do not accept generic documents at all, while others have strict rules about them. And be sure they are precise enough to be considered legal. In some states if the language in a homemade will is loose, or if a small detail, like the date, is missing or wrong, the entire will may be declared invalid. Finally, be sure the form fits your parent's specific needs. Generic forms are not customized, and may not accomplish what your parent hopes they will. Lack of clarity can lead to family arguments and even lawsuits over the terms, language and validity of a will.

**"**I had my mother-in-law write down all her specific bequests on a sheet of paper and sign it, right across the whole thing, and then I tucked that in with her will. It wasn't terribly official-looking, but it worked in her case. Everyone honored her wishes.**"** —NELLY O.

the family about these issues in advance. A letter of instruction might include:

♦ Wishes about how personal property, such as furniture, diaries, jewelry, military medals, letters— typically, possessions that have little monetary value and would not be specifically mentioned in a will— are to be divided.

♦ Instructions on what to do with business files, equipment and computer software, including a computer password.

♦ Funeral and burial instructions.

♦ Names and addresses of lawyers, doctors, brokers, accountants and other advisors. The location of all important financial and legal documents.

♦ An inventory and possibly an appraisal of personal belongings.

♦ Explanations or instructions regarding investments, income tax returns, outstanding debts, credit card accounts, other properties, mortgages, renters, insurance policies and death benefits.

♦ Special instructions on how to operate or maintain a house or other property. Your parent might include a list of regular maintenance people, such as the plumber, handyman, electrician, veterinarian or auto mechanic.

♦ Personal wishes, such as thoughts on how beneficiaries are to spend their inheritances, or how children should divide the estate if they can't come to an agreement.

## LEGAL HELP

The process of hiring a lawyer is described on page 274. If that's too expensive, your parent may be eligible for free or low-cost legal aid. Contact the state legal services office (which you can find through the local bar association or the area agency on aging). The American Association of Retired Persons runs a program called Legal Counsel for the Elderly (202-434-2152), which has legal advice hotlines in several states, including Arizona, Florida, Maine, Michigan, New Mexico, California, Ohio, Pennsylvania and Texas. Be sure that the lawyer you work with has knowledge of the issues that concern you, or the incentive to do some research with your interests in mind, as volunteer legal services are sometimes staffed by young, inexperienced lawyers.

◆ Any special messages to an individual or last comments to the family (although personal thoughts to an individual might be better conveyed in a private letter).

# Power of Attorney

A power of attorney doesn't give anyone the power of a lawyer. It is the document by which one person ("the principal") authorizes another ("the agent" or "attorney-in-fact") to act legally on his or her behalf—to sign checks, enter into contracts and buy and sell properties, for example. A power of attorney won't necessarily strip your parent of her own legal powers. She can still make decisions, vote and control her own legal and financial affairs. It simply names a deputy who can handle some or all of these matters as well, in case your parent is ever unable to handle them her-

## A LEGAL LEXICON

*A decedent* is a person who has died.

*A personal representative* is the general name for anyone overseeing the estate of a decedent—paying taxes and bills and then distributing property according to the terms of the will.

*An executor* (or *executrix*, if a woman) is a personal representative who is named in a will to manage an estate.

*An administrator* (or *administratrix*, if a woman) is named by the court to manage the estate when no will exists, no executor is named in the will or the executor named cannot serve.

*A fiduciary* is anyone acting on behalf of others. In the case of wills, a personal representative is acting as a fiduciary. In the case of trusts, the trustee who manages the trust is a fiduciary.

*Probate* is the court proceeding in which creditors are paid and an estate is divided after death.

*A grantor* is a person who establishes a trust.

*A beneficiary* is a person who is designated to receive funds, property or other assets from an estate, trust or insurance policy.

*A trustee* is a person who manages the trust for the beneficiaries.

*An attorney-in-fact* is a person who has the legal power to act on behalf of another person.

self or simply wants someone else to do the work for her.

Your parent needs to execute a document known as a durable power of attorney, which will remain in effect when she most needs it—when she is incapacitated. A regular power of attorney is useful if your parent wants to give someone short-lived legal authority—for example, to pay her bills while she is on vacation. But if she becomes incapacitated, this power will be revoked. A durable power of attorney remains valid until she dies.

Your parent should assign a durable power of attorney immediately because if she is deemed incompetent and unable to fully understand the legal ramifications of this document—for example, if she were to have a stroke next week—she would no longer be permitted to sign one. Without this fully executed document, your family might have to go to court to have her declared incapable of handling her affairs and have someone named as her legal guardian, an often lengthy, expensive and humiliating court procedure.

Power-of-attorney documents should be prepared by a lawyer to suit the specific needs of your parent and the laws of her state. Typically, the form includes the name of the person granting the power; the name of the attorney-in-fact and a back-up person to serve if the first person designated can't; a list of the duties and powers being granted; an explanation of when, for how long and under what circumstances the power is valid; and the proper signatures, which depend upon the requirements of the state.

**"***I told my mother how important it was for her to sign a durable power of attorney, and she said, 'No.' And that was it. No more discussion. She has always been controlling, but now that she is sick she is clinging more desperately to that control. She can't handle the idea that anyone else would ever manage her money or anything else in her life.*

*I didn't push it. It's her choice. I was upset for a while because I think she is making a mistake, one that may mean more work for me. But I realize that there's nothing I can do about it. And honestly, I don't want her doing something that makes her uncomfortable.***"** —DIANE P.

If your parent has assets in more than one state, she needs a durable power of attorney written for each state. Both the principal (your parent) and the attorney-in-fact should have copies of the document. The original should be filed with a county recorder's office, with your parent's attorney or in an office file where you both have access to it.

### Defining the Power

Your parent can give her attorney-in-fact broad powers—the authority to handle all financial and legal matters, as well as all personal matters, such as housing decisions—or limited powers, such as the authority only to sign checks from a single account.

Make sure your parent's wishes are clear on the form. Some states limit the powers of an attorney-in-fact unless specific provisions are written in, such as the authority to make gifts to others, to deal with the IRS and to transfer assets into or out of a trust.

A power of attorney is usually effective immediately, but for your purposes, it's best to file the document away, perhaps in a lawyer's office, until it is needed. Some states recognize a "springing" power of attorney, which kicks in at a predetermined time in the future—for example, when two physicians determine that your parent is no longer able to make decisions for herself. The idea sounds good, but in fact a "springing" power of attorney can cause trouble if there is any dis-

## YOU, TOO

This is a good time to get your own affairs in order. Do you have a will, a durable power of attorney, a living will and a health-care proxy? Have you thought about ways of protecting your estate from taxes and the future costs of long-term care? Do it now.

agreement over when the power takes effect—if one person thinks your parent is incompetent, and another believes that she can still handle her financial affairs, for example.

## TAKING THE REINS—EVER SO GENTLY

If you are designated as the attorney-in-fact for your parent and are taking over some or all of his finances, do so gently and with great respect for the power entrusted to you. Personal financial control is an important source of independence and pride.

Whenever you take over a new task, do so with your parent's consent or only when you determine that he is truly unable to handle it himself. Proceed slowly, keeping him in charge to whatever extent possible. You might start by getting his social security,

pension and other income deposited directly into his bank account (contact the social security office, bank manager or other agency representatives about this). Likewise, find out about having certain fixed bills, like mortgage, insurance premiums and some utilities, paid automatically from his account.

Let your parent retain whatever financial powers he still can. If he can't handle the important bills, he might continue to write checks for his weekly groceries, donations, gifts and other expenses.

So be wary. If your parent trusts someone enough to give them this power, she should trust them to know when to use it.

### Choosing an Attorney-in-Fact

Your parent should think very carefully about who to designate as her attorney-in-fact because this is a powerful tool. Having access to another person's money can be tempting when one's own finances are in trouble. The person should be someone whom she trusts completely, someone with whom others in the family feel comfortable, and preferably someone who lives nearby and can meet easily with lawyers, accountants, bankers or others. If there is no one she trusts, then she may be better off without this document.

# Advance Directives

When a person is too confused to make medical decisions or too ill to communicate his preferences, doctors usually confer directly with family members and rely on them to make decisions. Some states allow this by law, others permit it by practice. But sometimes family members disagree with each other or with the doctor, or they simply don't know what the patient would have wanted were he able to understand his condition and communicate his choices.

Advance directives—a living will and a health-care proxy form—are legal documents that enable your parent to explain in advance her wishes regarding medical care, and to name someone to make treatment decisions in her stead. These papers protect her, to a large degree, from getting unwanted treatment or from being refused treatment that she might want. They also give the family some guidance when making health-care decisions, and they reduce the chances of sibling fights and court battles.

Although most people have heard of advance directives and even think that they are a good idea, only a small fraction of the population has actually executed them. People put it off, or assume that advance directives are not really necessary *for them*. But these forms are not intended to cover freak incidences. At least one study suggests that more than 70 percent of deaths in hospitals occur after a decision is made to forgo life-sustaining treatment, and in most of those cases, it is not the patient, but the family who decides. In addition, many other treatment decisions that do not have to do with life support are routinely made by family members.

## LIVING WILLS

A living will states a person's wishes in the event that she is close to death and unable to make decisions about her medical care. Typically, it requests that the person be allowed to die free of pain and free of aggressive medical treatment when the end of life is in sight and there is no reasonable chance for recovery. Usually the terms are broad, but your parent can list specific treatments that are either wanted or not wanted in given situations. For example, a person may state that he does not want to be put on a respirator, but does want to receive artificial hydration.

Although it is not commonly done, a living will can also be used to express a person's desire to be kept alive with aggressive medical intervention. In fact, the National Right to Life Committee (202-626-8800) has drafted a Will to Live form with explicit instructions for life-sustaining treatment, regardless of the situation or prognosis.

While a living will provides assurance that your parent's wishes will be upheld, it has limitations. For example, in some states the documents are valid only when a patient is "terminally ill," which does not include situations in which a patient is in a coma or suffering from a debilitating but not terminal illness. Furthermore, living wills apply only to treatment that is life-sustaining, and some states exclude artificial nutrition and hydration unless they are explicitly written into the document. Be certain you know the laws in your parent's state. And urge your parent to sign a health-care proxy form in addition to a living will.

## HEALTH-CARE PROXY

A health-care proxy form covers a wider range of situations than a living will and it appoints a health-care agent, or proxy, who can make medical decisions on a person's be-

half, interpret written instructions and respond to changing health and medical needs. It should include a list of specific instructions and the powers that are granted. (While a durable power of attorney might empower someone to make health-care decisions, most states now require a power of attorney form that specifically encompasses health-care decisions.)

If your parent is going to have surgery, be sure she assigns a health-care proxy beforehand, as elderly people often become delirious briefly after surgery, and need someone else to make decisions about their medical care.

## SIGNING ADVANCE DIRECTIVES

Advance directives must be signed while your parent is competent, so don't wait. He needs specific documents that comply with all the rules of his state, and if he lives in more than one state—Maine in the summer and Florida in winter, for example—then he needs advance directives for each state.

His lawyer might prepare these advance directives when drafting his will, or you can get up-to-date, state-specific legal forms free from Choice in Dying (800-989-9455). The group will also help you fill out the forms (over the phone) and provide legal, medical and even some personal counseling.

Choice in Dying will store the documents for a nominal fee, or guide you on how to store them in your parent's state. (Certain states have rules concerning where advance

**❝** *My father had a bout in the hospital last year when things didn't look good for him, and after that I got much firmer. When he got out of the hospital, I said, 'Listen Dad, there are several things that we have to face head on, and one of them is a living will.'*

*My brother had said that we had to be delicate, but I said, 'I don't think we're going to have to be careful. I think we're going to find him ready for this.'*

*And he was. Ready, and even relieved to talk about it.* **❞**
—ELEANOR R.

directives are to be stored.) If the state has no stipulations, your parent should put the original copies in a safe place—an office file or strongbox—and inform other family members of its location, and copies should be sent to family members, agents, doctors, lawyers and others involved in her care. Your parent should also record information regarding the documents (where they are, and the name and phone number of her health-care agent) on an ID card, with other vital medical information, in her wallet. For help with making advance directives stick, see page 357.

## THE IMPORTANCE OF DISCUSSIONS

Now don't stop here. A living will and a power of attorney for health care should serve as a springboard for ongoing discussions about your parent's feelings concerning illness and death, so that when you have to step in, you have a good understanding of how she feels about these matters.

Don't make assumptions. *We don't need to talk. I know what my mother would want.* All of us have very personal, and often unpredictable, feelings about illness and death. Studies show that people named to serve as health-care agents are routinely wrong when they guess what the person they represent would want in a given situation.

So find out how your parent feels about these matters. She may simply say that she doesn't want to be hooked up to a lot of machines and leave it at that, but this is a broad statement applied to a vast number of possible specific scenarios, all of which are inconceivable to a relatively healthy person. You need to know more about her views, her wishes and her fears. Here are some of the issues you might discuss:

◆ If a friend or relative is hospitalized or has died recently, talk about the illness, the treatment and the outcome. How does your parent feel about the decisions that were made? How does she think the situation should have been handled, and why?

◆ What are her feelings about receiving life-saving medical treatment when she is terminally ill or severely incapacitated, and has no chance of regaining her health?

◆ Does she have religious beliefs about life, death and medical intervention? If so, what are they?

◆ What does your parent fear most about illness and death—pain, loneliness, lack of control, loss of dignity?

◆ What illness or permanent disability would be unacceptable to her—paralysis, mental confusion, loss of hearing, blindness, a condition that is very painful? Encourage your parent to talk about these issues purely from her own perspective, not how they would affect other people.

◆ What are your parent's feelings about receiving artificial hydration and nutrition? (Courts and medical associations consider these to be medical treatments, but some people view administering food and water, even when they are mechanically pumped into the body, as basic humane care, not medical care.)

◆ Does your parent trust her doctor's judgment about treatments? Has she expressed her philosophy and feelings about medical intervention to her doctor?

◆ What are her feelings about receiving only the comfort care offered by hospice—which offers no aggressive medical care—and dying at home?

◆ Which is more important to your parent, to be free of pain or to be mentally alert? (You may have to make decisions about the quantity of pain medication she receives.)

# A Question of Competency

Suppose that your father is too ill to speak except during brief moments. Or that your mother's dementia has gotten so bad that she doesn't know whether to wear a cotton T-shirt or a thick wool sweater on a hot, August day. Should he be making decisions about his medical care? Should she be allowed to handle her own finances?

These are not easy questions. There is no clear line between mental competency and incompetency, no simple test to determine your parent's decision-making ability. Competency is defined as the ability to receive and understand information, evaluate choices, make a decision that is consistent with a set of personal values and goals and communicate that decision to others. Certainly, just because your parent makes decisions that you consider foolish—he refuses a simple medical treatment or gives his money to a questionable cause—does not mean that he is incompetent.

Competency is not an all-or-nothing matter. Your parent may be quite competent in one area and not in another. Someone who cannot handle his own financial affairs may be perfectly able to make decisions about where he wants to live, for example. Or a person may be competent at one moment, during a phase of lucidity or when strong painkillers wear off, and incompetent at another.

If you have concerns about your parent's competency and are not sure whether you should step in and act on his behalf, get his doctor or a geriatric care manager to guide you. If someone has been assigned durable power of attorney, that person can step in right away. If not, you may have to go to court to have your parent declared incompetent and be named her legal guardian.

People often need guardianship to gain access to an ill parent's funds so they can pay bills, or to have a severely confused parent admitted to a nursing home against her will.

## SECURING A COURT MANDATE

Going to court is, obviously, a grave step and therefore always a

---

## THE GRIEF OF GUARDIANSHIP

Your father, who represented strength and vitality, who guided you through much of your life, is now unable to make basic decisions for himself. It's painful to see a parent become powerless and vulnerable, and even more painful to have to go to court to have him declared unfit. When it's over it may be very uncomfortable to be in the position of chief decision-maker.

❖ Be gentle with yourself. A lot is being asked of you right now. You are doing the right thing, and yet at times it can feel very wrong. Take time off from your job, if possible, to handle this new workload and to give yourself a chance to grieve.

❖ Move slowly, keeping your parent informed and in control as much and for as long as possible. When you make decisions, explain to him what is happening and why, even if you think he cannot understand you.

❖ Remember, this may be harder on you than on your parent. He may be relieved to let go of his duties and concerns, or he may be unaware of what is happening.

❖ If your parent has dementia and becomes angry with you for taking over, remember that his anger is, in part, due to the disease. Try not to take it personally. Remind yourself daily why you are doing this and how important it is that you take on this responsibility.

❖ During this time, everyone will have an opinion about what you are doing. The only "right" decision is the one that you believe is right. Trust your instincts.

last resort. If your parent is declared incompetent by the court, he will be stripped of some or all of his legal rights—the right to make decisions about his medical care or living arrangements, to handle his own finances, to write checks or buy or sell property, to vote, to marry or divorce, to drive and to enter into contracts. It is a potentially time-consuming and expensive process that can be draining for everyone involved, especially if your parent puts up a fight. But sometimes going to court is unavoidable and truly in the best interest of your parent.

States have different rules regarding guardianship, all of them, understandably, stringent. In most cases, you must retain a lawyer who files a petition with the court. A hearing date is set and an attorney is assigned to represent your parent, who is now referred to as "the proposed ward" (a troubling expression, but remember that it is only a legal term). A judge, or in some cases a panel or jury, interviews family members, doctors and others involved in your parent's life to determine if he is truly unfit to handle his own affairs and to what extent. In most states your parent does not have to be present at the hearing, but if he wants to fight the judgment, he may go to court.

If the court declares your parent incompetent, someone will be named to take over all or some of his decisions, duties and legal rights. This surrogate decision-maker, also called a guardian or a conservator, is usually a family member, but it can be an outsider, a group, an

*"After my mother died, my father's dementia got much worse. He started doing bizarre things and a couple of times he became violent. Eventually I had to establish a guardianship for him, and I can tell you, doing it was horrendous. My father has always been very proud and independent. He would never accept help from anyone. He fought the guardianship, and the court proceedings dragged on for almost five months. During all of that time he argued with me, screamed at me, and once he even threatened to kill me.*

*All the way through it I kept telling myself, over and over, 'This is for him. This is my gift to him. I am doing this for him.' Some days I believed it, some days I didn't. Some days it felt as though I was punishing him. He certainly saw it that way. But I know now that it was the right thing to do."* —RONA S.

agency or an institution. (The court will go outside the family if no family member is able to assume this role or act in the best interest of the ward.) Guardians can be granted total or limited authority. For example, you may be given the authority to handle your parent's personal care, while a bank trustee is assigned to oversee his financial affairs.

In most states a guardian must report back to the court at specific intervals or whenever a major decision is made, to show that he or she is acting responsibly.

# Estate Planning

The word "estate" conjures up images of the Great Gatsby, wide rolling lawns, pillared porches and polo fields. But in a legal context, an estate is simply a person's property and possessions, however large or small. Estate planning entails drafting a will (as well as a durable power of attorney and advance directives) and then structuring one's assets in a way that permits the instructions in the will to be carried out. (For example, a will is of little use if all the decedent's assets are held jointly and therefore do not fall under the jurisdiction of the will.) Estate planning can also reduce the taxes heirs will pay, and determine how various assets are to be managed and controlled.

Estate planning is most valuable for people with estates worth more than $600,000, the point at which hefty federal taxes kick in. You may not think your parent's assets are near that point, but if he has a house worth $250,000, plus a life insurance policy valued at $200,000, a retirement fund and some other savings, then he is probably pretty close to the mark. Older people often own more than they realize, as many rely exclusively on their incomes for living expenses and are not aware of what has accumulated in their bank accounts or what a piece of property is currently worth.

Even if your parent's assets aren't worth $600,000, estate planning can keep certain assets out of public and time-consuming probate proceed-

ings, reduce taxes on capital gains or give control to another person when your parent is incompetent.

Your parent may have already taken care of this, but if not and if questions arise, you may need to know about some of the basic legal tools available. Of course, a lawyer well-versed in estate planning should guide your parent and you.

## OWNERSHIP

Ownership should be a simple matter. Something belongs to one person or it belongs to another. But by law, an item can belong to one person, to another, or to two or more people in a variety of ways. The way in which a person owns a house, a stock, an account or other assets affects how vulnerable the property is to creditors, how it is passed on and how it is taxed.

### Sole Ownership

Sole ownership is fairly straightforward, but there are a few gray areas. For example, if your parent puts her house into your name, but remains in the house as a tenant, some states will still consider the house part of her estate. Likewise, if an item is in your parent's house, it is usually still considered hers. That is, in most states your parent can't write notes on the back of valuable objects ("This belongs to Connie," "This belongs to Anne") and assume that the objects are no longer part of her estate.

### Joint Ownership with Right of Survivorship

Married couples typically own a house and other assets as joint owners with right of survivorship. The primary advantage of this type of ownership, from a legal point of view, is that the property passes directly to the other person without going through probate.

Your parent might own something jointly with someone other than a spouse—for example, he might want to have a joint checking account with you so that you can pay his bills. Or sometimes a parent owns a house jointly with a child so the house will go directly to the child without probate and without substantial taxes (although in some states, property owned jointly between a parent and child is considered the property of the parent).

The most common concern of any joint ownership agreement is whether one owner can trust the other. When a bank account is owned jointly, all owners can draw on the account (even empty the account) without the approval of the others. The joint assets are also vulnerable to all owners' creditors.

### Tenants in Common

As tenants in common, the parties own property jointly, but there is no right of survivorship. Each person owns an indivisible share that is passed on directly to his heirs. For example, your father might own a business equally with two partners. When he dies his third would be

## SHRINKING AN ESTATE

If your parents want to shrink a hefty estate or if they simply like to be generous, they can give up to $10,000 per year to any number of individuals without paying gift taxes. They can make tax-free gifts in excess of $10,000 to an individual if the additional money is paid, on behalf of this other person, directly to an institution for medical care or education. That is, your parent can give you $10,000 and then send a check to the hospital to pay your medical bills, and not owe gift taxes on any of it. Your parents can also reduce the value of a large estate by giving away valuable

jewelry, silver, family heirlooms, paintings, etc. and by putting their life insurance policies into a trust. (If state taxes are going to be substantial, they might also change their primary residence to a state with lower estate and inheritance taxes.)

Don't let your parents be overly zealous about giving money away. They shouldn't give away so much that they jeopardize their own financial health. And they certainly shouldn't give away items that they still use and enjoy.

For the IRS publication, "Federal Estate and Gift Taxes," call 800-829-3676.

passed on to his heirs, not to the other business owners.

If your parents plan to pass on an estate that is worth more than $600,000—the amount exempt from federal estate taxes—each should maintain assets in his or her own names so each can pass on up to $600,000 free of taxes. Because a house is usually the most valuable asset and cannot be split like a bank account or stock portfolio, your parents might want to own it as tenants in common.

### "Stepped-up Basis"

When you sell something you pay a tax on the capital gain—the amount you receive minus the amount you originally paid for it. If you buy a house for $80,000 and sell it for $200,000, the capital gain is $120,000. But when something is passed on to an heir it is given a "stepped-up" value, and the new purchase price is the value of the item when it is passed on.

Here's an illustration: Your father buys his house for $80,000, and keeps it in his name. When he dies it is worth $200,000 and it is passed on to your mother, who sells it immediately. She has no gain to report because her purchase price, or the "base value" of the house, is the value it had when she inherited it. If your parents owned the house jointly, which is usually the case, your mother's gain would be nothing on your father's half and $60,000 for the half she owned.

In this scenario it would have been best if your father had owned the house—along with stocks and other assets—solely in his name so your mother would get everything at a stepped-up basis. To prevent people from switching titles around as soon as someone is diagnosed with a serious illness, Congress has invalidated any asset-shifting that occurs within three years of a person's death. Given this long waiting period, it's often best for couples to split assets. But if one parent is most likely to die first, then any assets that have appreciated significantly should be put into his or her name.

### TRUSTS

A trust is merely a way of holding money, property or other assets. Rather than having a bank account in your parent's name, the account is held in the name of a trust (for example, the John Parker Trust Fund). Trusts are not just for the rich. They are used to protect assets from estate and inheritance taxes, to keep property out of probate, to give a person some measure of control over someone else's assets or to keep money secure until an heir reaches maturity. They also offer greater privacy than bank accounts. Anything in a living trust (see chart on the following page) remains out of the public realm, whereas anything included in a will becomes public once it passes through probate.

Trusts fall into two broad categories: testamentary trusts, which are set up after a person dies, and living trusts, which are established while a person is still alive. Living trusts are either "revocable," which means that the person who set it up maintains control over the trust, or "irrevocable," which means that the person has no power to revoke or alter the trust in any way.

Don't be intimidated by the language of trusts. It's not as complicated as it sounds. The person establishing the trust is the "grantor" and the person appointed to manage the trust is the "trustee." The "beneficiaries" are the folks who eventually get the money or assets from the trust.

## Testamentary Trusts

A testamentary trust, which is described in a will and created after the grantor's death, is often set up to hold assets for a specific purpose, such as a child's education, or until a particular time (a child reaches 21 or gets married, for example). Testamentary trusts are also used to protect large estates from federal taxes.

Here's how it works: usually when a person dies all his assets go

*I was the executor of my mother-in-law's estate and it was an eye-opener, seeing how much money is paid out in taxes unless you do something to protect yourself. It's shocking. More than half of her estate went to Uncle Sam.*

*Having been through all that, my husband and I have made sure that our affairs are in order. We each have a will and a durable power of attorney and we have started to give our money to our children each year.*

*We learned the hard way, and we don't want them to have to go through what we did.* —NELLY O.

to his spouse, tax-free. Then, when the second spouse dies, all the assets go to the children or other heirs.

## THREE TYPES OF TRUSTS

| | Testamentary Trust | Revocable Living Trust | Irrevocable Living Trust |
|---|---|---|---|
| **When it is established** | Defined in a will and established after the grantor's death | Established before the grantor's death | Established before the grantor's death |
| **Who controls the assets in the trust** | The grantor retains full control of the assets during his lifetime | The grantor retains full control of the assets, usually until he becomes incompetent or relinquishes control for some other reason | The grantor specifies the terms of the trust, but cannot change those terms or revoke the trust |
| **Benefits** | • Holds assets until heirs mature<br>• Can reduce estate taxes | • Holds assets until heirs mature<br>• Can reduce cost and time of probate<br>• protects privacy because assets do not pass through probate<br>• Can avoid guardianship proceedings | • Can reduce estate taxes<br>• Can reduce cost and time of probate<br>• Protects privacy because assets do not pass through probate<br>• Can avoid guardianship proceedings<br>• Protects assets from creditors |

By setting up a trust, each mate can pass on up to $600,000 tax-free (saving more than $250,000 in taxes). When the first mate dies, the will dictates that up to $600,000 be put into a trust. Usually under the terms of the trust, the money can be used by the surviving spouse during his or her lifetime, but then is passed on to the children. When the second spouse dies, the children receive the trust from the first parent, and then up to $600,000 from this second parent is also free from federal taxes.

It is important to note that in order to accomplish this each spouse must have assets in his or her own name that can be put into a trust. Anything that is jointly owned goes automatically to the surviving spouse and cannot be put into a trust.

### Revocable Living Trusts

A revocable living trust is set up during the grantor's lifetime and can be changed or canceled at any time. The grantor usually acts as the primary trustee, managing the assets. A secondary or successor trustee, often a bank or other financial institution, steps in when the primary trustee becomes incompetent or dies, and manages and distributes the assets according to the terms of the trust. They are useful in a number of situations:

◆ For a person diagnosed with Alzheimer's disease or any progressive, debilitating illness, a living trust allows him to dictate, in advance, exactly how certain assets are to be managed, and even to monitor the actions of a trustee for a while. As he loses his ability to manage these matters, the trustee steps in and takes over.

A durable power of attorney offers much the same protection as a living trust—both give a second person legal authority to control assets—but a living trust provides slightly more protection and is useful when a person owns, say, a large stock portfolio or a number of properties. A living trust includes detailed instructions about how assets are to be handled, and the trustee has a legal responsibility (known as "a fiduciary duty") to manage the trust carefully and in the best interests of the beneficiaries. If the

## A LIVING TRUST IS NOT A WILL

Some people call living trusts "substitute wills" because a trust dictates how assets will be distributed, just as a will does. However, it is virtually impossible to put all assets into a trust, so there will always be some part of an estate left under the terms of a will. Therefore, regardless of any trusts that are established, your parent should still have a will. She should also have a durable power of attorney, to give someone the authority to manage assets that are not in the trust, to sign contracts and to handle other legal and financial affairs.

beneficiaries question the actions of the trustee, they can challenge him or her in court.

If your parent likes the idea of establishing a trust, but is reluctant to put any assets into it right away, an attorney-in-fact can often be authorized to put assets into a trust at a particular time, for example, when the grantor becomes incapacitated.

◆ A revocable living trust is also a good idea any time there is potential for arguments over some portion of a will. While a will can be contested, the terms of a living trust cannot.

◆ A living trust can, in some cases, reduce the time and expense of probate, since its contents are not subject to a will or to probate (they are still subject to taxes, however). Trusts may be especially valuable in states that have onerous probate proceedings; when something about an estate would make probate particularly complicated; or when a person has assets in several states and wants to avoid multiple probate proceedings.

◆ Because courts have no control over living trusts, they are sometimes preferable to testamentary trusts, which often require an annual accounting.

### Irrevocable Living Trusts

Setting up an irrevocable trust, which can be neither changed nor destroyed, is a serious step that requires a good deal of thought. Irrevocable trusts should be established only under highly unusual circumstances and only by people

## CHOOSING A TRUSTEE

A trustee, like an attorney-in-fact, should be a family member who is at ease with finances and respected by the beneficiaries of the trust, or a professional trust manager or financial advisor. A relative can be appointed in conjunction with a professional, which makes a good mix—the heart and soul of a family member combined with the business instincts and neutrality of an outsider. (For an irrevocable trust to be excluded from an estate, the outsider must be able to outvote a spouse.)

Because some bank trust officers are overly conservative or unskilled investors, it's a good idea to plan a regular review of the accounts if the trustee is in charge of investing the trust's funds.

with a very large estate.

Irrevocable trusts are sometimes used to reduce estate taxes. As long as your parent is not a beneficiary of the trust, then she is no longer considered the owner of the assets and they are not considered as part of the estate. The trust would still be subject to gift taxes and capital gains taxes, but these are generally far less than estate taxes. (Anything that was placed in an irrevocable trust within three years of a person's death, however, is still considered part of the taxable estate.)

Irrevocable trusts are sometimes used to shelter a life insurance policy so the proceeds are not included in the estate or to protect assets that are expected to appreciate significantly.

# Probate

Probate, the legal process of settling an estate, has a nasty reputation, some of which is deserved. It can involve enormous amounts of paperwork, long periods of time and thousands of dollars in legal fees. But estate administration, as it is sometimes called, isn't always so onerous, and sometimes it is far easier and cheaper than anyone expects.

During probate, the decedent's debts are paid, the estate is inventoried and assets are doled out according to the terms of the will. The process usually lasts at least six to twelve months, but it can go on for years—the amount of time it takes depends upon state laws, the practices of the presiding judge, the complexity of the estate, the clarity of the will, the efficiency of the executor and whether the will is contested. Small estates, or those that contain only a small amount of probate property, may qualify for a streamlined version of probate, called small estate administration or summary administration. In this case, the transfer of assets is handled through an affidavit, or court order, that takes no longer than a few months to complete. If property is owned in more than one state, each state will conduct its own probate proceeding. Experienced local at-

*"My mother-in-law died almost a year ago and I am still in contact with the lawyer almost weekly. I thought her financial situation was simple, but it turns out she made a number of gifts years ago and never paid any gift taxes. And she has property in a couple of states. It's a nightmare. I think she named me as her executor so she could torture me even after she was gone."*

—Susan V.

torneys can usually expedite probate proceedings, but it is possible in some states to do it yourself. A probate clerk can guide you through the process.

# Dividing the Estate

Most wills note only that property be "divided equally" among the children. So it's up to siblings to find an equitable way to split up possessions. If not done with great care, this can severely damage family relationships, especially if a will is poorly written or siblings are not on good terms. The division of valuable items, family photographs, letters and other such mementos can lead to bitter disagreements and hurt feelings. Your father's high school sweater or your mother's old diary may suddenly become an invaluable icon. Even those who thought that their parents' assets weren't particularly valuable, that the family's relationships were strong, or that their

> **"The hard part was cleaning out the house. We came across all these little reminders, bits and pieces of our childhoods and memories of Dad. That was upsetting. My sister and I took care of it at our own slow pace. We met at the house three or four times over the course of a month or more, taking one room at a time. Then we would always go out for a beer when we were done. There was a lot of crying and a lot of laughing that went on. Dividing things up didn't divide us. If anything, it made us closer."**  —ALICIA B.

own hearts were generous, can be drawn into battle.

So, when you divide your parent's belongings, do it ever so carefully. And before you start, agree upon some ground rules.

♦ If possible, wait a few weeks until the grief has subsided. Emotions won't be so volatile and perceptions so askew.

♦ Try to gain some perspective before starting. Each person should weigh the value of their relationships with siblings against the value of the items in the house. What will matter in the long run?

♦ Assign some value to each item so everyone knows its relative worth and walks away with items of roughly the same cash value.

♦ Before heading to the house,

have each person write down three items that she or he most wants, in the order of preference. What is most important to one person may not be particularly important to another. If this is so, the crucial items can be divided without contest.

♦ Ask an outsider—a friend or professional—to monitor the division of the estate if you can find someone whom everyone trusts and if the person is a good mediator.

♦ Decide together who will be present when items in the house are distributed. Are spouses invited? Children? Friends? You may not want in-laws putting in their two-cents worth.

♦ For those who cannot be present, you might photograph or videotape items in advance and let the absentees make a list of their preferences. They might have a relative or friend stand in their place.

♦ Select items in some order—you might draw straws to determine who goes first—and then take turns choosing. You might rotate the order so each person has at least one chance to choose first in a room.

♦ Plan several breaks if the house is large or if there is a potential for disagreements.

♦ If beneficiaries are unable to agree, the executor usually divides assets in "approximately equal shares." If there are irreconcilable differences, then the property is sold and the heirs receive cash.

## FOR MORE HELP

❖ **The area agency on aging** has information on state laws concerning the elderly, as well as names of local legal aid societies that offer low-cost or free services. To find the area agency on aging in your parent's community, call the Eldercare Locator at 800-677-1116, or the state unit on aging, listed in Appendix A, page 377.

❖ **The American Association of Retired Persons** (800-424-3410) has information on a number of legal issues facing the elderly.

❖ **Legal Counsel for the Elderly** (202-234-0970), a program of AARP, makes referrals and supplies information on trusts, wills, nursing home regulations, advance directives and other legal issues. In some states the group runs a hotline which offers legal counsel to older residents.

❖ **Choice In Dying** (800-989-9455) has up-to-date advance directive forms for each state, and information about advance directives and patient rights. It also offers support and guidance to people who face difficult end-of-life decisions.

❖ **The National Academy of Elder Law Attorneys** (520-881-4005) offers some limited information on hiring a lawyer and other legal issues, but it does not make referrals.

❖ **The Internal Revenue Service** (800-829-3676) has publications on probate and taxes.

# Chapter Fifteen

# THE AGING BRAIN

*What is Normal? • Getting Tested • Alzheimer's: What to Expect • Other Dementias • What Now?*

A PILE OF UNOPENED BILLS SITS ON YOUR MOTHER'S DESK, which is odd because she's always been punctual about paying them. Now that you think about it, you've noticed a number of unusual things about your mother recently. She missed two lunch dates with you. There was that silly incident over the dog that enraged her. And last week she called and asked you to come over right away, but when you got there she couldn't remember what was so urgent.

A cold wave passes through you. *Could it be . . . ?*

When elderly people become forgetful or confused the possibility of Alzheimer's disease looms ominously, and for good reason. Alzheimer's is a cruel disease and caring for someone with dementia is overwhelmingly painful and difficult. But don't be too quick to assume that your parent's waning awareness or inability to concentrate is caused by irreversible brain disease. Mild forgetfulness and confusion may be benign side effects of old age and mental inactivity, or they may be symptoms of a treatable disorder. Before you panic, urge your parent to see a doctor who is well-versed in such matters and find out exactly what is wrong and what can be done about it.

# What Is Normal?

The human brain, a chunk of jelly weighing about three pounds, is comprised of a hundred billion nerve cells, all interconnected to form an elaborate communication web. But just as skin sags and bellies protrude, this fabulous control center reflects its age. Sometime after adolescence, nerve cells and their support cells begin to atrophy and die and linkages are severed. By the time a person reaches 70 or 80, the brain may have lost up to ten percent of its original mass.

But a few million brain cells more or less doesn't necessarily alter a person's intellect. In fact, some people remain sharp, imaginative and productive all the way through their old age, despite the changes in the brain. And many are affected only mildly, in inconsequential ways. They may need an extra few minutes to remember a person's name or what it is they came into the kitchen to get, they may have some trouble balancing a checkbook or following a long story. But a little forgetfulness is nothing to worry about. Up to half of people over 65 say they have more trouble remembering things than they used to. After 80, almost everyone experiences some decline in their mathematical, verbal and spatial skills. It's what doctors call age-associated memory impairment or benign senile forgetfulness—"benign" because it's harmless and not going to get significantly worse and "senile" because

it occurs in old age. (In our culture the word "senile" has such negative connotations that it is often dropped from the phrase.)

While the decline in the size of the brain may be largely to blame, other factors certainly play a role, including poor vision and hearing, hormonal changes, physical illness and the effects of medications. Sometimes older people shift their brains into low gear because others expect less of them, or because they lack intellectual stimulation. If a vibrant and brilliant woman loses her job and has little to do during her day, her mental engine is bound to slip into idle.

Be patient with your parent. Help her cope with her absent-mindedness. (See Chapter Eight for tips that can help any forgetful mind.) Help her see some humor in her slip-ups. Assure her that forgetfulness is normal and nothing to be overly concerned about. In fact, worrying about memory loss may only exacerbate the problem. Most important, urge her to use her mind more, not less.

# Dementia

The word dementia comes from the Latin *de*, meaning without, and *mens*, which means mind. Dementia is not a specific illness, but rather a group of symptoms which have dozens of causes, in the same way a fever and chills may be caused by the flu, meningitis, malaria or other illnesses. The symptoms of dementia include severe memory loss (especially short-term memory), confusion, disorientation, delusions, personality changes, and difficulty with language, math and visual-spatial relationships (seeing and understanding three dimensions).

Most researchers agree that dementia is not an inevitable part of aging, but the result of disease, infection, injury or another ailment. But it is common in the elderly, especially in the very old. At least five percent of people over 65, and twenty percent of people over 85 have some form of dementia. (One frequently-cited study suggests that nearly ten percent of people over 65 and fifty percent of those over 85 suffer from dementia.)

About 60 percent of all cases of dementia are the result of Alz-heimer's disease. Perhaps 15 to 20 percent are caused by a series of small, often unnoticeable, strokes that produce what is known as multi-infarct dementia, and another 15 to 20 percent are caused by a combination of these two. Less than 10 percent of dementia cases are due to other causes, such as alcoholism, brain damage and brain tumors, or Creutzfeldt-Jakob, Huntington's, Parkinson's or Pick's disease. (If your parent has Parkinson's disease, don't assume that dementia is a future certainty. Most estimates suggest that less than half of these patients will develop dementia, and it tends to affect memory and the speed at which one thinks rather than language skills.)

## MENTAL HYGIENE

The adage "use it or lose it" applies to the brain as well as the body. Studies show that elderly people who continue to read, work, travel, learn new skills and pursue intellectual interests maintain a higher level of mental functioning than those who do not. In fact, those who exercise their minds can slow, and in some cases actually reverse, the effects of time, recovering mental abilities they had ten or twenty years earlier. Those who continue to be active, interested and engaged may also slow the progression of Alzheimer's and other forms of dementia.

So encourage your parent to use his mind more. If he is mobile, get him to take continuing education classes, to join senior trips or to volunteer. If he is less mobile, get him to read (or listen to books on tape), to play bridge or scrabble or to discuss politics or sports with a companion.

Your parent needs to keep the rest of the package fit too, as there is convincing evidence that low blood pressure, good overall health, exercise and a general sense of personal control all contribute to a keener mind.

## DEMENTIA OR OLD AGE?

In the early stages, it is difficult to distinguish between dementia and benign aging. The symptoms of dementia can be fairly innocuous at first and most people compensate for minor mental slip-ups with reminders and notes, or they find excuses for their errors. *Oh, I'm sorry about our date. I was sure we said Tuesday.* Social skills are usually the last to go, so during short visits a person with early dementia may seem perfectly fine. He may chat about old times, and remember who's who and what's happening. Families and friends, who don't want to believe that something might be wrong, are more than happy to dismiss a slightly disheveled appearance or a few memory lapses.

At some point, however, the problems become hard to ignore. The dementia begins to interfere with relationships and the details of daily life, such as shopping, paying bills or selecting clothing. Your parent might lose a particular skill—an avid crossword puzzle fan may have trouble filling in the blanks, a lifetime golfer may fumble over selecting the proper clubs.

If you suspect dementia, think carefully about what your parent was like before. Are these problems really new or did you simply fail to notice them earlier? All of us are far more aware of memory slips in older people than in younger ones. When Grandpa loses his hat repeatedly an alarm goes off, but there isn't even a second thought when a teenager keeps losing his.

Generally, in dementia, a per-

> **&&Mom would forget something on the stove, or forget what she just did, and I'd think, 'Well, she's getting older. Maybe I'm just looking for problems.' But finally I said, 'No, something is not right.'**
>
> *She would wear the same clothes over and over and not care if she took a shower or washed her hair or anything, which is really out of character because she used to be immaculate. She would say 'No, I didn't wear this yesterday,' or 'I washed them,' when I knew she hadn't.***
>
> —LINDA K.

son's memory doesn't just slip, it disappears. He doesn't simply miss an appointment, he insists he never had one. He doesn't just lose his glasses, he forgets that he wears glasses. He doesn't forget who spoke at a meeting, he doesn't know he ever went to a meeting.

In addition to memory problems concerning specific facts, a person with dementia may easily become lost or disoriented, even near his home or in another familiar place. He may have trouble with language, so he will grope for the right word, use the wrong word or resort to gibberish. His emotions may become heightened and irrational, and unpleasant personality traits can become amplified. He might also become accusatory, critical or uncharacteristically aggressive. He may have trouble sleeping. And he is likely to have trouble concentrating, reasoning and making decisions. Whatever the symptoms, they usually grow progressively worse.

# Getting Tested

If you suspect dementia, urge your parent to consult an experienced doctor or medical team for a diagnosis. Why bother? Well, for a number of reasons. First of all, your hunch may be wrong. If not, between five and ten percent of all cases of dementia are at least partially, if not fully, reversible. And the sooner they are diagnosed, the easier they are to treat. Reversible causes include overmedication or adverse drug reactions, malnutrition, an overactive thyroid (which skews the body's hormones, causing anxiety, irritability, depression and confusion), and a disorder called normal pressure hydro-cephalus (in which spinal fluid builds up in the brain, causing memory loss, incontinence and an unusual, shuffling gait). In the elderly, depression can also mimic the early phases of dementia, causing a disorder known as pseudodementia.

If your parent's illness cannot be cured, doctors may be able to slow the progress of the disease through medications (antihypertensives, for example, in the case of mini-strokes), treat particular symptoms, such as anxiety or insomnia, and take care of any medical problems that may be exacerbating his confusion. In follow-up consultations, a social worker can counsel your family, teach you about lifestyle changes that will help ease the symptoms and lead you to community agencies and Alzheimer's groups that provide services and support to patients and their families.

A diagnosis will also force your family to face what is happening and to plan for the future while your parent can still be part of that planning. And learning the biological reasons for your parent's behavior should give you all a little more patience, empathy and tolerance.

Convincing your parent to have an evaluation is another matter, of course. It will be easy if he has noticed the problems and wants to know what is happening to him. But if your parent is like most people with symptoms of dementia and denies there are problems, insists that it's just old age, believes that nothing can be done and resents any suggestion that there is some-

**❝My mother had severe memory loss that hadn't been diagnosed. I discovered a stubborn streak in myself and insisted on her being tested. Memory loss, incontinence and a very awkward walk—those were her symptoms. She couldn't remember how to set the table or how to put her stockings on. But she always recognized us and there weren't any delusional aspects.**

**It turned out she had a treatable condition, normal pressure hydrocephalus. It was corrected with a shunt when she was eighty, and that was the closest thing to a miracle I've ever seen. She woke up, smiled at me and said, 'I haven't seen a Broadway play in a long time. Let's get tickets.'❞          —BARBARA F.**

## SIGNS OF DEMENTIA

The symptoms of dementia represent a change from how a person used to be; they are persistent and grow steadily worse.

❖ Memory loss—information is forgotten frequently and permanently

❖ Confusion—simple tasks are difficult to perform

❖ Disorientation—the person gets lost even in familiar places

❖ Poor grooming—personal hygiene is neglected and clothing may be soiled or inappropriate for the event or the weather

❖ Mood swings—the person easily becomes upset, agitated or angry

❖ Language difficulty—words are forgotten, misused or garbled

❖ Math difficulty—counting or balancing a checkbook is a challenge

❖ Poor judgment—a person makes unsafe or unusual decisions

❖ Repetition—the person says or does the same thing over and over

thing wrong, then you have a challenge before you.

Wait for the right moment, when your parent is calm and at his most lucid. Discuss your concerns as delicately as possible, touching on some of the changes you have noticed, without criticizing or alarming your parent. If he refuses to believe there is anything wrong, try the do-it-for-me approach: "It would really put *my* mind at ease if we could be sure." Or ask your parent's doctor to recommend an evaluation.

If your parent absolutely won't budge, make an appointment for yourself with a geriatric social worker or someone from the local Alzheimer's Association to discuss your parent's symptoms, issues that concern you and ways to make life a little easier for both of you.

### WHERE TO GET AN EVALUATION

Your parent's primary doctor should be able to rule out reversible causes of confusion and may even be able to diagnose the cause of the dementia. But if the doctor dismisses these concerns as part of old age or prescribes drugs for the symptoms without looking for the cause, consult another doctor. Look for a geriatric specialist or neurologist, or find out if there is a geriatric assessment center nearby. For a referral, call the local chapter of the Alzheimer's Association, a large municipal hospital or other medical professionals.

## WHAT HAPPENS IN AN EVALUATION

Alzheimer's can be diagnosed with certainty only by studying the brain during an autopsy, but doctors can rule out other possibilities and then make a diagnosis by the process of elimination. This may seem like a crude technique, but it is a surprisingly good one in this case, accurate nearly 95 percent of the time.

Doctors take different approaches in an evaluation—aggressively calling in specialists and ordering a number of tests, or focusing on the family's immediate needs and doing more listening than probing. In general, a thorough evaluation takes at least two or three hours and may include some or all of the following:

**A mental status exam.** The doctor will take note of your parent's appearance and speech, and ask about his moods and any psychiatric problems, such as hallucinations, obsessions or phobias. Most doctors will conduct what is known as a Mini Mental State Examination. This fifteen-minute test assesses your parent's ability to perform simple tasks, recall new information, think abstractly, calculate and communicate. He might be asked, for example, to count backwards, name the current President, follow a simple instruction (fold this piece of paper and put it on that table) and perhaps draw some familiar object like a clock. Incorrect answers do not mean that a person has dementia, and doctors take into account the patient's education, age, degree of nervousness and previous abilities in judging the results.

During these questions, your parent may be frightened or embarrassed if she has trouble answering them. If you are present, don't give clues or advice, but do offer some quiet reassurance and comfort.

If your parent does poorly on this test, the doctor will try to determine when the problems began and how they have progressed over time, and may order a neurological exam and laboratory tests.

**Neurological exam.** Looking for physical signs of illness or injury, a doctor will test your parent's reflexes, sensory and motor function, gait and coordination.

**Laboratory tests.** Blood and urine samples will be examined for the presence of a variety of disorders that cause or contribute to confusion, such as infections, anemia, kidney and liver disease, thyroid abnormalities, heavy metal or drug poisoning, vitamin B-12 deficiency, syphilis and AIDS.

**Scans.** Imaging technology, CAT, MRI and PET scans, take pictures of the brain to detect damage from seizures, strokes, blood clots, tumors, bleeding or a build-up of spinal fluid. (If the suspected ailment is not treatable, there may be no reason to have the scan.)

**Spinal tap.** A spinal tap, in which the doctor inserts a slender, hollow needle into the spine and draws a small sample of fluid, is usually used only if the doctor suspects an infection or disease of the nervous system. Current research suggests that spinal fluid might be used in the future to diagnose Alzheimer's.

**Psychiatric exam.** A psychiatrist will examine your parent to identify any reversible causes of dementia, such as depression, as well as anxiety, paranoia or other mental illness.

---

*"My parents were married for fifty years, and about five years ago my mother started to be really horrible towards my father. She went through these wild ups and downs when she would yell at him or become terribly depressed and not want to go out or do anything. I think she finally exhausted him, because he died two years ago.*

*We all blamed her, and for a time I would have as little as possible to do with her. I was so angry at her for being so cruel to Daddy. Then, last year, she became so depressed while visiting my brother in Florida that he took her to the hospital. They said she had been having mini-strokes.*

*Oh boy, did I feel badly. I mean, she didn't know what she had been doing. She couldn't control her rage or depression or paranoia. I'm just glad that I know now so that I can take care of her and stop resenting her so much. She really has no idea what she is doing."* —MARGE W.

# Alzheimer's Disease

While dozens of diseases cause dementia, by far the most common causes are Alzheimer's disease and something known as multi-infarct dementia. Alzheimer's affects more than four million people in this country, and multi-infarcts affect at least two or three million.

In Alzheimer's disease, brain cells degenerate and the brain becomes littered with telltale debris, known as plaques and tangles. *Neuritic* (or senile) *plaques* are blobs of dead or damaged tissue surrounding a protein known as beta-amyloid, and *neurofibrillary tangles* are twisted bits of fibers found within brain cells.

What causes this destruction is unknown. In fact, scientists are not even sure if Alzheimer's is a single disease with a single cause, or a number of related diseases caused by a variety of factors. In other words, different paths may lead to the same type of brain damage and symptoms.

Alzheimer's seems to be genetic in about half of all cases, but if your parent has Alzheimer's, don't become overly alarmed about your own future health. The disease may require that you inherit a faulty gene from both parents. Or you may inherit only a propensity for the illness, and some second assault, such as an injury or exposure to environmental toxin, may be necessary for the disease to develop.

Beyond genetics, researchers are

## THE STAGES OF ALZHEIMER'S DISEASE

Although people with Alzheimer's react uniquely to the illness and follow an unpredictable course, experts have tracked a few of the more common symptoms of the illness. The stages described below are only a rough outline of what *may* occur over the course of a person's illness, which typically lasts eight to twelve years.

**Stage I:** A person with the disease is usually still alert and social, and may be very much enjoying life, although he may know that something is not quite right. Frustrated by the forgetfulness and afraid of what is happening, some people become anxious or depressed, which only exacerbates the memory loss and confusion.

❖ Short-term memory fades. A person has trouble remembering recent events, learning new things, retaining information and concentrating.

❖ Speech is slightly impaired. A person confuses one word for another or can't find the right word.

❖ Hygiene is neglected. Clothing may be soiled or disheveled, and bathing and grooming forgotten.

❖ Judgment is hindered and thinking abstractly is difficult.

❖ Emotional responses are erratic and exaggerated. A person may become easily upset, anxious, angry or depressed, often in response to the changes taking place.

**Stage II:** The signs become obvious. A person may exhibit bizarre behavior, such as getting lost on the way to the bathroom, hiding away food or other items or becoming outraged for no apparent reason.

❖ Short-term memory is gone. A person is unable to learn new information or skills.

looking at a number of other possible causes for Alzheimer's, including toxins in the environment, an abnormal response by the immune system in which it attacks the body, prior brain injury, a slow-acting virus, or simply worn-out brain cells that run amok. The notion that aluminum causes or contributes to Alzheimer's has received little support recently, but is still under study.

# Multi-Infarct Dementia

Up to 40 percent of all cases of dementia are thought to be wholly or partially caused by a series of strokes so small they can occur unnoticed. Blood flow is blocked to some part of the brain, usually because of a clog, clot or rupture,

❖ Coordination is poor, creating a risk for falls and accidents. A person may require assistance with bathing, eating and dressing.

❖ Complex tasks that require any decision-making or a series of steps are overwhelming.

❖ Agitation, wandering or pacing is common.

❖ Moods are even more exaggerated. A person may be uncooperative, hostile or aggressive, although some people become serene and peaceful. (They are less frustrated by the illness because they don't remember what they used to do.)

❖ Language and speech troubles worsen.

❖ Ability to add, subtract or do other calculations is lost. (The checkbook may be overdrawn or bills left unpaid.)

❖ Sleep cycles fall out of sync. A person may sleep at odd hours and wander at night.

❖ Repetition. Stories or actions are repeated monotonously.

**Stage III:** At this point, patients are totally dependent and require constant care.

❖ Confusion is acute. Most long-term memory is gone, in addition to all short-term memory.

❖ Physical rigidity and seizures may occur.

❖ Hallucinations (seeing or hearing things that don't exist), delusions (irrational or unfounded beliefs) and paranoia (in particular, a belief that others are trying to kill the person or that a spouse is cheating) are all possible.

❖ Patients are totally incontinent.

❖ Eventually, patients are unable to speak, get out of bed or feed themselves. They become susceptible to malnutrition, infections, pneumonia and other illness.

leaving behind a pocket of damaged or dead tissue. With each successive stroke, the brain loses more and more of its ability to function.

People with multi-infarct dementia (also referred to as vascular dementia or chronic cerebrovascular lesions) generally are at risk of stroke because of diabetes, high blood pressure or other cardiovascular disease. Doctors can spot the disease with an MRI or CAT scan.

While the symptoms are similar to those described for Alzheimer's, multi-infarct dementia often affects physical abilities before it affects the mind. A person might become weak, lose some vision or become incontinent before he becomes forgetful or confused. Symptoms typically appear suddenly, growing worse in spurts, and sometimes even disappearing for intervals. In Alzheimer's, the decline is more progressive.

If diagnosed early, the progression of multi-infarct dementia can sometimes be slowed by lowering the risk of stroke. This is done by administering medications that treat high blood pressure, high cholesterol or vascular disease; instituting better diet and regular exercise to improve circulation; and improving the management of diabetes.

# Dealing with the Diagnosis

Under normal conditions, doctors meet privately with patients to discuss a diagnosis, and then let the patients decide how much, if anything, they want to tell their families. But dementia derails everything in life, including the doctor-patient relationship. Quite often doctors confer with the entire family, which is helpful because every family member is affected by this illness, but this should be done only with your parent's consent. And the doctor should never discuss the diagnosis *only* with the family, bypassing your parent completely.

No matter how confused your parent is and no matter how painful the news may be to him, he should be told about his diagnosis. When it comes to an individual's health, honesty is always the best policy. All of us have a fundamental right to know what is happening to us, regardless of the severity. Knowledge

## FORGIVE YOURSELF

If you have been snapping impatiently at your forgetful father or yelling at him for being disruptive or rude, you may feel guilty once you understand that his behavior is due to an illness. Forgive yourself. You reacted perfectly normally under the circumstances and have nothing to feel guilty about. In fact, even now that you know the diagnosis, you are sure to have plenty of angry moments in the future. It would be almost impossible not to, given the nature of this disease. Give your parent as much love as you can, forget about what happened yesterday and focus your energy on today.

about our own health allows us to retain some control over our lives, to plan for the future and understand the present.

People with dementia usually take the news far more calmly than their families expect. Of course it is upsetting, but they already know something is wrong, even if they don't want to admit it. At least a diagnosis lets them know why their world is so askew.

### BREAKING THE NEWS

When you talk with your parent about a diagnosis of dementia, try to understand what she may be experiencing. In addition to feeling devastated, she may be afraid of losing dignity and respect, and of becoming a burden to the family. Listen, share her concerns, offer warmth and support and reassure her that she will not be left alone. Tell her that you all, as a family, are going to get through this together. Without dismissing her fears, focus on all she can still do and on the good times she and her family can still have together.

Of course, you will have your own turbulent emotions to contend with as well. You may have suspected Alzheimer's and now realize you were totally unprepared for the truth. You may feel shock, horror, anger, grief and helplessness. You may feel even more sorry for

---

*"When the doctor told me it was probably Alzheimer's I just kept saying, 'It's got to be something else. It can't be right.' Here was a woman who was such an active person. She raised eight of us by herself. She was completely independent. I just couldn't believe that her mind could be affected like that.*

*I was very frightened. You read and hear so much about people with Alzheimer's. My first thought was, she's going to become like a baby, like a vegetable.*

*So far, I've been managing. It's a challenge, that's for sure. We have good days and bad days, but somehow we get through them all."*
—LINDA K.

---

yourself than for your parent and afraid of the work that lies ahead. You may secretly hope that the disease runs its course quickly. These are all normal reactions. Don't be ashamed of them. You have a great deal to comprehend and to come to terms with.

## NOW WHAT?

The doctor or a member of his or her staff should talk with your family about the future and set you up with a social worker who can provide referrals and counseling. If you ask for this assistance and none is offered, do some research on your own, because a diagnosis by itself is of little use. You need help. Call the Alzheimer's Association, which has local chapters throughout the country that run support groups and provide referrals to local services from housing and legal aid to financial and medical assistance. Call other local senior service organizations as well, for further guidance and information.

## PLANNING FOR THE FUTURE

Because your parent is going to need extensive care, and at some point will be unable to make decisions for herself, your family needs to plan now for the future. If she has not already done so, your parent should name a durable power of attorney and/or set up a living trust, sign a will and advance directives (see Chapter Fourteen), compile important documents and notify family members where these items are

## ON THE LOOKOUT FOR OTHER PROBLEMS

If your parent has dementia, be aware of other problems that can exacerbate the symptoms (or cause symptoms of dementia on their own).

**Depression.** Depression may have the appearance of early Alzheimer's and goes hand in hand with dementia in about 20 percent of all cases. Frustrated by the symptoms of dementia, the person becomes depressed, and the depression then worsens the symptoms. Identifying and then treating depression—and it is extremely treatable (see page 106)—can alleviate confusion and memory loss substantially.

**Delirium.** While it typically comes on suddenly—in a matter of days or even hours—delirium is sometimes confused with dementia or may coexist with it. Symptoms vary widely but often include disorientation, inattentiveness and changes in personality. It is often reversible, but must be treated immediately.

**Medications.** Antidepressants, heart medications, anti-inflammatory drugs, sleeping pills, ulcer medications, insulin and cold medications can all cause confusion, agitation and other symptoms. Your parent's doctor should be aware of all drugs that he takes, including nonprescription ones.

**Alcohol.** While prolonged, heavy use of alcohol can cause permanent brain damage and dementia, even moderate drinking can worsen confusion, agitation and depression.

**Vision and hearing impairments.** Make sure that your parent gets his eyes and ears checked regularly, as poor hearing or blurred vision can make his world even more confusing.

**Vitamin B-12 deficiency.** Medications or age can impede a body's absorption of vitamin B-12, causing fatigue, depression, anxiety, memory loss and other problems typical of dementia. The deficiency is treated with injections of the vitamin.

kept, and determine how future medical and living expenses will be paid. Your family also needs to discuss her care and living situation.

While a diagnosis like this forces one to think about the future, it can also make clear the value of the present. Talk with your parent about her priorities. If your mother is still relatively lucid, find out if there is anything that she wants to do while she still can. Does she need to resolve an old conflict or visit a distant friend?

Has she always wanted to take a trip to San Francisco? Try Thai food? Go back to a childhood home? Remember, while it's hard to believe, life is not over, either for you or your parent.

# Treating Dementia

For now, and perhaps even after new drugs are developed, the best treatment for dementia will come from you, not the doctor. Your parent needs a safe and familiar environment, simple stimulation, a lot of reminders and cues, good physical care and plenty of love and encouragement. (See Chapter Sixteen for specifics on living with dementia.) Your parent may be able to receive this care at home, at least for a while, but eventually most families deplete their financial and emotional resources and have to look for some other housing situation or a nursing home.

## MEDICATION

Unfortunately, scientists have had little success in developing drugs that can bolster an ailing memory or give new life to a slowing brain. But some drugs, as well as ginkgo and vitamin E, do appear to slow progression of the disease. And doctors can treat symptoms, such as agitation, anxiety, aggression and insomnia.

Drugs are invaluable when symptoms become severe, but be sure they are used with extreme caution and discretion. Antidepressant, antianxiety and antipsychotic drugs are powerful substances which have not been well tested in elderly patients, especially elderly patients with fragile mental makeups. If not used correctly, they can cause serious side effects.

Remember the rule, "low and slow"—start with a low dose and then slowly increase it as necessary. Once a drug has had the desired effect, ask the doctor when your parent might be weaned off of it, to see if it is still needed. People with Alzheimer's change quickly—a jumping bean who needs something to calm her down can turn into a couch potato as the disease progresses, making a drug unnecessary and dangerous.

Psychotropic drugs also do not mix well with alcohol or a number of other drugs, including over-the-counter pills found in most household medicine cabinets. The combined effect on the brain may cause greater confusion, agitation and disorientation. Be sure to consult her doctor before your parent takes any new medicine, even if it is apparently harmless.

## MEMORY EXERCISES

If your parent has irreversible dementia, she will not regain mental abilities that are gone, but if she is still in the early stages she may be able to slow further loss and make the most of what abilities still exist. Mental stimulation—learning, reading, travel or anything else that exercises the mind—is the best preventive medicine.

The value of formal memory exercises, which are sometimes prescribed for people with dementia, is debatable. These exercises use computer tests, flash cards and games to teach patients to remember things through repetition, practice and mnemonic devices. *I'll remember her name is Martha because that was my cat's name and they both have orange hair.*

These exercises may be helpful for people who have only mild forgetfulness, are in the earliest stages of dementia or have lost some mental function because of a stroke or accident. But once a person is seriously confused and unable to remember virtually anything, these devices may be only exercises in frustration, reminding a person of what she can no longer do. If a doctor recommends them, leave it up to your parent to decide if she wants to do them or not. Don't push it.

## FOR MORE HELP

**Alzheimer's Association**
**800-272-3900**
**800-572-6037 (in Ill.)**

**Alzheimer's Disease Education and Referral Center**
**800-438-4380**

**National Institute of Neurological Disorders and Stroke**
**301-496-5751**

# Chapter Sixteen

# LIVING WITH DEMENTIA

*A New Approach, for Yourself and Your Parent • Tips for
Everyday Living • Coping with Problems of Behavior*

.................................

I F MARRIAGE, CHILDREN AND ILLNESS TEST ONE'S FLEXI-
bility and patience, then caring for a person with dementia
is the final exam. Rarely is one asked to give so much only to
receive so much aggravation and anguish in return. Dementia
doesn't just take away a person's ability to remember names,
calculate numbers or tell a good joke; it steals his personality, his
endearing quirks and his beloved memories. You are left to care
for a hauntingly familiar stranger, someone whose physical features
and occasional glances are heartwarming, but whose behavior and
personality, more and more, seem to belong to someone else.

For you, as the child in this relationship, witnessing such a
transformation in a parent is particularly unnerving. The person
who had the wisdom of longevity, the person who made vital
decisions, the person who was once your primary caregiver, is
increasingly dependent, incompetent and childlike. Your father
may throw tantrums, have trouble feeding himself or forget his
way home. He may become slovenly and self-centered. And you
may be called upon to care for him in ways you never imagined,
sometimes against his wishes or without his understanding. And
while you still love the person you knew, you may feel resentment
or even disgust toward the person he has become. It's a confusing

mix of emotions that can wear you down very quickly.

The cruelty and heartbreak of this disease can't be avoided. Nevertheless, you can help diminish some of the symptoms, learn tricks for coping with others and get outside support, all of which will make this rough ride a little smoother for both of you.

# Helping Yourself

Dementia calls for a stronger-than-usual arsenal of self-preservation measures. This illness takes an enormous toll on family members. And in this situation especially, your own care and your parent's care are inseparable.

If you are caring for your parent with any regularity, his mental state will reflect yours. If you are always on the verge of exploding or crying, he will feel the pressure and become that much more anxious and bewildered. Life together can swirl into a downward tailspin. But if, on the other hand, you are calm, your parent will be more capable and composed.

Attend to your own needs, if only to help your parent. Join a support group. (The Alzheimer's Association can refer you to a local one.) Schedule breaks away from your parent. Review the chap-

ter, "Caring for the Caregiver," page 27, and try the suggestions outlined below.

## ACKNOWLEDGE THE SITUATION

Early in this disease it's natural to believe, on some level, that your parent will wake up one day and be the person she used to be. That kind of hopefulness gets people through the day. But it also leads to frustration and despair.

If your parent has progressive dementia, she will not get better. She will not be able to do things today that she couldn't do yesterday. She will probably be even less capable tomorrow. Acknowledging the situation and accepting these harsh realities is extraordinarily painful, but it is the only way to move forward and to appreciate what you still have.

## REMEMBER THAT DEMENTIA IS A DISEASE

With dementia, there are no physical signs of illness. Your mother looks the same as she always did, so it's natural to expect her to be the same. But she is not. She cannot control her behavior. She is not repeating the same questions over and over

❝*Sometimes it's as if my mother were dead, the woman who raised me, the one that I used to go to for comfort. I don't have her anymore, and I miss her terribly.*❞

—LINDA K.

# A SAFETY CHECKLIST

Dementia creates new hazards, which means taking extra precautions, beyond those listed on page 137.

❑ Turn the temperature on the water heater down to 120°F. and label all hot-water faucets clearly with large, red letters. A person with dementia may not test the water temperature, and when it's too hot, he may not realize immediately that he is being burned or he may not react quickly enough to escape injury.

❑ Place an identification tag in your parent's wallet or on a necklace in case he gets lost.

❑ Post by every phone a clearly-written list of emergency numbers (police, fire, poison control, doctor) and instructions for calling 911.

❑ Install handrails and grab bars throughout the house, as dementia affects coordination and balance.

❑ As your parent grows more confused, lock (or install child-proof latches on) any cabinets that contain household cleaners, solvents, medicines, matches, liquor, knives, scissors or other dangerous items. Check for hazards outside the house as well, such as paints, clippers, saws, grills and lighter fluid.

❑ If your parent is apt to wander, put locks on doors leading outside. Place them high or low on the door where he won't easily find them. Remove bedroom and bathroom door locks that are operated from the inside so he can't accidentally lock himself in.

❑ Your parent should not smoke when unattended. He might forget a burning cigarette or drop a smoldering butt in the wrong place.

❑ If your parent has trouble operating the stove, remove the knobs or encase them so he can't leave the burner or the oven on. Or put the electric stove on a timer so it can be operated only between certain hours. Ask an electrician for other stove safety tips.

to exasperate you: She cannot force herself to remember the answers any more than someone with a broken leg can force himself to walk.

If you can keep the thought planted firmly in your mind—and repeat it daily, almost like a mantra—that your parent's behavior is caused by the disease, not the person, it will alleviate some of the frustration and help you to keep some perspective.

## PUT YOURSELF IN HER SHOES

Imagine being given a colossal assignment, one that you simply cannot do. You are overwhelmed by the challenge and humiliated by your lack of ability. Making matters worse, someone is standing over you growing increasingly impatient and annoyed as you struggle and fail. The pressure and embarrassment make it harder for you to think, so you fumble even more.

For your parent, getting dressed or eating a meal that involves several foods and an assortment of utensils may be formidable tasks now. She can't remember what to do next or why she is doing this at all. If you criticize her, hurry her or become annoyed, she will only become more anxious and confused, and less able to perform. But if you can muster some patience and compassion, she will actually be more successful with the task at hand.

## FORGET LOGIC

Of course bananas should not be put in the oven and hair should not be combed with a toothbrush.

---

*"Sometimes, she says something—a little joke or a comment—that shows me she is still there. Buried under that disease, a piece of my mother still survives. It's that little piece that remains, the memories of who she was and those soft, familiar hands that keep me going."*

—MARGE W.

---

But if you attempt to explain why to your parent, you will be wasting your breath. She is living in a world where everything is changing. Nothing is familiar and nothing makes sense. You can't reason with her, so stop trying. Instead, laugh with her, give her a hug, and hand her the hairbrush.

## VENT YOUR ANGER— SOMEPLACE ELSE

Your worst anger may erupt during the early stages of the disease, when you are still fighting what is happening, trying to hold on to the person your parent was and struggling unsuccessfully for a logical explanation. You go for a visit (or to another part of your house) and, before seeing your parent, you promise yourself that today you will be patient. But within minutes of walking in the door you find yourself snapping, "Mother!! What have you done? How many times have I told you not to rip up the mail? *Why do you do this to me?*" Minutes later you hate yourself for getting so irate, and you hate her, or this disease, for turning you into a shrew.

Welcome to dementia. The disease distorts the personalities not only of patients, but of their caregivers as well. People who never used to swear seem to learn every vulgar word in the book. People who were kind become crabby. People who love their parents dearly suddenly want them to disappear.

The problem is that while dementia breeds anger, it also feeds off of it. Yelling at your parent or yanking his shirt off because you can't stand to wait while he fumbles with each button may trigger a wild, emotional tirade. If you can back off and cool down, things will go more smoothly and you may actually get him dressed and fed faster.

When you can't cool off, vent your anger elsewhere. Make sure your parent is safe, and then leave the room. Take a few deep breaths. Stretch your muscles, yell out loud or punch a pillow. And always have a list of friends or support group members you can call when you need to release some steam.

> **❝**I have said things that I would never have dreamed I could say to my mother. I yell and scream at her. I've cursed her. Sometimes I hate her. I was brought up to know that you don't do those kinds of things. But you get to a point where you just don't know what else to do. I'm usually a pretty controlled person, but with this, you don't have any control. Or I don't.
>
> I don't like these sides of myself. I don't like what's happening to me. Every day I pray for patience.**❞**
>
> —LINDA K.

When you do slip and lose your temper with your parent, which you are bound to do now and then, don't hate yourself. You acted naturally, and if there is anything positive about this disease, it's that your parent will forget that you ever even raised your voice.

## BEWARE OF ABUSE

When a parent has dementia, the stress can become overwhelming, and you may find yourself lashing out, shaking, pushing or even striking your parent. If this happens, get away from him *immediately*. Drop whatever you are doing and walk away. Call a neighbor, a relative or a friend to take over for you. You need support and you need a break—right now.

Call the local chapter of the Alzheimer's Association. Most chapters have Help Lines that can get you through the moment of crisis and help arrange emergency respite care.

## FOCUS ON THE GOOD TIMES

Embrace any passing moments of intimacy or apparent awareness. You may not get them toward the end, but earlier on there may be breaks in this storm when your parent returns to you. Suddenly, there is a moment of singing or dancing or hugging, or maybe your parent tells an old story or gives you a familiar look or thanks you for all you are doing. Savor it. Remember it. Make a note of it and pin it to your wall. This is a shot of strength and pleasure that you may not get again.

## DON'T ASSUME HE'S MISERABLE

Early on, when your parent is still aware of what his abilities used to be, he may be extremely upset about what he can no longer do. But as the disease progresses, he may become perfectly content in his mixed-up, timeless world. He may not know that life used to be different. No matter how active he used to be, he may be happy just sitting, stroking a pet, watching the leaves blow in the breeze or listening to a favorite song. It may seem sad to you, but this may be all he needs.

*"I had everybody here for Easter a few weeks before my mother died. I thought, 'What did I get myself into?' because I couldn't give my attention to anything else. She needed all my time.*

*But she really enjoyed herself. My niece is a psychologist and they were trying to trigger her memory, asking her lots of questions, mentioning composers and songs. She loved music.*

*I asked her that night if she had enjoyed her company. And the way she smiled at me I knew that it was a very, very successful day."*
—SALLY T.

## REMEMBER YOUR SENSE OF HUMOR

If your mother thinks you stole her stockings so that you could wear them over your head and rob her

*"Over the years we tried to convince my father to use a cane when he became unsteady on his feet but he always refused. He'd say he got around much better than any of us or he'd get angry and change the subject. When his dementia got worse, he also became much frailer, and one day I took out the cane we'd gotten for him and tried to slip it into his hand. Before I could do it, he looked at me with a concerned expression on his face and said, 'Eric! I didn't know you used a cane!'"*
—ERIC S.

it's sad, but it's also a bit amusing. Help her look for her stockings and assure her that you are not going to rob her, but when you repeat the story to your sister, go ahead and laugh about it. (*What was I going to steal, her dentures?*)

You need to grieve, of course. You are losing your parent in a very painful way. Yet despite the gravity of the situation—and because of it—you have to give yourself permission to laugh. Let go. Who knows, maybe your parent will see the humor too.

## GIVE YOURSELF SOME CREDIT

It may not feel as if you are doing a good job. In fact, most of the time it may feel quite the opposite. You may lash out at your father. At times, you may wish that he would die. You would have to be a saint to do otherwise. Give yourself some credit. If it helps, write a list of all that you are doing for your parent and put it someplace where you will see it regularly. Then stand in front of the mirror and tell yourself that you are a good person. You are. In fact, anyone caring for someone with dementia is an unsung hero.

And remember, if you are in a support group or have friends in a similar situation, don't compare yourself to them. Their parents may have different symptoms of dementia, they may have a very different relationship with their parents, and their lives may hold entirely different pressures.

## USE RESPITE CARE

To preserve your sanity and health, take regular breaks away from it all. Before your parent is accustomed to a routine that includes only you, get her used to a companion, a day-care program or another caregiver. (See Chapter Nine for information about these services.) The longer you wait to take a break, the harder it will be for her to accept change, a new place or unfamiliar people. Once you arrange for some sort of respite:

◆ Don't ask your parent if she wants to go to day care or if she wants to have a particular person care for her, because she'll say no. Tell her what is happening. Don't make it her choice.

◆ Ease into the arrangement gradually. If you are having a new companion or aide come to the house, or if you are taking your parent to day care, and your parent clings to you, stay with her for the first day or two. Then leave her for an hour, working up to half a day, and so on.

◆ Schedule the changing of the guard for a time of day when your parent tends to be calm. Don't have a new companion or aide come in the late afternoon if that is when your mother is most anxious and confused.

◆ Provide detailed instructions about your parent's daily routines and habits, and suggest ways of dealing with outbursts, wandering, accusations or other difficult behavior. If possible, have the aide watch you in action once or twice, so he or she can follow in the same path.

◆ Make it clear to your parent when you will return. (She may ask for you every five minutes.) Put a calendar or clock, depending upon how long you will be gone, on the wall, marking the day and time that you will return. The companion or aide can draw an X through each hour or day as it passes.

◆ Remember to keep a regular schedule. Your parent should go to day care at the same time each day, or have a home-care worker come to the house at the same time each day, if possible.

◆ If your parent says you are abandoning her, accuses the aide of stealing, refuses to go to day care, or locks a visiting nurse out, consider any underlying reasons she might have for behaving this way (not that there is necessarily any logical reason). Maybe she is afraid you are leaving her for good, or worried that this other person is going to hurt her. Find a way to help her overcome her fears (for example, leave a large picture of yourself and a note saying that you love her and will return soon).

◆ Be committed to this arrangement. Give yourself a month or so to put up with the fussing that may accompany it. Don't give in. The longer the new arrangement is sustained, the easier it will become for your parent to accept it.

*❝I tried to leave my mother at a day-care program and the next thing I knew she was running after me. I'd spent so much time finding a situation that would be right for her, and I was very upset that she refused to cooperate.*

*Several months later I tried again, at a new place. But this time I got my mother there early, before anyone else. It was like starting somebody off in kindergarten. We began with one day a week until we had worked up to four days. It was all very gradual. When my mother got anxious the staff put a sign up: 'Sally will be here to pick you up at four.'*

*She came to love the place. That's the funny part. She looked forward to it. Of course, as soon as she got off the van, she couldn't tell me where she had been or what she had done. But while she was there she was happy, that's all I know. And that's all I cared about.❞*

—SALLY T.

## SOCIALIZING WITH YOUR PARENT

Social isolation is one of the more serious side effects of this job and exacerbates caregiver burnout. You must find ways to meet both your need for change and companionship and your parent's need for an unchanging environment. Get out on your own regularly, but if you need to include your parent in your socializing:

❖ Keep gatherings small. One or two people may be manageable, but a large party may confuse your parent.

❖ Whenever possible, socialize around a regular daily activity. Invite people over for a meal during your parent's regular mealtime, or have friends join you on your parent's daily walk.

❖ Invite people to come to your parent, rather than moving her to a new environment. This way she will be more settled and can choose to go to her room when she gets tired.

❖ If your parent has odd habits or troubling behaviors—your mother burps loudly throughout dinner—warn guests in advance. Everyone will be more comfortable and most people will understand and be supportive when they know what to expect.

# Helping Your Parent

J ust as keeping your cool will help your parent remain calm, making life simpler for him will make life more manageable for you. Give your parent a simple and predictable environment. Adjust your expectations and learn what makes him anxious, what helps him to relax, what distracts him and what reassures him.

## GIVE HIM RESPECT

Respecting your parent, and treating him as an adult can be challenging when dementia strikes. But even when you are cutting his food or helping him bathe, remember that your parent is not a child and shouldn't be treated like one. He has lived a long life and has well-formed opinions, dreams, likes and dislikes—even if he can't remember what they are. Help him maintain a sense of dignity. Address him with the same respect you always have.

Make sure that your tone of voice is not condescending. Don't scold him. He hasn't done anything bad; it's the disease that is making him behave badly. Refrain from talking about him as if he were not in the room or unable to comprehend your words. Protect his self-esteem and modesty and ask others who care for him to do the same.

## LET HIM DO ALL THAT HE CAN

Whatever his limitations, your parent should be encouraged to do all that he can. Day-to-day it may be easier to do things for him, and it may seem like an act of kindness, but the truth is that people with dementia who are encouraged to do things for themselves retain their capabilities and their independence much longer than those who are not.

Think of tasks that he can manage on his own or with minimal help. Have him polish the silver, stir the orange juice or water the grass. Ask him to read from the cookbook while you make dinner. And then tell him how helpful he has been. You may feel it's demeaning to have your father cut out coupons, but the task may be quite enjoyable to him—at least more enjoyable than sitting on the couch alone. Of course, letting your parent help may at times require more work from you and others (the laundry may need to be refolded, the spilled juice wiped up), but it's a small price to pay for a little contentment and pride.

If your parent has become helpless and demands that you or someone else do everything for him—a common response to dementia—do not fall victim to his demands. They may stem from your parent's frustration and fear, they may be an attempt to regain some control, or they may be a cry for attention and reassurance. Do reassure your parent, but don't respond to his orders. Trust yourself to know when he really needs your help and when he can help himself.

## SIMPLIFY HIS WORLD

The simpler your parent's world —his house, his tasks, his conversations, his visits—the better. But your parent may not realize that the volume is too loud or the lighting too bright or the room too crowded. He just knows that he is unhappy and becomes agitated. So it is up to you to learn what upsets him and try to rectify it. Here are a few guidelines:

◆ Get rid of knickknacks, colorful rugs, mirrors, piles of papers and clutter, especially in the room where your parent lives.

◆ Furniture should be simple, and placed so that it can be easily used. Pathways should be clear. Once you arrange the furniture, don't rearrange it.

◆ Buy handrails, grab bars, sturdy chairs with wide armrests and a walker if necessary.

◆ Keep the noise down. You may not notice that the television is blaring, but it may confound him.

◆ Use signs wherever necessary—on the bathroom door, bedrooms, cabinets and bureau drawers ("socks," "shirts," "pants," etc.). If your parent can't figure out which item in the refrigerator he should eat, write LUNCH across his sandwich bag. Use symbols if written words don't work.

◆ Get phones with large pushbuttons, which are easier to read and easier to use.

◆ Offer simple choices. Don't ask your parent what he wants for dinner. Say, "Do you want chicken or fish?" Or just tell him what you're going to have for dinner.

Simplifying the world is particularly important if your parent's coordination and mobility are impaired. He may know what move-

## SUPPORT FOR PATIENTS TOO

There are hundreds of support groups for the families of people with Alzheimer's and other forms of dementia, but only recently have there been support groups for the patients themselves (because of the assumption that patients didn't understand their illness or didn't want to acknowledge it). It turns out that patients, at least those in the early stages of the illness, are relieved to talk about the difficulty of becoming dependent, the aggravation of forgetfulness, the hardship of losing a driver's license and other emotional issues and practical problems.

To find out if there is a patient support group near your parent or to get some pointers on how to start one, call the local chapter of the Alzheimer's Association, or call the national headquarters at 800-272-3900.

ment is necessary to carry out an action and have the muscle power to do it, but the signal from the brain to the muscle is interrupted, so he can't execute the motion. His walk may be unsteady and awkward and simple tasks may take forever.

If this is the case, eliminate unnecessary steps and then offer instructions that require only single movements. For example, instead of asking him to bathe, walk through each step with him, one at a time: "Unbutton your shirt. Take the shirt off. Step into the shower." And so forth.

## STICK TO A ROUTINE

Create a schedule that works for your parent, and then stick to it. If she is most lucid in the morning, schedule complex activities, like bathing, for that time. If she gets restless and fidgety in the middle of the day, create a calming task for her to do every day at that anxious hour. If she is most confused in the evenings (a common syndrome called "sundowning"), keep the evenings quiet and soothing. (Sundowning is sometimes lessened by turning on all the lights in the late afternoon, before the sun starts to set.)

Likewise, plan your visits for the same time and the same day every week. Or if your parent goes to day care every weekday, then try to follow the same routine on the weekend by getting her up and dressed and then giving her some activity to do that is similar to what she does in day care. She won't remember the schedule, but she won't be surprised by it either.

## DIVERT HER ATTENTION

Sometimes forgetfulness can be used in your favor. When your parent is about to do something, or is already doing something that you don't want her to do, it's easy to divert her attention.

When your mother starts into a tantrum or begins to tell a repetitive story, change the subject or suggest a new activity. Have her look at a photo album, sip a cup of tea, go for a walk, knit, listen to music, sing a song, play a tune on the piano or flip through catalogues. Or engage her in a chore she enjoys.

If she gets riled up in the middle of a task that has to be finished, like getting dressed, divert her from her frustration. Pause for a moment and sing a familiar song or tell an

> *I've learned that I have to think ahead and make it look like I really don't want my mother to do something, and then she'll do it.*
>
> *I came home Thursday afternoon to find her physically wrestling with Mildred, the aide who takes care of her while I'm at work. It was raining and Mildred wanted her to go inside, but she wouldn't do it. I suggested that Mildred tell Mom to sit outside, that she didn't want her to go in the house. Then Mom wanted to come inside. You learn to do whatever works.* —CAROL G.

old family story. It should calm her down and when you return to the task she may forget that this is something she didn't want to do. A short break may calm you as well.

## IGNORE SOME THINGS

Avoid correcting your parent repeatedly. It is demeaning and confusing for him (he may not understand what it is he is doing wrong), and it is exhausting for you. Instead, try to ignore some things, as long as they aren't dangerous or harmful. Does it really matter if your parent remembers the dog's name or if he talks about his late wife as though she were still alive? Who is it hurting if he wears socks that don't match or if he wants to eat eggs for dinner and turkey for

**"When my mother was in the nursing home, I used to visit her at lunch time and feed her. After she had eaten, I would hold her hand and talk about the past, and she would lie there and listen. She never really said anything, or at least anything that made sense.**

*One time I was flipping through old photos and she reached out and touched my cheek and there was a warm and connected look in her eye when she stared up at me. She said, 'They're all gone, aren't they?' I said, 'Yes, they are. But I'm still here and Polly is still here.' And that was it. She was gone again. But I don't think I'll ever forget that moment.* **"**
—GLORIA C.

breakfast? You have enough struggles in the day. Some battles just aren't worth fighting. Ignore his mistakes and agree with him sometimes even when he's wrong.

When you need to correct him, say something that will get him back on the right track without being critical. *You probably did take your medication, but let's check your pill box just to be sure.*

You may also find that ignoring certain habits helps to curtail them. If you can stay out of a struggle, maybe not even look up, your parent may stop the behavior. This technique works best if you pick just one behavior to ignore and alert everyone else caring for your parent to the plan.

## TRY A HUG

Warmth and love are potent healers. When your father gets riled, discombobulated, anxious or depressed, stroke his hand or cheek. A gentle touch will help both of you get through the next few minutes—and a few minutes of peace can be a saving grace at this time.

# Tips for Everyday Living

Managing day-to-day requires imagination, ingenuity and perseverance. Every week, and sometimes every minute, brings a new challenge. Unfortunately, there are no standard rules or answers. You simply have to try different tacks and see what works. Here are a few of the more common issues that arise and some possible ways of coping.

## BATHING, GROOMING AND DRESSING

When the smallest things become herculean battles, it's tempting to let things go. But your parent's grooming affects her dignity, as well as the feelings of others who spend time with her.

◆ Allow her to do tasks according to her own habits, not yours, and encourage her to do them the same way every day. For example, your mother might always brush her teeth before bathing, or she may like to wash her hair in the afternoon. A routine and predictable order should help in getting these things done.

◆ If baths or showers don't work, sponge baths are fine. Remember, she only needs to bathe about three times a week.

◆ Use simple-to-wear clothing, such as slip-on shoes or sneakers that close with Velcro, elastic-waisted pants or sweatpants, shirts that pull over the head or snap up the front and tube socks, which don't have a front or back. (See Appendix E, page 416, for a list of easy-to-wear clothing catalogues.)

◆ In addition to clearly labeling dresser drawers, mark the front and back of clothing. For example, sew a tag into the back of your father's pants that says BACK.

◆ In the morning lay out your parent's clothes in the order of how they go on.

◆ If your parent wears old clothing or bizarre outfits, you might just get rid of the ratty outfits and put away clothing that is inappropriate for the weather. Then give in to her choices.

## EATING

Some people with dementia fail to eat because they think they have just eaten, and others forget they've just eaten and insist on having another meal. Some forget what to eat, and have a box of chocolates for lunch. Even those who want to eat properly often have trouble getting the food from the kitchen to the plate or from the plate into their mouths.

◆ Make it easy. Be sure your father has food that is ready to eat (sandwiches, stews, soups) or link him up with a meal-delivery service. (See page 174.)

◆ Keep the kitchen stocked with bite-size finger foods, such as chicken nuggets, cut-up fruits and vegetables, tiny egg rolls, stuffed mushrooms and tea sandwiches. You can buy some in the gourmet section of a grocery store. This sort of food is easy to manage—it needs no utensils and there's little chance of spilling. And if your parent likes to pace, he can take finger foods with him as he strolls.

◆ All sorts of utensils, plates and cups that make eating easier can be found at a medical supply store or ordered from a catalogue (see page 416).

◆ If you are dealing with a constant eater, place a mark on the clock, showing what time the next meal will be served. Or simply keep some low-calorie snacks in the house—carrots, celery, cucumber, raisins, low-salt crackers or butterless popcorn. Instead of arguing with your parent about whether he did or didn't just eat, give him a plate of healthful food.

***

**“**My mother will eat with each member of the family as they come and go. Sometimes on Sunday mornings my daughter's boyfriend will get her coffee and an egg sandwich before he leaves, and she won't say anything to anyone about it. Then she'll eat breakfast again with my husband and me an hour later. It's not a big deal, I guess, but how much can one person eat?

She got four boxes of candy for Mother's Day and ate all of them single-handedly. I keep imploring people, 'Please don't give her candy,' but they don't listen. Now I sometimes hide the candy or even throw it away. She doesn't remember it existed.**”**              —CAROL G.

***

◆ The snack approach is also helpful for a non-eater. *I just ate two minutes ago. I'm not eating another meal now!* Instead of forcing your father to the dinner table, put a plate of filling snacks in front of him—a milkshake, chunks of cheese, crackers with a hearty dip or a flavored diet-supplement drink like Ensure.

◆ If your parent is alone at mealtimes, have meals ready for her in the refrigerator. Call her or set a timer to go off when it's time to eat.

## SLEEPING

Restlessness, confusion and a disrupted internal clock all make getting a good night's rest difficult. Studies show that some people with dementia wake up at least twice every hour.

If your parent is wandering the halls at 2 A.M., tossing and turning at 3 A.M. and hunting for the bathroom at 4 A.M., here are a few sleeping tips specifically for people with dementia:

◆ Since her internal clock isn't dependable, your mother has to rely on external clocks. Schedule naps and bedtime and then stick to the schedule. And don't let her go to bed at 7 P.M. or she'll want to start her day at 3 A.M. Try to keep her awake until other people in the household retire.

◆ Make sure your parent gets outside in the fresh air for at least a short time every day.

◆ Guide her to activities that are calming before bedtime—doing a puzzle, reading, listening to music. You might even help your parent get into her bed clothes half an hour before bedtime so she can calm down from the effort and isn't flustered on retiring.

◆ Make sure your parent has gone to the bathroom before going to bed.

## MEDICAL ALERT

As the dementia grows worse, your parent may no longer be able to tell you when she's feeling ill or has pain, so you or someone else must be on the lookout. Sudden changes in behavior—increased confusion or agitation, unusual exhaustion or lack of appetite, for example—may be signs of illness or medication problems. Be aware of such shifts in behavior, and when you note one, alert the doctor that something is wrong.

◆ Don't lay out clothing the night before. Your parent might wake up in the middle of the night and think it's time to get dressed.

◆ Make sure your parent feels safe. Keep familiar furnishings and photographs near his bed.

◆ Be sure there's a night light in your parent's bedroom and put reflector tapes in the hallway.

## TELEPHONES AND MAIL

If your parent lives with you and you aren't getting your bills or are wondering why there are never any messages on your answering machine, it is time to make some changes.

Get a post office box or put a latch on your mailbox that is a little difficult to undo. If you live in a suburban or rural area, you might be able to work out a plan with your mail carrier to leave the mail on a shelf in the garage or in the neighbor's box. Ask the phone company for a call-forwarding service so your calls can follow you, keep the answering machine in a locked drawer (so your parent can't turn it off), or turn the ringer on the phone and the volume on the answering machine off. You might want to install a second phone line for your parent to use.

If your parent lives alone and is having trouble handling the mail, arrange with creditors to have her bills sent to your address.

*“Last week Mom raced me to the mailbox and I actually had to wrestle the mail away from her. She had it all stuffed under her sweatshirt, and I knew I would never see it again. Finally I put a bungee cord on the box. She can't figure out how to get it off. The mailman has a little trouble with it too, but he's getting better at it.”* —CAROL G.

## MONEY

Even if your parent used to be thrifty, you may find that he is suddenly spending money recklessly. Or if he can't count anymore, you may discover that he's giving the checkout person 20 dollars for a bag of candy that costs 70 cents and walking away without any change.

If you have control over your parent's finances (and by this point, you should), let him carry some cash, but only as much as you are willing to let him lose. If he doesn't go to the store often, you might also leave him with his credit cards, or perhaps only the expired ones.

## DRIVING

The question of when to give up the car keys is a sensitive subject with any older person (see page 153), but it can be explosive when a parent has dementia. When you express your concern, your parent may have no idea what you are talking about, despite his several recent fender-benders. Or when you steer him away from the ignition, he may accuse you of holding him captive.

Try to talk with your parent about driving early on in this disease, before he needs to quit. If he is already a danger and needs to be stopped immediately, you have to take action regardless of his response. (Remember, this is not only about your parent's safety, but the safety of everyone on, or near, the roads.) If possible, get rid of the car so there is no threat of his driving. If the car is needed, get an auto mechanic to show you how to remove the distributor cap so the car won't start. When you need to use the car, you can easily put the cap back on.

## TIME AND ORIENTATION

To help your parent track the hours and days, keep clocks and calendars in sight. When you go out, put colored tape on the clock where the hands will be when you return, with the words, "Janie will be home at this time." A timer may be helpful, to remind your mother when to take her medications.

Your parent may be aware of her lost ability to track time and, as a result, be constantly worried about doing things at the wrong time. She may get nervous that she is late for an appointment that isn't scheduled until next week. Or she may be concerned about wearing out a welcome and say it's time to go just minutes after she's arrived for a visit. Try to understand her concerns. Imagine how confusing it would be if you had no idea what day it was or how much time was passing. If large clocks and notes don't help, reassure your parent that you or someone else will help her get to where she needs to go on time.

## COMMUNICATION

Over time, dementia tends to skew communication in a number of ways. People may talk fluidly, but the words may have no meaning. They may have trouble with grammar or finding the right word. They may be able to formulate and write words and sentences but have difficulty pronouncing them. They may not be able to find the right word for an object and say instead, "that thing that you play music on." Or, they might jumble their words, so that "needle" becomes "beedle," or "food" becomes "fide."

Your parent may not only have trouble expressing herself, she may also have difficulty understanding what others say. She may be able to read a sign, but have no idea what it means. She may understand what

# A PLACE IN THE PAST

A person with dementia may have trouble remembering not only the day and the hour, but the decade. Many people with dementia become lost in the past, talking about people who are long dead or a job that they left many years ago. This can be extremely upsetting for you, not only because it is a stark reminder of just how confused your parent is, but also because you may want to talk about today when your parent can talk only about yesterday. You may want to tell your father that you love him, but he is lost in 1930, a time when you didn't even exist.

As hard as this is on you, keep in mind that the past may be a very comforting and safe place for your parent. It is a place he can remember and a time when he was fit and able. In any case, trying to bring him into the present may only disorient and upset him. So don't frustrate yourself by trying to pull him into your world. If he is happy in the past, let him stay there. When he says that he is going to visit Wayne, a friend who died ten years ago, don't try to convince him that Wayne is gone. Instead, try something like, "Wouldn't it be nice to see your friend Wayne. Tell me about how you met him, Dad."

---

you say in person, but not what you say over the phone. She may be able to repeat a message, but not interpret it.

When communication fades:

♦ Have your parent's hearing checked and be sure she has no dental problems that might be hindering her speech.

♦ When you talk together, find a quiet place and do it at a time when you won't be interrupted or distracted.

♦ Use simple words and sentences. Speak slowly and deliberately. Use a calm, but amply loud voice. A deep voice is better than a high-pitched tone, which can be more difficult to understand and may suggest that you are upset.

♦ Supplement your words with nonverbal cues. Point to things, use photographs, pantomime and touch.

♦ If you are giving your parent instructions, don't assume she understands what you are saying, even if she assures you that she does. Double-check by asking her to repeat the instructions and explain what they mean. (And remember, if the instructions pertain to something in the future, she may not remember them, even if she understands them.)

◆ Listen carefully when your parent speaks. Give her your complete attention. Be patient, look directly at her and above all, do not interrupt her.

◆ When communicating becomes more difficult for her, listen for words that are repeated or seem especially meaningful, and respond to those. As you look for meaning in her words, be aware that common themes people with dementia try to express are loneliness and fear, concern about family and a desire to be well again.

◆ Let your parent talk even if she is making no sense. She thinks she's making sense, and the sound of her own voice may be calming and reassuring for her.

Late in the disease, your parent may lose all ability to communicate. It's hard to know which of the many losses of dementia is the most difficult or the most painful, but when the lines of communication fall silent, you may feel shut out completely. Your parent, no longer able to relay his needs, his pain, his fears or his wishes, becomes isolated. Caring for him becomes even more challenging and very, very lonely.

You or other caregivers should monitor your parent's comfort and health more carefully now because he can no longer explain when something is amiss. Make sure his bedroom is clean, well-ventilated and at a comfortable temperature. Check to see that he eats, inspect him occasionally for sores and be aware of any signs of pain or illness.

"Eventually my mother couldn't express what she was feeling. I would say, 'What's wrong?' and she really didn't know. One time she said, 'I want to be free,' and I understood that she wanted to leave, to be free of the disease, to go back to some other part of her life. Later, it was about her mother. She wanted to go home and she wanted to go to her mother who was waiting for her, she said. And that made me very sad because I figured she was preparing to die.

I realized that she wasn't sad. In fact, I think she was quite ready to go. I was projecting my own sadness, my own sorrow onto her."
—MARY W.

And keep talking to him. He may still understand what you are saying, and your presence and the sound of your familiar voice will bring him comfort that he may not be able to express.

At this point, be sure to watch your parent's body language carefully. Facial expressions, like a smile, a grimace or a frown, or body movements, like a clenched fist or a turn of the head, can all be revealing.

## INCONTINENCE

When your parent becomes incontinent, it may not be caused by a problem in her urinary tract, but by a disruption in the brain's messages, in which case Kegel exercises and toileting schedules are unlikely to be effective. Some of the tips on page 99 should help, especially making sure the bathroom is clearly marked with bright letters or a picture on the door, that the path to the toilet is clear, and that she empties her bladder or her bowels regularly even if she thinks she doesn't need to. Also:

◆ If your parent confuses other objects, such as buckets, wastebaskets and flower pots, for toilets, put lids on them, move them out of your parent's path or label them.

◆ Look for cues that your parent has to go to the bathroom. He might play with his fly, suddenly become fidgety, or look toward the bathroom without actually getting up and going. If he has speech trouble, he may say, "I have to key." Or he may revert to childish words, such as doo-doo or poopie. Listen for any such hints that he needs to go to the toilet.

◆ Once you have helped him to the bathroom you may need to find ways to help him use the toilet. You might leave the room to give him privacy, or encourage his urination by turning on the tap water. But don't hurry him. Give him all the time he needs.

◆ Try not to be angry with your parent when there is an accident. He cannot help it. Set up his house or living area with plastic liners or other protection. If this doesn't suffice, he may need to use diapers or a catheter. Talk with his doctor.

# Coping with Behavior

No matter what your parent is doing today that is making your life miserable, keep in mind that it will probably change—maybe in a week or two, perhaps in a matter of months, but it will change. A person who is agitated and aggressive often becomes calmer and quieter with time. A person who is always poised on the edge of danger, turning the gas burner on high and hiding scissors under the couch cushions, will eventually lose interest in such things. A lot of patience, a list of strategies, and the knowledge that this too shall pass will help you cope.

## LOSING, HIDING AND HOARDING THINGS

If your parent is hoarding food, money or other items, and it is not harmful, let him do it. People with dementia sometimes hoard things because they are afraid that they will have to care for themselves in the future, that they will be abandoned, or that people are trying to harm them. It may give your parent some peace of mind to squirrel things away. If possible, offer help. Provide a tin for food or a safe hiding place for other items. When hiding, hoarding or pilfering get out of hand, talk with the doctor because there may be medications that can help.

## A "LOSING" STRATEGY

Losing and hiding things is par for the course with dementia. Be prepared:

❖ Keep two sets of anything that's important—eyeglasses, keys, dentures, hearing aids.

❖ Attach small items to large key chains so they can be found more easily.

❖ Get in the habit of checking wastebaskets before emptying them.

❖ Attach house keys or glasses to a string that hangs around your parent's neck.

❖ Check all pockets carefully before clothing is laundered or dry-cleaned.

❖ Keep important things in the same place, always. The house keys hang next to the door, the dentures go in the glass by the sink, etc.

❖ Limit hiding places by locking cabinets and closets.

❖ Keep a neat and orderly house if at all possible, so there are fewer places to lose items.

## AGITATION

Your parent picks up a magazine. Puts it down. Lies down. Gets up. Goes to the bathroom. Lies down. Asks you what she should do. Goes to the bathroom again. Asks you again what she should do. Sedatives start to look tempting, and they are sometimes necessary, but they are not the best solution.

Try some of the tips offered already, particularly giving her small tasks to channel her energy, and reducing noise and commotion. And keep yourself as calm as possible. Some other ways to calm her nerves:

◆ Try to get at the cause of her restlessness. Sometimes agitation is prompted by some unspoken concern. Your mother may be wringing her hands or pacing because she is worried about being late for an appointment or about getting home safely from a visit. If you can figure

❝For somebody whose mind is deteriorating, she does really well. She's fast. She'll snatch things off the table and put them in her pockets faster than you can see her.

I made hot cross buns for Easter and by the end of the meal her pockets were filled with them. I think she's saving in case of a flood—I mean, we have more than enough to eat. Nobody goes hungry around here, and she certainly eats well. She's always putting food away as though she might not get another meal. I keep asking her, 'What are you doing that for?'❞ —CAROL G.

out what's worrying her, you may be able to calm her fears.

◆ Make sure your parent isn't consuming any caffeine or drugs that contain stimulants.

◆ Encourage your parent to exercise (see page 155) so she'll use up some of the nervous energy. If she wants to pace, let her pace. Or get someone to go for a regular walk with her.

◆ Try relaxation techniques, such as massage or therapeutic touch, and soothing music.

## WANDERING

People with dementia often start out on an errand and forget where they are going or where they started from. Or they just amble aimlessly out the door and into the night. Even if your parent has never wandered before, be sure he wears an identification bracelet or necklace. Lock the doors with

## GRANDPA DOESN'T KNOW IT'S ME

A dearly beloved grandfather with dementia says bizarre things, or is mean or rude. He wets his pants or makes a mess of his food. It's hard enough for an adult to understand, but this disease can be frightening for children. It also leaves them with unhappy memories of someone who is dear to you.

Explain that Grandpa's brain is sick and that he doesn't mean what he says and can't remember what's just happened. Assure them that Grandpa still loves them, even though he may not be able to show it now. And encourage them to discuss their feelings about this with you. If you ache for your children to know your parent as he was, perhaps you can offer them a glimpse into the past with stories of your childhood and old photos.

Once they understand what is happening, children can be wonderful company for an older person with dementia, and a big help to you. They are often more forgiving than adults, and in this case they may be able to play at the same level as your parent. A child might like to sing songs or play games that are manageable and calming for his grandparent.

For help explaining dementia to a young child, get the book, *Grandpa Doesn't Know It's Me,* by Donna Guthrie (Human Sciences Press). It describes the loving relationship between a little girl and her grandfather, and the bewilderment and fear she feels as he becomes afflicted with Alzheimer's disease.

bolts placed high or low on the door, or use plastic childproof knobs. If wandering becomes a regular problem:

♦ Attach a bell to the door so it rings and alerts you or others when it is opened.

♦ Look into motion-sensitive and pressure-sensitive alarms that alert you when your parent moves about or gets out of bed. You should be able to find them in medical supply stores.

♦ Some caregivers find it helpful to put a sign on the door: "Jack, Do Not Leave." But this may work only for a week or two.

♦ Install a sturdy fence around the property.

♦ Along with an ID card, put a card in your father's pocket with instructions to him: "Dad, stay calm. Find a phone. Call this number." Be sure he always has a quarter.

♦ Alert the local police to the situation. Have photographs of your parent on hand so that if he does get lost, you can hand them out.

♦ Sign up with a tracking service such as Safe Return (888-572-8566), Care Trak (800-842-4551) or Care Electronics (303-444-2273).

♦ If nothing else helps, consult your parent's doctor about the possibility of using medications to control the wandering.

## REPETITION

Repetition is the Chinese water torture of dementia. The first few drops land on the head with little impact, but as the minutes and hours pass, each drop, each repeated tale or movement echos more irritatingly and painfully than the last. Other people can't understand why you are getting so angry, and neither can you. But you are certain that if your parent says or does the same thing one more time, you'll scream.

Sometimes, like pushing the needle on a broken record, you can nudge your parent out of whatever behavior is bothering you. Diversions may help you here, or if she asks the same question over and over, either stop answering it or reply in a different way. (She asks, "When's dinner?" and instead of telling her again that it's at seven, you say, "We'll have dinner after Charlie comes home.") If the problem is a repeated motion, touch often works better than words. If your parent is constantly rubbing one elbow, touch her other arm or a leg.

When nothing works, focus *your* attention on something else. Tune her out. Try to ignore her motions. Don't respond to her questions. Be creative about diverting yourself.

## ACCUSATIONS AND INSULTS

Dementia doesn't obliterate people's personalities, it rearranges them. Certain traits become more pronounced, others fade away, and oddly enough, new traits can appear. It's not uncommon for people with dementia to become mean and insulting. Your parent might complain that you never visit, that you don't feed him enough, that his wife is cheating on him or that you've hid-

## MY FATHER DOESN'T KNOW ME

As dementia moves through your parent's brain, destroying his abilities and his memories, it will eventually get around to that cherished pocket that holds his memories of you. He may know who you are at one moment, but not at another. He may know your name, but forget that you are his daughter. This is the heartbreaking nature of dementia.

Suddenly, you no longer exist for your parent, and it may feel as if part of you has died along with those memories. The magnetic forces that drew you to care for your parent during this time, and kept you at it when things got rough, are weakened or gone. Your father doesn't look at you with the same familiar gaze, full of knowledge and memories, but with the blank look of a stranger or the angry glare of a victim.

With all that you are losing, this is a debilitating blow. But your parent needs you now more than ever. Not only does he need you to protect him because he can no longer fend for himself, but your warmth, your gaze and your touch are powerfully reassuring, even if he can't say so. Your parent has nothing left to give you now, and he needs everything from you. It is a lot to ask. Love him with whatever tiny reserve you have left, for even though he doesn't remember your name or your past, you may be his entire world now.

---

den things from him (which you may have, and for good reason). He might call people names, or he might be rude to strangers on the street, leaving you to apologize for him.

Given all that you are doing to care for him, such attacks can shatter the patience and control you are trying so hard to sustain. No matter how confused he may be, a parent's criticism hits a nerve, and the insults may be virtually impossible to shrug off.

But shrug you must. Whenever your parent makes a biting remark, remember that he doesn't know what he is saying, or mean what he says.

Try hard not to take such comments personally. Think of yourself as one of those blow-up clowns that you punch and they pop right back up— the blow was meaningless and did no harm.

Also, consider what might be behind your parent's comments, especially if the same criticism is made repeatedly. For example, people with dementia often accuse others of stealing things because it explains why they can't find something. Your parent might claim that someone is keeping him prisoner because he is losing his independence and can't understand why. He might insist that you are mean because he feels frightened, alone and insecure. Or he might accuse a spouse of infidelity because he feels inadequate as a mate.

So next time your father accuses you of stealing his clock, rather than bristling, you might simply accept the blame: "I probably did lose it. Let's see if we can't find it together." And rather than arguing, "I am not cruel to you!" console your parent and address his real fears: "I know the world feels cruel to you now. I don't like this either. But we have each other and we will get through it together."

Remember, don't try to reason with your parent. Simply do what you can to reassure him that people love him and that he is safe. Your father may not stop making the comments, but if you understand why he makes them, you will be better equipped to put up with them.

# Special Problems

Certain behaviors and actions—incontinence, violence, inappropriate sexual behavior, hallucinations—can easily become too much for caregivers. If you encounter these problems, try some of the tips outlined here, consult a geriatric social worker or other specialist (call the local Alzheimer's Association or your parent's doctor), but if nothing helps, you may have to look for other housing and care for your parent. (See Chapters Ten and Eleven.)

## AGGRESSION AND VIOLENCE

Some of your parent's anger and aggression is understandable; life has taken a terrible turn, and each day now is a series of failures, losses and frightening experiences. But some of it is due to damage to the brain which can abolish inhibitions and disable all emotional controls. As a result, your parent may not only behave badly, he may not realize that anything is wrong with his behavior. Family members who no longer like this angry imposter, but who still have to care for him, face an agonizing conflict.

Accept that little you do is going to change your parent's behavior, but try to derail his outbursts as best as you can. Look for cues that set off the rage and be ready to jump in and divert his attention. Try to

**"**My mother went through a violent stage, which was the scariest part of her dementia for me. She was a different person. It was horrible. She would yell, scream and swear—at me, at the rest of the family, at the doctor. She would come right up to my face and threaten to hit me.

When we were in public, she would get frustrated and there was no controlling her. I would take her to church and if somebody moved their head in front of her or talked, she would say, 'When is he going to shut up?' very loudly, you know.

She would never have done that before, never be rude. It was horrible for all of us.**"**    —LINDA K.

keep things calm, as yelling back will only escalate his anger.

While it's rare for a person with dementia to become physically violent, it happens. Remember to remove or lock up potential weapons (knives, guns, baseball bats, umbrellas, scissors, etc.) and to post emergency numbers by the telephones. Don't put yourself or others in danger under any circumstances. If your parent tries to assault you or someone else, do not try to disarm him or fight with him. Get away from him as quickly as possible and call the police. When your parent can't be calmed down in any other way, aggression can be treated with medications, so talk with your parent's doctor.

If an outburst is physical but not dangerous—if your parent is storming around the room cursing violently, or banging his fists on the bed—let it happen. You might even provide a safe environment where he can explode, in a room where there are no sharp edges, glass or other dangerous items. He'll tire himself out quickly.

## INAPPROPRIATE PUBLIC OR SEXUAL BEHAVIOR

Inappropriate public behavior is common with dementia; inappropriate sexual behavior is not. When either one occurs, decide first whether the behavior is worth making a fuss about. Sometimes what is construed as sexual behavior, such as sitting outdoors naked or rubbing one's crotch, may simply be an effort to get comfortable. It may be hot outdoors, and the crotch may itch. If your parent's behavior is not hurting anyone—if your father is masturbating alone in the living room—try to ignore it, if you can. It's painful and bewildering, but you cannot force him to adhere to social norms that have disappeared from his mind. Ignoring him, whether it stops the behavior or not, will certainly save you a lot of aggravation.

When your parent's behavior does need to be curbed, try to head it off before it starts. If he tends to play with his genitals in public, be sure that his hands are busy with something else. If he urinates in unusual places, buy him trousers without a fly (elastic-waisted pants or sweatpants), which are slightly more difficult to open. Then as soon as you see him struggling with his belt or waistband, steer him towards the men's room.

Also, stay one step ahead of your parent. See if something in particular triggers the unwanted behavior so you can intervene early. If you know that a long line or a wait at a restaurant will set your father off, for example, tell the waiter that you need to be served quickly. As soon as your mother starts berating a stranger or unbuttoning her dress on the street, suggest a diversion—one that she really enjoys, like having ice cream or visiting a grandchild.

Most important, don't make a fuss when your parent embarrasses you in public as that will only draw more attention. Instead, gently convey the message that your parent is ill. Rather than lashing out at him, get him back on course, console him and calm him, apologize to anyone he offended, and exit quickly, if at all possible.

## DELUSIONS AND HALLUCINATIONS

Your mother says that someone is trying to poison her. Your father tells you that he just spoke to Vanna White. As if you didn't have enough to worry about.

Delusions—believing something that is not true—are common in people with dementia largely because they tend to misinterpret what is happening around them. Your father may no longer understand the difference between a person on television and a person in real life. Your mother believes she is being starved because she can't remember her last meal. Hallucinations—seeing things or hearing things that don't exist—are less common, but some people with dementia experience them. Your father says that there is a camel in the corner of his room or he tells you that elves speak to him.

You can no more convince your parent that these things aren't true than someone could convince you that what you see is not there. Don't argue with your parent. In fact, it's better to do just the opposite. If the hallucination is not frightening—and some are actually amusing or pleasant—let your parent tell you more about it and accept her word as true. If a delusion is not causing

> **❝***My mother would wake up in the middle of the night screaming, 'Get them out of here! Get them out of here!' She would say she saw people, little children, at her bedside. I didn't know what was going on.*
>
> *At one point I had a minister come and talk to her. I didn't know what else to do. I thought maybe he could help get rid of any demons or spirits in her life but it didn't help.*
>
> *One day it just stopped on its own. She stopped crying out. I asked her later about the little children, if she had seen them lately, and she didn't know what I was talking about. She told me I was nuts.***❞**
> —MARY W.

any trouble, go along with it or ignore it.

If the beliefs or visions are upsetting your parent, assure him that he's safe, that the goblins are friendly ones or that you will shoo the camel away (or feed it and make it a pet). Take a bite of any "poisoned" food first or let your parent keep her own closet of food if she feels she is being starved. As with other troubling behaviors, look for any underlying meaning—when he says that his bed is on fire, find out if the electric blanket is on too high. If all else fails and the delusions or hallucinations become a serious problem, talk with the doctor.

# Chapter Seventeen

# IN THE END

*Talking about Death • Caring for Your Dying Parent
• How Much Medical Care • Hospice • The Face of Death*

A T SOME POINT IT BECOMES CLEAR THAT YOUR PARENT is neither invincible nor immortal, that despite all your labor and love, the best efforts of doctors and the prayers of friends, he will not be around much longer. It's a deeply painful thought. Inconceivable, even. How can this person who has been with you from the start, cared for you and guided you, ever be gone? No matter how sick your parent is, no matter how much or how little he can say or do now, he is still there and still your parent. How could it ever be otherwise?

For most of us, the death of a parent is too painful to think about, too awkward to talk about and certainly too traumatic to witness. But as your parent nears the end of his life, keep in mind the wise words of Dr. Sherwin B. Nuland, author of *How We Die.* "Death belongs to the dying and to those who love them." This death, your parent's death, belongs not to hospitals, doctors and nurses. It belongs, in part, to you.

This doesn't mean that your parent should not be in a hospital or under the care of a doctor. It means that wherever your parent is, you, your family and he have some control over his death—not perhaps over its cause or timing, but over how he dies and what sort of life he lives until that point. You can choose which medical treatments will be used and which refused, where and how your parent's last months or days will be spent, who will be with him, what comfort and support will be given and, finally, what sort of memorial will honor his life.

Death is a process, a final passage of life, that demands both practical and emotional involvement from everyone who is near. You and other family members are facing a great loss, but you can still cherish this time with your parent and help him find some comfort and peace. Death is not simply a grim and heartbreaking betrayal. No, when we are willing to see it, death is also a potent reminder that despite all of the aggravations in a day, life is precious—very, very precious. To whatever extent you are able, acknowledge this dying process and, in doing so, celebrate life.

# Beyond Denial

Although you know your parent has only a limited time left to live, you may find that you are tiptoeing around words like "terminal," "hospice" or "death" and avoiding any discussion of a funeral. You may find yourself saying, "Everything is going to be fine, Mom," when you know full well that it won't be. That's understandable. It's as if by saying the word "death," we might make it happen, and by dodging the word, we can hang on to hope.

But whether you say it openly or not, your parent probably knows what is happening. She understands that she is incurably ill and that her life is drawing to a close. In fact, she may be doing just what you are doing—avoiding the subject of death for fear of upsetting you. How sad to spend these last days in silence,

when both of you might welcome the opportunity to share your fears and sorrow.

Break the taboo and talk with your parent about her illness and dying. Ask about her concerns and needs, and share your own grief. Talking may help ease her emotional pain, which is often far worse than any physical pain that comes with dying.

For you, such discussions are an opportunity to express your love and appreciation, make any apologies, share an intimate time with your parent and start saying your goodbyes. This is your chance to say all the things you never said—things that later you may wish you had said. Talking about death will expose you to more pain, but it will also expose you to more love and help you, in the long run, to heal.

Acknowledging the severity of your parent's illness has practical benefits as well; it allows the two of you to discuss any unfinished bus-

## PRESERVING THIS TIME

You may want to keep a journal of all that is happening and all that you are feeling now. If you don't want to write in a diary or don't have the time, buy a small tape recorder and keep it in the car, in the bathroom or by your bed. Talk into it about whatever is on your mind. Record the painful emotions, the memorable comments, the tender looks and loving embraces. As unforgettable as this experience seems now, many of the details and much of the intensity will be lost if they are not recorded, and you are sure to want to remember them in the future.

iness, as well as her wishes concerning pain medication, medical treatment and hospice care.

## BROACHING THE SUBJECT

You may be able to grieve and talk about death with friends and family, but unable to talk about it with the person who is in fact dying. It's too close, too stark, too massive. Even if you knew what to say, there's the problem of saying anything without getting all choked up, or saying the wrong thing or bursting into tears—although there is really no "wrong thing" to say, and tears can be helpful, too.

The first time you say the word "death" aloud or suggest a future without your parent is the hardest. Once the door is open, it will be easier to talk about it (and you should leave the door open for more conversations). If you don't want to be direct, you can raise the subject gently with an open-ended question that lets your parent lead the conversation. For example, ask your parent what the doctor has told her, or if there is anything she wants to talk about.

Quite often this conversation arises on its own, at an unexpected moment and in an indirect way, and that is the moment for which you need to be prepared. Your parent might suddenly say, "I'm going to miss you." Or she may be more roundabout, and say, "I've got to get my finances in order," or "Open your present now because I won't see you on your birthday." People in the late stages of illness sometimes broach the subject in even more cryptic ways. Your parent may talk about a relative or a friend who is dead, or

> **"**I asked her about dying. I said, 'Do you think about dying much?' And she said, 'No, I really don't.' And that was it. That was the end of the conversation.
>
> I was blunter than I usually am, but I wanted to give her a chance to talk about it. I didn't get anything, but I know it didn't offend her either. We're just different. I enjoy introspection, thinking about life, and she doesn't. She's always been that way.**"** —BETTY H.

**❝** *I knew Dad was extremely sick and that he probably wouldn't make it through the year. But we didn't talk about it. We talked about his illness and treatments, but not about his dying.*

*About three weeks before he died I noticed that he wasn't eating and I mentioned his lack of appetite. He said, 'That's what happens in the terminal stage of cancer.' It was as if a window shattered. There was a silence that seemed to last several seconds. Finally I said, 'Are you afraid of dying?' And he said, 'No. I want to be sure that your mother is going to be all right. But I'm not afraid.' And that was it. We didn't say anything else. I just wrapped my arms around him and we held each other.*

*That was the only time the word was said, but it was enough. It was as if a veil was removed. After that, every look, every touch was so intense and so close because we both knew, and we knew the other knew.* **❞**          —MARJORIE C.

he might make references to traveling—getting tickets, packing bags, going on a boat or leaving someone behind.

Be ready for these moments because you can easily be caught off guard and find yourself shutting your parent off by saying something like, "Oh Mom, don't say that. There's no reason to be afraid." Be careful not to change the subject, disagree, try to cheer your parent up or dis-

count her fears. Instead, offer her a safe place to expose her feelings and concerns. More valuable than anything you say is what you allow your parent to say.

If you reflexively jump away from an opening, don't worry. You did what most of us do. There will be another opportunity. Simply bring the subject up later—"Do you remember when you told me that you would miss me?"—or listen carefully for another opening. But try not to wait too long, as time may be short now.

## WHEN COMMUNICATION IS GONE

If your parent is too sick to speak, you can do the talking. Talk about the emotions you think she might be feeling or the issues she might be worried about, and watch for her response in her facial expressions or other body language. Reassure her, console her and share with her. Do it even if you think she can't understand or hear you. You can never be sure how much an ill person comprehends, and even if she doesn't understand your words, she will be calmed simply by your presence and your voice.

## OPTING NOT TO TALK

Despite your best intentions, it may not be possible for you to discuss death with your parent. Don't be hard on yourself. For some people, this kind of candor comes naturally, and for others, it's too much. Talking about death requires that you accept that your parent is going to die. It means leaving the safe harbor of denial, and exposing yourself to a whole set of razor-sharp emotions—shock, anger, despair, helplessness and profound sadness.

But before you decide to skip this conversation, consider the pros and cons carefully because you may not have another chance. What is the worst thing that might happen if you speak candidly? How will you feel if you say nothing? What might such an honest gesture mean to your parent? How might it help her? How might it help you? Whatever you decide, be sure you are comfortable with your decision.

If it is your parent who doesn't want to talk—if you open this dialogue and your parent repeatedly changes the subject—then you should respect her wishes. In this case, silence is a way of honoring your parent, of letting her deal with death in her own way.

You don't have to use words to let your mother know that you love her and that you will miss her. The look in your eyes, your embrace, your tears and tenderness will tell her what she most needs to know.

# Your Parent's Perspective

To care for your parent now, you need to understand some of what he is going through. Of course,

## PLEASE DON'T GO

You may find that you are not only having trouble talking to your parent openly about death, but that you are doing just the opposite. When the subject comes up, you find yourself stating emphatically that she will get better. Or you plead desperately with her not to die, saying that she mustn't leave you.

In your own way, you are telling your parent that you love her and that you will be sad when she is gone. Your words are meant to be kind and affectionate, and your parent probably understands this. But

be aware that such denial shuts your parent out, for it leaves her no way to share her feelings with you. Worse, it puts her into the role of protecting you. In addition to dealing with her own grief, she must now worry about you and your future.

If you want to tell your parent that you love her, that you wish life wasn't this way, that you will miss her, do so. But if you find yourself pleading with her or denying the truth, think about how your words are affecting her and try to take a different approach next time.

*"One afternoon I was wiping my father's face with a damp washcloth, to cool him. I was exhausted and he was barely conscious. He was very thin and pale, but I could still see my father there, the young, strong man that I knew. I stroked his forehead, his cheekbones, the hollows and curves of his neck. His skin was always so soft.*

*He was there, still there for me, but he wasn't going to be there much longer. I knew that. I could still love him and touch him and hug him, but just for now. For this moment. But maybe not again. And at that moment I loved him more than I have ever loved anyone in my life.*"

—MARJORIE C.

without facing death ourselves, it is almost impossible to imagine. Elisabeth Kübler-Ross, a pioneer in the field of death and dying, provides some guidance. She has mapped out five emotional responses that she found to be common among terminally ill patients.

Keep in mind that the reactions noted here are by no means universal. We react to death as individually as we react to life. Also, while these responses are presented as sequential stages, many people bounce among them, moving, for example, through a period of denial, a few days of anger, and then back into denial.

**Denial.** Denial is the brain signal that says, "This cannot be happening. It is not possible. There must be another explanation." It is a normal, protective response to an unbearable reality. Don't encourage your parent's denial, but allow it, especially early on. Urge him, gently, to face the truth, and don't lie or fudge the facts. But don't try to force it. If he insists that he is going to get well when the doctor has told him otherwise, at some point you have to let him believe what he wants to believe.

If your parent remains in denial (as is the case for many people), you may have to make some plans and decisions for your parent. It's a lonely place to be, but one that you have to accept.

**Anger.** Once your parent realizes that he is indeed dying, he may become angry—angry at himself for being ill, angry at others who are not ill, angry at God for letting this happen, angry at doctors who bring the bad news, and angry at family and friends for any reason or no reason at all. Your parent may express his anger loudly, in fits of rage, or he may bottle it up. Again, allow him his emotions. You might even encourage him to express his anger, because this may prevent him from withdrawing into a bitter silence.

**Bargaining.** People who are terminally ill often go through a period of mental bargaining, usually with God or whatever higher power they believe in. *Let me get well, and I'll be a good person from now on.* Your parent may be bargaining for time—perhaps he wants to be around for a specific event, such as an anniversary, a birthday or a celebration—or for comfort, for health or for love. You probably won't know the specifics of the deal, but you may notice that he is taking an active role in his health care, doing everything he can to prolong his life.

Learn if there is a particular goal your parent has in mind. If he wants to see a loved one before he dies, help bring that about. If his bargaining involves lifestyle changes, such as eating well, exercising and dealing with psychological pain, encourage it, not as a way for him to cure his illness, but as a way for him to gain some control over it.

**Depression.** Realizing that there is no escaping death, no bartering with God, your parent may begin to mourn the loss of life and the loss of those around him whom he loves. He may mourn things he failed to do in the past and dreams he will not be able to fulfill in the future. He may feel helpless, powerless and deeply saddened. He may worry terribly about being a burden to you and other family members.

Kübler-Ross describes two types of depression: reactive and preparatory. Reactive depression encompasses specific concerns—*Will the children be okay? Will I be in pain? Will I be alone in the end?*—and the loss of self-esteem due to the illness. Such concerns can often be eased with reassurance. But in the second type of depression, when your parent may be preparing for death and grieving the loss of life, reassurance usually is not helpful. A dying person cannot "cheer up," and must be allowed to have this sorrow. He may want to share his sad-

ness, but it's more likely he will be silent. You can share your parent's grief without words, perhaps by touching him tenderly or just sitting quietly by his side.

**Acceptance.** The last stage is a calm, almost peaceful, time when the person accepts that death is approaching. That is not to say that he welcomes death, but he is relieved that the struggle is over. He is no longer trying to extend his life or to get well. He is no longer de-

---

**❝***My father had a wonderful death. That's a funny thing to say, but his whole countenance changed. He was a difficult and demanding man, and he made a lot of people angry during his life. But when he learned he had only a few months to live, he walked back through his life and reviewed it all. He became very sweet and tender. The minister came frequently to see him, and prayed with him. It made him very genuine and real, and you could say anything to him. We were very close during those weeks. I spent a lot of time up in his room, sitting at a card table trying to write. It was a lovely, sort of profound, relationship.*

*The minister told me much later that he'd never seen a person prepare himself for death as beautifully as my father had. I don't know where it came from, but I hope that I can do the same. It was a tremendous gift that he gave us all, at the end.***❞**
—BETTY H.

pressed or angry. Instead, he may just be weary. And he may be preparing for his departure, seeking simply comfort and serenity.

This stage is the easiest for your parent but it may be the most difficult for you, especially if you have not reached a similar stage of acceptance. You may sense that your parent has given up when you think that he should still be fighting. You may feel his separation and long to bring him back.

But he is ready to go, and he may already have begun to sever his ties to those he loves. As a result, he may want to see fewer and fewer people, not for any lack of feeling for them, but because he has said his good-byes already and is at peace with that. Saying good-bye again would require too much energy from him. He may choose not to see certain people who he knows have not yet accepted his dying; their denial may be too much for him to handle now.

If your parent refuses visitors, respect his wishes. If he chooses not to see you, try to understand his response and be happy for him that he has reached this stage of readiness. It is time to let him go. If you can, give him your blessing.

**Other issues.** In addition to these common responses to terminal illness and death, a number of more specific issues often arise. They too are important to understand as you care for your parent and try to share this time with him.

◆ People are often more afraid of dying than of death. They are afraid of the process, of the un-

known, and, more than almost anything else, of being alone. Your parent needs affection and assurance that you or others will be with her throughout this time.

◆ People who are dying are afraid of pain. Straightforward information from a doctor about what is to come and how pain will be controlled should alleviate much of this fear.

◆ Some people are afraid that they will be a burden to others as they grow sicker. Your parent needs to know that you or another loved one will gladly take care of her directly, or continue to oversee her care in a hospital or a nursing home.

◆ Death forces people to review their lives—what life has meant, what its value has been, and how they will be remembered. They want to know that their lives have been valuable, that they have accomplished certain things and that people liked them. They are more apt to die in peace if they feel that they have lived successfully. Encourage your parent to review all the good things in her life—friends, jobs, milestones, successes. Let her know that her life has been worthwhile and, in particular, that you respect, love and admire her. Tell her that the lessons she taught you and the memories of her life will be passed on to future generations.

◆ Those who are dying also want to know that their affairs are in order, their dependents cared for, their battles reconciled. They want to know that nothing crucial will be left unsettled or unfinished. If your parent feels that she has left something undone, help her to bring it to conclusion. Urge an estranged relative to speak to her, or help her dictate a note to someone she has distanced herself from.

Also, let your parent know that you will miss her terribly, but that you and others will be able to go on after she is gone. As the end draws near, let her know that it is all right for her to go; give her permission to die peacefully.

# Caring for Your Parent Now

Whether your parent is in a hospital, a nursing home or at home, there is much that you can do to care for her now:

◆ Be aware of her mental and spiritual health. In addition to talking with you, she should have the opportunity to talk to a counselor, social worker, psychiatrist or clergyman. (Even if she can't communicate, she might be consoled by their reassuring words.)

◆ Make the most of your parent's days. Think about what she might most appreciate. Does she want to be left in silence? Does she like to listen to music, the television or radio? Would she like someone to tell her stories about old times, read her poetry or sing her favorite songs? Would she like to watch birds come to a feeder outside her window? If she can be moved, would she like to be driven along a waterfront, or would she like to lie on a lounge chair in the sun? Or would she simply like someone to sit quietly with her and stroke her? Focus your attention as much on providing emotional comfort and pleasure as on any physical care and pain relief she may need.

◆ Treat your parent with respect and dignity and ask others to do the same. Keep her informed about what is happening and give her as much control over decisions as possible. Respect her modesty, even if she seems unaware of such matters. And ask people around her to call her by the name or title she is used to.

◆ Give your parent lots of affection. Touch is a powerful tonic—for both of you. Hold her hand, stroke her forehead, rest your head on her arm, kiss her cheek or give her a gentle massage.

◆ Even if your parent can't express her thoughts, or if she seems oblivious to what is happening, assume that she hears and understands what is going on around her. Hearing is the last sense to go, so take private conversations out of the room and don't talk about your parent as if she were not there. Talk to her as you or others turn her, bathe

*"I don't know where she ends and I begin, our lives are so intertwined. Part of me is very much looking forward to losing her and being free. But frankly, I think that when she goes I'll feel like, 'Oh my God, I'm going to die now too.'"*
—SASHA L.

her, feed her. *I'm going to lift your right arm and put a pillow under it.*

◆ If your parent is bedridden watch for bedsores. As she becomes frailer and spends more time in bed, her skin will become increasingly thin and fragile. The pressure and friction on bony spots—elbows, heels, buttocks, the back of the head—can cause sores that, if left untreated, are very painful. (See page 82 for more on bedsores.)

◆ Make sure her room smells fresh, and if she is at home, keep linens, commodes and other items clean.

◆ As your parent becomes sicker, take stock of your own emotional state, as well as hers. Death is a consuming process—for everyone involved. You and other family members need to get away from the preoccupation with illness and death and talk about other things. You need to eat well and get some sleep. And you should meet, even if it's only briefly, with a counselor, social worker, member of the clergy, hospice nurse or another person trained in grief counseling and bereavement. If anyone involved becomes extremely anxious or depressed, he or she should see a psychiatrist or his own personal doctor. These problems can be treated effectively with medication and counseling.

## IN A HOSPITAL

Most people today die in institutions—80 percent, according to some estimates. In the hospital, your parent gets complete medical attention and round-the-clock nursing care, which is usually covered by public or private insurance. The reality of death seems less stark, and the kind of hands-on care required of you is far less rigorous than if your parent were to die at home.

But hospitals have drawbacks. Your parent is in a relatively impersonal and unfamiliar place that imposes some physical and emotional distance between her and her

## DO NOT RESUSCITATE

When a person becomes severely and irreversibly ill, the family and doctor (or the patient) may draft a Do Not Resuscitate order. This means that if the person's breathing or heartbeat should stop, there will be no attempt to revive her. DNR orders are usually made when the family, patient and doctor believe that resuscitation would only delay the inevitable and leave the person severely and permanently incapacitated. Keep in mind, the chance of an acutely ill, elderly person surviving resuscitation is about 15 percent, and the chance of that person ever leaving the hospital is between 0 and 5 percent. (See page 357 about enforcing such directives.)

## A NOTE ON PAIN

Pain is no simple matter. It radiates from, and is compounded by, a number of sources—the disease's symptoms; chemotherapy, surgery and other medical interventions; emotional anguish, exhaustion and fatigue; and the fear of pain itself. Dreading what may come, we tighten our muscles, clench our jaws and, as a result, become physically and psychologically overwhelmed by the first twinge of pain.

Determine the roots of your parent's pain and address them. Be sure his questions about illness, dying and pain medication are answered. Let him talk about troubled relationships or spiritual questions. Easing his emotional pain will in turn ease his physical pain.

Whatever else you do, be adamant that your parent receives ample pain medication. Although doctors say that they believe in sparing patients from pain, they commonly limit narcotics for fear that patients will become addicted—an absurd concern when the patient isn't expected to recover. Or they fear that heavy pain medication will hasten death, which it sometimes does. But your parent should be comfortable, even if it means that death comes a day or two sooner.

It's best to receive medication at regular intervals before the pain begins (alleviating pain is more difficult than keeping it at bay in the first place), and extra doses of medication should be available at any indication of pain. Ask the doctor about a morphine pump that gives regular shots of pain relief while allowing the patient, if he is able, to push a button for additional doses when necessary. Studies show that patients who control their own pain medication actually use less medication and report less pain than those who do not have such control.

loved ones. You can't be there as often as you might like or at the times you might like, and when you are there, the hospital machinery and other routine intrusions get in the way of your having intimate time together. Furthermore, you and your parent have less control over her care. But there are things you can do to increase the intimacy and regain some control, even in a hospital. (See also Chapter Seven on how to care for your parent in the hospital).

◆ Unless you want all-out medical treatment for your parent, try to keep her out of the intensive care unit. The staffs in these units will keep your parent alive at almost any cost (physical, emotional and monetary), and the units are not de-signed to make patients and their families comfortable. The beeping monitors, bright lights and bustle of personnel is unsettling, and it hinders the kind of communication and physical contact which is so desperately needed now. Many ICUs also have rigid rules about visiting hours and the number of visitors, further impeding intimacy and solace.

◆ Be sure that your parent's liv-ing will or other directives are filed in her medical record and that the nurses and doctors overseeing her care are prepared to follow them.

◆ Be diligent in getting your parent the attention and care she needs. As she becomes sicker, she (as well as the rest of the family) may receive less and less attention from the hospital staff. Medical pro-fessionals are taught to treat illness and injury; they are given little or no training in how to provide gen-eral comfort or to tend to the emo-tional needs of dying patients and their families. Just like the rest of us, nurses and doctors have their own fears of death and tend to keep their distance. Whether conscious-ly or not, they may avoid or ignore a chronic patient out of a sense of helplessness or failure. It falls on you to search out and then persist in sus-taining adequate care.

◆ You might also find a hospi-tal social worker or chaplain, both of whom are generally better equipped than medical staff to address the emotional and spiritual needs of your parent and family.

◆ Visit regularly, but keep your visits short if they tire your parent. Remember, she may want you to simply sit quietly with her.

◆ Make sure your parent is get-ting all the pain relief she needs. There is no reason to limit med-ication if it can make her more comfortable.

◆ Ask the nurses if you or an-other family member can spend the night. Some hospitals have units where family members can sleep, while others may allow you to sleep in an extra bed or cot in your par-ent's room.

◆ If your parent is afraid of be-ing left alone or you don't like the thought of her being alone but can't always be with her, hire a compan-ion or find a volunteer who will sit by her side.

## AT HOME

If your family decides that ag-gressive medical treatment is futile and unwanted (see page 355), and you find the hospital too impersonal and clinical, your parent can come home to die, with the help of a hos-pice or visiting nurses and, most of all, you and other family members.

By making this choice, you give her the comfort of home, and keep her free from unwanted medical treatments, intrusions and the oth-er indignities of hospital life. She is surrounded by the people she loves, and has some control over what she wants to do—sip a glass of sherry, watch television at three in the morning, have some quiet time alone

> **"**In the hospital, they neglect the people who are old and very sick. I know they are short-staffed, but my mother was not a demanding person. That was her big thing, not to bother anybody. But when she called for a bedpan or painkiller, the nurses responded very slowly. One afternoon I was there and she wanted to walk, and the nurse said she would have to wait until later. But 'later' never came.
>
> That did it. I said, 'I've had it. Let's get her home.**"**      —NELLY O.

or listen to Mozart. You also create the opportunity for intimacy, as there may be times when your parent is lucid, when the narcotics have worn off or she has a small burst of strength, and you can share a treasured moment of warmth and humor. At home, you will be able to grieve, love, hurt and care for your parent freely, privately and completely.

All this intimacy comes at a price, however. Such an undertaking often entails sleepless nights and challenging days of changing diapers, keeping track of medications, lifting and shifting your parent to prevent bedsores and providing other heavy and demanding physical care. Even if health aides and nurses are enlisted to do the physical work, the constant proximity to death can be enormously draining. These are long days and nights, spent watching your parent become sicker and weaker and closer to death.

Caring for a dying parent at home can be rich and rewarding, but it is not for everyone and you should not feel pressured to take it on unless it is right for you. When considering home care, think about how you react to illness and whether you will be able to handle such intense immersion in the dying process. Would you do better at caring for your parent while she is in a hospital or a nursing home, where you are buffered from some of the indignities of death and can physically remove yourself from the situation when needed?

If you are interested in caring for your parent at home, call a local hospice organization. They can tell you what to expect, what help they can provide and what your role will be.

## HOSPICE CARE

Hospice, the philosophy and practice of caring for the dying, is based on the belief that death is a natural and inevitable part of life and that at some point, rather than battling illness and trying to ward off death, all efforts should be focused on enhancing whatever life remains.

There are more than 2,100 hospice organizations across the country. Most offer home-care services and respite care. Hospice organizations typically have a medical director, nurses, home health aides, social workers, psychiatrists, nutritionists, speech and physical therapists, clergy and volunteers, all of whom work with the family and patient as needed. Whatever a family's specific needs, staff members are usually available 24 hours a day to answer questions or to make personal visits if there is an emergency.

A few hospices operate residential centers where patients can receive care for short periods, or stay when home care is not an option. The others can make arrangements for respite care by moving a patient temporarily into a nursing home, or can arrange for nurses and aides to fill in at home while a family takes a break. Nearly half of all hospices have contracts with hospitals so that patients can be transferred if they need more extensive medical care to control symptoms or get through the final stages of dying.

With the help of a hospice a person who is incurably ill and close to death is removed from the fast pace and machinery of the hospital and brought home—or in certain cases to a homelike setting within a nursing home, or at a hospital or a free-standing hospice center—to die more comfortably and peacefully. Hospice nurses and doctors do not try to cure or rehabilitate patients, and in general they discourage the use of life-support systems and aggressive medical treatments such as ventilators, feeding tubes, chemotherapy, radiation and surgery. Instead, the focus of care is palliative, aimed at relieving pain and symptoms such as nausea, dizziness and constipation. (Hospice care occasionally includes aggressive medical procedures to ease pain or treat some secondary illness—for example, radiating a tumor to ease pressure on a nerve.)

Hospice nurses, who often work

*When we brought my mother home from the hospital there was all this equipment that had been delivered. We had a back-up generator in case the electricity went out, and tanks of oxygen. We had a commode and a special bed. I thought, 'What am I doing?'*

*But we saw an improvement in her, almost right away. She perked up, being at home. She started her crocheting again. She could walk down the hall—she refused to use the walker—and sit in my room in the sun. She seemed so much happier. And I knew that what we were doing was right.*        —NELLY O.

with a patient's primary physician or hospice doctor, are extraordinarily adept at managing pain without causing unnecessary grogginess. There is no getting around the fact that serious illness and the treatments aimed at combating it cause physical agony as well as mental anguish. But once under hospice care, patients generally do not suffer severe pain, except in rare circumstances.

As important as the physical care is the social, psychological and spiritual support the hospice staff provides to both patients and their families. Nurses, aides and social workers guide families through the daily regime and discuss the dying process, grief and other emotional and practical issues with family members and the patient. They help resolve conflicts; offer financial guidance, pastoral support and be-

## FOR MORE HELP

**The Hospice Helpline
(800-658-8898)**

**The Hospice Association
of America
(202-546-4759)**

**The Cancer Information
Service
(800-422-6237)**

reavement counseling; and in some instances even assist in planning funerals. Almost all hospice services, from companions to nurses to medical equipment, are covered by Medicare as long as the agency is certified, and most are.

### Hooking up with a Hospice

Before a patient is accepted for care, some hospices require that a doctor determine—as much as such a determination is possible—that he has less than six months to live. The timing is important, because this is when Medicare and other health-care coverage typically begins to cover hospice care. Nevertheless, most hospice organizations will begin working with a patient and family as soon as they decide that the focus of the patient's care should be palliative rather than curative.

If you are interested in hospice care, contact the local hospice organization as soon as possible so your family can build a relationship with the staff, gather information and start to make arrangements. If there is a choice—many urban areas have more than one—ask about certification, staffing, credentials and admission requirements (some accept patients who are less ill than others), and find out if the hospice has a contract with a hospital or nursing home to offer inpatient care.

If you are interested but there isn't an established hospice organization in the area, don't despair. Hospice is not just an institution and a group of people, it is a philosophy of care. You can still take care of your parent at home; you will just need to do a little more legwork and organize your own support system. Call a home-care agency to inquire about visiting nurses and home health aides and say that you are interested in hospice care. More and more home-care agencies are offering palliative care to the dying, whether or not it is presented under the title of hospice. Talk to your parent's doctor and contact a social worker, member of the clergy or a psychotherapist who specializes in bereavement.

*«Would we do it again? Yes, she was my mother! She was Michelle's grandmother. It's wearying, but it was a special time, during those months. There was an incredible closeness and tenderness among all of us. I was worried about Michelle because she's just a teenager, but she developed a bond with her grandmother.»*                    —TERRY C.

If your parent is in a hospital or a nursing home and you are not able to care for him at home, ask if the institution can offer hospice-type care, or if hospice nurses can work with him within the institution. Sometimes hospitals or nursing homes have wings specifically for hospice care, or are willing to turn a room into a hospice-type facility, low on medical gear and high on homeyness.

## PREVENTING BURNOUT

Whether you realize it or not, you are emotionally living this death almost every minute. Even during a break, sitting in another room, you may hear your parent's raspy breathing, feel the health aide's presence or smell the soiled bed sheets. Your sleep may be interrupted, and you may have little time to eat, or appetite for food. This kind of caregiving takes a tremendous toll on a person, but you may be so caught up in it that you aren't aware of how it is affecting you. If you want to keep caring for your parent, you have to take care of yourself, even through this intensely demanding time.

Get help early. Tell the hospice nurse that you would like to get a home health aide or a companion for your parent. Most hospices provide aides directly, and, if not, they will arrange for one. And recruit friends and relatives to take shifts, make meals, run errands or do anything else that might be helpful to you now.

When others are caring for your parent, get away. Go for a walk, see

*"We felt we had to do it all ourselves, so we took shifts. I would stay with Mom until midnight and then my daughter would sit with her. My sister would come during the day, and if she couldn't come, then one of my aunts would come. We were on this round-the-clock schedule, which was fine as long as everybody showed up for their time slot. It got to be, 'Okay, we've made it through today. Now let's hope everybody's in place again tomorrow.'*

*In the end, that last week before she died, I found that I couldn't deal with it. I totally broke down. I hadn't had any sleep. I was exhausted. I started crying and couldn't stop. I called the hospice and they sent someone over right away."* —SUSAN V.

a friend, run errands, sit on the beach or go for a drive. If you don't pace yourself and remove yourself from your parent occasionally, at least for short periods, you will not last long at this undertaking. If you are concerned about leaving, consult the hospice nurses, who can often tell whether a dying person has weeks, days or only hours to live. If it's hours, then stay, of course. If it's more, then go.

When your parent's hospice care continues for more than a month or two, use respite care. Nearly all hospices provide it or know how to get it. Your parent can be moved into a nursing home or a hospital temporarily, or you can hire round-the-clock aides to care for your parent at home. Take a week or a long weekend and get away. Tend to your own needs and to other important relationships. Get your mind on something else. And get some sleep.

If you feel that you can't leave the house at all for a day or two because your parent is close to death or for some other reason, at least get out of earshot occasionally and get your mind on something else. Take a nap or a long, hot bath, call a friend on the phone, flip through a magazine or have a good meal. (Caregivers often forget to eat during this period, or they eat only junk food, which wears them down more quickly.)

And even during this grim time, don't be afraid to laugh. It may seem disrespectful, but it is not. Watch a comedy or read a funny book. Your emotional core needs strength, and laughing is a great recharger.

If you run out of stamina, if your parent continues to live for longer than you expected, if the emotional drain is too much or the care becomes too demanding, don't be ashamed to tell the hospice nurses how you feel and talk with them about possible solutions. Many terminally ill people who are cared for at home die in a hospital, a nursing home or another institution because their families simply become overwhelmed by the task. It's not surprising. While providing hospice care can be a fulfilling lesson in living and loving, it is always an extremely exhausting lesson in dying. Give what you can, but recognize and respect your personal limits.

# Decisions About Medical Intervention

Throughout your parent's illness everyone has wanted her to get the best medical care available, barring nothing. But at some point the question may arise, does getting the best medical care available mean getting *all* the medical care available?

Aggressive medical treatment is intrusive and, in some cases, even violent. If it offers no real hope, but represents only some vain effort—for example, jump-starting an elderly patient's heart with electric jolts and starting intravenous lines when there is virtually no chance of recovery—then the treatment is not only futile, but inhumane.

It's not always clear, of course, when medicine is futile and when it stands a reasonable chance of improving matters, or when a procedure will be more harmful than helpful. Whether or not to perform cardiopulmonary resuscitation on an old and dying person may be a clear-cut choice, but how does one know when a cancer treatment is no longer useful, when a dialysis machine should be turned off or when continuing to treat a case of pneumonia no longer makes sense?

As a general rule, if a treatment cannot improve the quality of your parent's life or extend a life that will be reasonably comfortable—that is, if it only prolongs or exacerbates pain and suffering—the treatment should be stopped or refused. But "pain and suffering" and "reasonably comfortable" are difficult phrases to define. For one person, being immobile and hospitalized without hope of recovery may make life unbearable. Another person might want to hang on, regardless of the pain or indignity, to see an anniversary, the birth of a grandchild, or simply because the will to live has not yet been diminished by suffering or exhaustion.

If your parent is alert and able, she will decide whether to accept or refuse medical care. She may want your help or opinion in deciding, or she may not.

However, if your parent is too ill to make choices about her own treatment, the decision will rest with you and others in the family. If your parent has given you power of attorney for health care and you have discussed her views at some length, then the question of what to do may be clear—never easy, but clear. If you haven't discussed these issues, then you must trust your own good judgment.

Take your time. If that means keeping your parent hooked to a machine for a few extra days, then go ahead and do so. You need time to make this decision and then to accept it.

Make sure you fully understand your parent's state, prognosis and options. Get a second opinion from another doctor if you need more perspective. Talk with family members and to an outsider, preferably a professional with experience in these matters, such as a social worker. And think about who your parent is and what she valued in life.

> **"** *The nurse called me at work and said that my mother was vomiting and had diarrhea. The nursing home needed my permission to start an IV line for fluid and nutrition. I was about to say yes when I stopped myself. Was this really what she would want? No. I knew my mother wouldn't want it. So I said, 'No. Give her whatever she will take on her own.'*
>
> *It was a very, very long day and I didn't sleep at all that night. I live far away and I'd been back and forth twice that week already so all I could do was wait by the phone. She died the next day.*
>
> *Do I regret my decision? Not at all. Could I do it again? I hope so.* **"**
> —CARL L.

You and your siblings know her best. You know better than anyone else what she could tolerate and what she could not, what she would consider acceptable, how she felt about medical treatment and how she felt about death.

Remember, if you choose to withhold or stop a medical procedure or treatment, you are not killing your parent, the disease is. That sounds simple, but you need to believe it in your heart. And you need to know that your decision is not causing your parent to suffer. In fact, it is likely that you are reducing her suffering.

If you focus your attention on making the remainder of your parent's life comfortable and full of love, if you think about what's best for

## WHEN THERE'S DISAGREEMENT ABOUT TREATMENT

If your family can't decide what to do about your parent's medical care, or if your wishes regarding treatment clash with those of the doctor and you have no power of attorney giving you the authority to make decisions about her health care, contact the hospital ombudsman, the social worker or the hospital's medical ethics committee. You can also call Choice in Dying (800-989-9455) or the National Right to Life Committee (202-626-8800) for counseling, legal advice and support. (The former group works to protect patients' wishes concerning medical treatment, whatever those wishes may be. The latter opposes euthanasia and will help you keep your parent on life support or secure aggressive medical treatment.)

her and what she would want rather than what's easiest for you, you will make the right decision—whether that means ending treatment or continuing it.

### MAKING ADVANCE DIRECTIVES STICK

If your parent has signed advance directives, how do you ensure that they are carried out? Doctors frequently overtreat dying patients and ignore written requests to withhold life support. They have a powerful drive to treat illness, as it is all they are trained to do.

To make sure your parent's requests are honored, you or he should talk to his doctor as soon as possible. Be sure the doctor understands your parent's wishes, respects them and is willing to carry them out. Be sure, too, that every family member understands and is willing to abide by them. If even one sibling disagrees with a decision to withhold care, a doctor may

insist on providing full medical treatment.

If your parent is in a hospital or nursing home, be sure that his advance directives are on file there, and speak with any doctors, nurses or aides who are involved in his care. Find out exactly what they will or will not do in an emergency. Be persistent in assuring that his wishes are honored.

*We didn't have a hard time making the decision to stop my father's treatments. He was quite ill—the cancer had spread rapidly, and he'd had a small but jarring stroke—and the doctor said it was time to call hospice. We didn't question his opinion. We knew this was the right thing to do. Intellectually it was easy, but emotionally it was the hardest thing I have ever done. It's a devastating step to take, to let go of the hope and accept that nothing more can be done.* —MARJORIE C.

If you are caring for your parent at home, decide in advance what you will do if his breathing stops. If he doesn't want to be resuscitated, then you shouldn't call an ambulance because in most states paramedics must, by law, start resuscitation efforts. Admittedly, it's difficult to refrain from making such a call. In that frightening moment, people often find that they aren't quite ready to allow a parent to die, despite advance directives, and they have an overwhelming desire to "save" him. It will help if you can prepare emotionally and practically for such an event. Think about what you would do and how you might say good-bye. If you are worried that someone in the household might, in a state of panic, call 911, see if you can get a non-hospital DNR order, a legal document which releases paramedics from their obligation to resuscitate. (You can obtain a DNR order only through your parent's doctor.)

## COMAS AND PERSISTENT VEGETATIVE STATES

The neat border between life and death becomes blurred when most of the brain, but not quite all of it, is damaged or destroyed, and a patient falls into the twilight zone of a coma or a persistent vegetative state. It may be easier to cope with the emotional turmoil if you understand the biology of what has happened.

In older patients, these states usually are caused by stroke, heart attacks or Alzheimer's disease. When a person is in a coma most

*"My mother was in a coma for ten days in the hospital. I knew we were finally saying good-bye because I saw her dying before me, little by little, and I just wanted her to go. I wanted it to be over. After all those years of watching her be strangled by this disease, I knew she was finally going to be set free."* —SALLY T.

of the brain no longer functions. The comatose person behaves much like someone under heavy anesthesia. She does not respond consciously to stimuli, such as shouting or poking, although she may be able to breathe on her own.

Once in a deep coma for more than a month or two, patients usually enter what is referred to as a persistent vegetative state. Few recover from this, and none fully. In the case of an older person, the chance of recovery is virtually nil. At this point the brain stem, the most rudimentary portion of the brain which controls basic bodily functions, is all that remains alive. The lungs take in oxygen, the heart beats and the body eliminates waste, but the person has no consciousness, no self-awareness, no thought process. Studies using sophisticated scanners that measure brain activity show that patients in persistent vegetative states do not feel pain, though they may jerk reflexively when pinched.

The situation is sheer hell for family and other loved ones. The person is there, soft and warm to touch and hold, and, in some sense, alive. She may even have normal sleep-wake patterns and her muscles may react involuntarily. Her eyes may open and blink. She may cough or yawn. Her lips may even curl into a smile. Because of such signs of awareness, it's almost impossible for families to believe that this person can't think, feel or communicate. It's a horrifying trick played out by medicine and human biology. With the advanced technology available today, it's possible for a person to remain in a persistent vegetative state for many years.

The last stage of this contiuum between life and death occurs when the brain completely stops working, a state that doctors sometimes refer to as brain death. Although the term seems to leave room for doubt or hope, there is really no difference between this and death. The term "brain dead" is often used when a person remains hooked to a respirator, heart machine and other gadgets that keep blood oxygenated and pumping, usually so his organs can be used for transplantation. The brain, however, is no longer functioning and the person is, in fact, dead.

## A NOTE ON SUICIDE

If your parent is interested not only in ending treatment, but wants to speed up the dying process by committing suicide, you need to be absolutely certain that he is not suffering from any sort of dementia, depression or other mental disorder. His own doctor or, better yet, a psychiatrist, can determine whether he is fit to make such a decision. (Doctors often fail to diagnose depres-

sion, especially in patients who are terminally ill.)

Be sure that your parent fully understands the course of his disease and the scope of pain relief and comfort care available. Most people who choose suicide do so to avoid pain, humiliation and disability. But often their visions of the future are inaccurate. Pain can almost always be conquered and feelings of humiliation can often be spared when loved ones speak openly to one another. Have your parent talk at some length to a hospice nurse or other medical professional who is well-versed in issues of death about what his future holds and what care is available.

If you conclude that his desire to commit suicide is based on reasoned thinking and full information, then you are left with little recourse but to support him as best as you can. Doing so may horrify and anger you. You may feel painfully helpless. But even if you do not agree with his decision, stay with him. Don't abandon him. Your parent needs you now, and you will surely regret it if you fail to support him.

Although physician-assisted suicide is generally illegal, some doctors will help a patient commit suicide if the patient is terminally and incurably ill, and is deemed to be mentally competent to make such a decision. Some will supply ample doses of narcotics without comment, while others will provide directions for and even personal help in using them. (The Hemlock Society USA in Denver, Colorado, provides information on assisted suicide and other forms of euthanasia.)

# What Death Looks Like

What does death look like? How do you know when the end is near? What can you expect to see? What will your parent experience?

In wonderful old movies, a dying person is propped up on clean, downy pillows, her hair is in place, her face is tired but still attractive, and she gazes lovingly at someone before gracefully lowering her lashes and heaving a last sigh. In the real world, death is a lot less picturesque. The scenario is different for each person. Some people die slowly, some go unexpectedly in their sleep, some lapse into a coma and others are alert right up to the end. Generally, death from an illness is not a dramatic moment, but a slow process, a gradual departure.

As a person becomes sicker, he gets weaker. He becomes less mobile and usually becomes incontinent. Many dying people have trouble swallowing and eventually refuse nearly all food and drink. As the person eats less and less, he becomes thinner and thinner, until his face is quite sunken and sallow.

It's horrible to watch, but this failure to eat is probably causing you more pain than your parent. Very sick patients, who grimace because of an infection or a broken bone, do not express any such discomfort as a result of being disconnected from nutrition and hydration tubes. In fact, forcing food and fluids into a body that can no longer handle them

*"During the last week, Dad couldn't talk or respond. The hospice nurses told us that he had only hours to live, but five days passed like this. The tension of thinking every moment, 'This is it,' for such a long time got to be too much.*

*A hospice worker told us that we had been spending so much gratifying time with Dad—talking about what he meant to us, about experiences we'd shared and how much we loved him, and reading his favorite Robert Frost poems—that he was fighting to stay alive. She said, 'He's going to hang on as long as this stuff keeps coming. He's loving it. There is so much energy here. You have to leave him; only then will he be free to leave.'*

*She suggested that each of us go in and say good-bye. And rather than clutching him close to us, that we stroke him very lightly, moving from his head, down his arms and out beyond his body into the space of the room. This was a very physical way of letting go. Each of us did this and we went to bed around midnight, more calm ourselves. Around 2 A.M. he died very peacefully.*
—Ruth S.

can overload these systems and cause a number of problems, including a backlog of water into the lungs and severe constipation.

Make sure your parent's mouth is always fresh and moist. Give her ice chips or small amounts of water and wipe her teeth, gums and tongue with a damp cloth, or use disposable mouth swabs.

Several other symptoms, such as breathing difficulty, nausea and vomiting, constipation, confusion and infections, are common as death nears, but most can be treated so they do not cause severe discomfort or pain. If you are aware of such symptoms, alert the doctor or nurse. Your parent may also become achy and stiff from being in bed, so it is important to move him regularly—over on his side, to a chair, sitting up, lying flat, with legs elevated, and so on.

Your parent will become less aware of what is happening—because of both the illness and pain medication—and he may drift in and out of consciousness. Sleep patterns are often disrupted, so he may stay awake at odd hours of the night and sleep soundly in the middle of the day. Communication may be limited. At times your parent may stare off as though he is thinking about something, his eyes may look glassy and you may not be able to draw his attention.

Some dying people appear to have what has come to be called a near-death experience. They see and chat with people who have died, or talk about being in some distant place. This may startle you, but usually these experiences are quite pleasant, or at least not unpleasant. Your parent may also twitch or jerk occasionally, but this is nothing to worry about. It is usually not a sign of pain, just a restless muscle.

In the last days or hours, your parent's fingers, toes, elbows, nose, lips and other extremities may feel cold and turn a bluish gray. At the same time, his temperature may rise and he may have bouts of sweating (be sure to sponge your parent off and keep the sheets clean and dry).

His breathing may be labored and, if mucus that he is unable to cough up has collected in his throat, he may make a gurgling sound when he breathes, something known as a death rattle. It sounds a little like someone sucking up the last bits of a drink into a straw, a noise that can be disturbing, even frightening, if you have not been forewarned. Eventually there may be gaps in his breathing—he will stop breathing for a few seconds (and so will you), then gasp for another breath and continue breathing normally for a while. Near the end, these pauses will become longer until the breathing stops altogether.

The final moment is often quiet and uneventful, though a few biological reactions can take place that will be less upsetting if you are prepared for them. Sometimes the bowel and bladder release. The eyes and jaw may remain open. Sometimes people let out a howl or yell, not a cry of pain or despair, but simply a last muscular spasm of the voice box. In a few instances, people make a last, energetic effort just before they die—sitting up, trying to stand, gasping for another breath—which may upset those who are watching, but you should know that such activity is largely reflexive, and not a conscious effort on the part of the dying person.

If you are aware that your parent is dying, it's hard to know what to do during these last hours, minutes and seconds. You may feel paralyzed, awkward and intensely helpless. You may feel shock. Focus your energies on making your parent feel loved and safe. By now he will have little, if any, ability to communicate, but it is likely that he can still sense your voice and your embrace. Give him a peaceful exit. Speak gently to him and let him know that you are there, that he has nothing to fear, that he is safe, that you love him, that he has had a good life and that he is free to go. Hold him or touch him, and give him all the love in your heart.

# The Moment of Death

Your parent has taken his last breath and you are standing beside him. Whether you are weeping or numb with shock, you face the question of what to do next.

Actually, you don't have to do anything. If you are in the hospital, you don't need to call for a nurse. If you are at home, you don't have to contact anyone right away unless you want to. There is no need to whisk the body away.

If you want, you can just sit with your deceased parent, hold him in your arms, touch his hands and face, say good-bye or weep. You may want to wait for other family members to arrive so they, too, have this moment to say good-bye. You may want to pray, take part in another

**❝**At about 1 A.M. my sister woke me and said, 'She's choking. Something is happening.' I ran in and found my mother dying. I held her for a moment and then she died. And that was it. She was gone.

Bonnie and I just looked at each other and looked at Mom. We didn't cry right away. We just stood there. It had been a long haul. And now it was over. She was dead. It seemed very matter-of-fact, almost anti-climactic.

We pulled a blanket up, tucked her in, and then we made some tea and sat in the living room. It hit us both at the same time and we just started to cry. The exhaustion, the reality of this death, looking around that familiar room. After all we had done, our mother was gone.**❞**
—SUSAN V.

religious ritual, or tend to your parent's body in some way. You can pick out clothing for his burial (which most funeral homes require) or, if you choose, dress him or even bathe and groom him. Some people find that such a task is actually a healing and tender final gift. Do whatever feels right for you. This time and these acts belong solely to you and your family.

When you are ready, call the hospice or your parent's doctor. You may want to call a member of the clergy. Don't worry if it's the middle of the night. Most clergy would rather come when they are needed than on the following morning when the crisis is over. Also, call a funeral home. Once your parent has been declared dead by a doctor, nurse or coroner, the funeral home can pick up his body and begin the process of filing a death certificate and preparing the body for burial or cremation. (If it's late at night, they may not come until morning.)

As soon as you are able, call the members of your parent's immediate family. Do not hesitate to "bother" someone who is on vacation or at work. Most people want to be told as soon as possible, and feel cheated or deprived if they are not notified of the death until hours or days after it has happened. If the family is a large one, make a list of people to be called and ask other family members to share the task. Most people will want to know whether a funeral or a memorial service has been scheduled and will understand when you keep the conversation brief.

Over the next few days, call your parent's (and your) closest friends and relatives. You don't need to call others beyond that, as news of the death will travel quickly on its own.

(See Appendix G, page 423, on what needs to be done after your parent's death and how to plan a memorial service.)

## WHEN YOU ARE NOT THERE

If you had hoped to be with your parent when she died, and weren't—whether you were far away or just made a quick trip to the store—you may feel cheated out of something or guilty that you didn't extend your last visit. It may ease your mind to hear an account of the last days or moments of her life, so ask the doctor, nurses or whoever was in the room at the time, to tell you about every detail while the memory is still fresh in their minds.

Beyond that, don't berate yourself for not being there. Your parent may have chosen, in some way, to die when you weren't. This is something you will never know. But you did nothing wrong. You gave your parent love and care long before that final moment, and that is what really matters.

# GOOD GRIEF

*Stages of Grieving • Growing from Grief
• The Surviving Spouse • Reviewing Your Relationship
with Your Parent • Children and Grief*

.........................................

YOUR PARENT IS GONE. HE WAS OLD AND SICK, AND IT was probably time. Yet the loss is jarring. Your world has changed. A big piece is missing.

Grief rolls in like a series of waves, washing you in sorrow, confusion, anger, relief and regret. It may pulse through you evenly or crash down on you when you least expect it. If you were close to your parent, you may feel as though your very core has been assaulted and that life will never be the same again. In fact, it won't be. With time, the hole will grow smaller and less painful, but a bit of it will always remain.

You can't control your grief, shake it off or speed it up, and you shouldn't try. Grief is a necessary and valuable process that allows you to accept this loss, say good-bye to your parent and move on with your life and other relationships. It is not something to race through or escape from. Allow yourself to feel it in your own way and at your own pace.

# Stages of Grief

W hile each person's grief is unique, psychologists have mapped out a number of common reactions. You may experience only a few of them and do so in no particular sequence, bobbing from one emotion to another and then returning to old feelings you thought had long disappeared. But these descriptions should assure you that your reactions are normal, and also give you some insight into the feelings of others who may be mourning your parent's death.

**The immediate impact.** Numbness, denial, disbelief and shock are often the first reactions. There is a sense that this didn't happen or couldn't have happened. The truth that your parent is dead seems real only at certain moments.

In the immediate days after a death, some people feel intense pain, while others respond with cool detachment. Some become disoriented and have trouble making decisions, while others become adept organizers. Some are unable to do much, while others are hyperactive, restlessly pacing, scrubbing kitchen counters, cleaning out closets and losing themselves in other physical tasks. Your reaction is not a measure of how much you loved your parent. Each person's response is simply one way of coping with this loss.

As you digest the reality of your parent's death, you may feel angry at him for leaving you or overcome by guilt for things you said or did or failed to say or do. And you may feel resentment or jealousy toward others who still have their parents.

Acute grief causes physical repercussions as well, weakening the immune system, tipping hormones out of balance, upsetting one's appetite and disrupting sleep. Some people become physically sick in the early stages of mourning, and suffer from chronic headaches, the flu or other illnesses.

In the days and weeks after your parent's death, take time off from work and other responsibilities to care for yourself if you can. Spend time with family and good friends. The more support you have, the better you will cope. Be willing to ask for a shoulder to cry on when you need it. Most people want to help and feel complimented that you trust them enough to ask.

Resist the temptation to be stoic about your loss. No matter what your relationship with your parent was like, you have suffered a great blow. At the same time, don't force it. People may tell you to "get it out," let yourself cry and feel the hurt, but dragging painful emotions to the surface before you are ready may not be helpful. Your heart and soul need time in order to heal. Experience only as much as you want to, and at your own pace. Some people like to immerse themselves in

> **"**My mother died nine years ago and I still wonder, 'Where is she? Where did she go?' I can't seem to let go of this feeling that she is still there, somewhere.**"**  —BARBARA K.

> **"**After my father died, we went into the living room and collapsed on the couch and, to be perfectly honest, we started laughing. That sounds horrible, I know, but we were completely exhausted. We had worried so much and cried so hard that I don't think we had any other emotions left.**"**                    —TINA R.

memories of the deceased parent so they can grieve more intensely, while others prefer to avoid such hurtful reminders.

**The aftershocks.** In the weeks after the funeral, family members return to their homes, friends no longer offer words of condolence and employers run out of sympathy. Everyone may think it's time for you to be your old self again, but you may still be grieving and unable to carry on with business as usual. Give it time. Some people experience grief only after the formalities and commotion subside. For others, the initial pain gives way to despair, hopelessness and depression. Some become irritable, and some become anxious and restless.

Unless you welcome them, say no to invitations, extra assignments and social obligations. Continue to make yourself a priority.

You may find yourself yearning and searching for your parent, visiting his grave or his favorite spots, trying in some way to stay close to him. Some people adopt the habits and mannerisms of the dead person and, in a few cases, even the symptoms of the person's final illness.

(Such an obsession, along with its symptoms, will pass.)

It's common to have dreams about the deceased person, which are usually upsetting but may also be reassuring. For months after the death, you may think that you see your parent out of the corner of your eye, or sense for a moment that you hear her come into the house. You may forget she is gone and pick up the phone to call her.

Your parent's death may cause you to reexperience other losses in your life, of loved ones who died, friends who moved away, close relationships that were severed. This compounds the pain and adds to the confusion. And yet, if those losses weren't fully mourned when they happened, this may be an opportunity to grieve and let them go, too.

After a loved one dies, people often speculate about the phenomenon of death, the meaning of life and their own spiritual or religious beliefs. It may help to talk with a member of the clergy even if you have no connection with a particular religious institution.

Having said all this, it is quite possible that you are not grieving at all now, that instead you feel

> **"**I have kept myself so busy since she died, perhaps because there has been so much to do, perhaps because I want to be distracted. But now I find myself crying sometimes when I'm driving home from work. During that quiet time alone the reality sets in that she's not here anymore.**"**                    —NELLY O.

## NO REGRETS

When a parent dies and there is no longer a chance to do more or do differently, people sometimes feel guilt. Perhaps you got angry at a father who was confused, or fed up with a mother who needed a lot of care. Perhaps you didn't visit as often as you think you should have, or maybe you wished for your parent's death.

Be realistic. Put in the same situation again, it is likely that you would think the same thoughts and behave in the same way. And honestly, would a slightly different approach or a few more visits have made a genuine difference in your relationship or your parent's care? Certainly any thoughts you had about your parent's death did not hasten or affect his dying.

Remember all you did for your parent, how much you gave and what you shared. Think about the days of worry, the calls, the care, the unending love and support. Now that this time is over, you have only to be proud.

relief. Don't feel guilty about any lack of sorrow. If your parent was sick for a very long time, in great pain, or lost to dementia, you may have finished your grieving process some time ago.

**Letting go.** Sleeping or eating problems, crying bouts, despair or depression may persist, but to a far lesser degree. This tends to be a time of reflection and growth. With the acute pain gone, people often review their relationship with the parent they have lost and reminisce about time spent together. Friends and mates may try to get you to focus on the present or the the future now, but this review is an essential part of saying good-bye.

Recognizing your parent for who he truly was and reconciling, or at least accepting, your differences will help you detach. It may also help you sort through your own personality traits—in what ways you are like or unlike your parent and how you might change.

Logic suggests that the more you loved your parent, the more deeply you will grieve his death, and conversely, that a troubled relationship means you will grieve less and perhaps even welcome this departure. While that may be, often just the opposite is true. If the relationship was full of conflict, you may be left with unresolved anger and dueling emotions of love and hate. But now there is no one to confront. You will have to reconcile the relationship on your own. If the turmoil persists, a support group or psychotherapy can be invaluable in

**❝**In the beginning, I welcomed the pain I felt when I thought about my mother. I wanted to remember her, to think about her, and I thought that as long as I felt the pain, she was still with me, still alive in some way. I was afraid that when I stopped hurting, she would be gone. It seemed like a betrayal to stop mourning.

Now I realize that it's okay not to grieve. The memories have faded, but they never go away. She'll always be with me, a part of me.**❞**
—BARBARA K.

resolving such a struggle. Mental health centers, hospices and community centers sometimes offer bereavement groups and counseling.

**Moving on.** Now life begins to return to normal. If you have allowed yourself to grieve, accepted the loss and adjusted to the changes in your life, you should be able to face each day with more energy and spirit. You won't think of your parent as often. In fact you may go through many days without thinking of him at all. Sorrow may come only at rare moments now—at a wedding, a celebration of a new job, the birth of a child and other important events your parent cannot witness. And your memories of your parent should be more pleasant now—memories of her as a younger, more vital woman, instead of those visions of how she was at the end of her life.

# Growing from Grief

The death of a parent can arouse far more complicated emotions than the death of a friend. It is not simply a matter of feeling sorrow and then getting back into the old groove. Life will never be the same. Whatever sort of relationship you had with your parent, your life is different now. In some ways it may be worse, and in other ways you may find that it is better.

**Newfound independence.** Whether you are 17 or 70, when your only surviving parent dies, you become an orphan. That may leave you feeling, at least for a time, afloat, rootless and profoundly alone. You

## DRUGGING GRIEF

Think twice before using drugs or alcohol to dull your emotional pain. Grieving is a necessary and natural response to a loss, and dulling the pain may only prolong or postpone it. Sleeping pills in particular can cause dependency and severe reactions. If you are suffering from clinical depression or from sheer exhaustion because you can't sleep, medication may be necessary for a short time, but be sure to use it in low doses and only under the supervision of a doctor.

**"**_I had a very difficult relationship with my mother. I struggled in those last years to get close to her, to build some sort of loving mother-daughter relationship, and nothing ever worked. We were never close._

_Given how little we had together I was amazed at how much I missed her. After she died there was a big hole, this big, empty hole in my life that I couldn't seem to fill or escape. I am still trying to figure out what that is about. Do I miss her, or do I miss the relationship I never had with her?_**"**
—JANE M.

may have lost a safety net, a confidant or a link to your childhood. The awareness that you are truly on your own, that you are no longer someone's child, can be a crushing and unexpected aspect of grief, but with time it can also be an impetus for new growth and bolder independence. If your father guided you financially or your mother fed your ego, you will have to learn to do these things for yourself now. And if you had a stressful relationship with your parent—if your mother was domineering or your father always made you feel inadequate—the loss can actually be liberating.

**A clearer view of one's self.** A parent's death brings you face-to-face with your own mortality. You don't have a buffer against the future anymore. You are now the older generation, and therefore the next in line to go.

You may have already studied your own wrinkles and white hairs. You may have settled into retirement and your "golden years." You may have even contemplated your own death. _Will I be like she was? Will my children care for me? Without children, who will care for me?_ With the death of your parent, these ruminations and questions become a little more stark.

This confrontation with mortality can depress you, but it can also serve as a clarion call to recognize how precious life is and to make the most of it—and perhaps to do better in old age than your parent did.

**Redirected energy.** The job of caregiver, although draining, may have given you a sense of purpose as it consumed your days. The loss of that role can mean some adjustment. If you have been at it for some time, you may have distanced yourself from friends or cut back on your hours at work, and become accustomed to a superhuman pace. Now there is a void.

Slowing down, finding new meaning in your life and reestablishing broken ties will take time. It requires patience and awareness. Find worthwhile tasks for yourself, and be careful not to fill the vacuum by taking over the care of yet another person, such as a surviving parent who is managing all right on her own.

**Changes in family structure.** Certain family patterns and rituals may disappear with your parent. You no longer know what your sister is up to because your mother isn't there to spread the news. Holiday plans are now open because Thanksgiving

## REVIEWING YOUR RELATIONSHIP WITH YOUR PARENT

After your grief has subsided, you may find it helpful to explore your parent's life and to consider any unresolved issues between the two of you. Approach these projects only when you are ready and only if doing so feels right for you.

❖ **Write.** Set aside time when you won't be interrupted to keep a journal or write letters to your deceased parent. Tell him whatever is on your mind. Say all the things you never had the nerve to say. Tell him how he angered you or what you appreciated about him. And when you are ready, tell him good-bye.

❖ **Interview.** Talk with your parent's relatives and friends about his life, his childhood, his professional life, his relationships. Pursue whatever interests you and delve into areas that you may have avoided when your parent was alive.

❖ **Commemorate.** Create rituals to honor and remember your parent. Visit her grave, frame photos, return to a favorite spot, plant a memorial tree or garden or have a family gathering on the anniversary of her death.

❖ **Join.** Get involved with a support group or attend seminars on grief (hospice organizations sometimes hold or know about such meetings). It will give you a chance to talk about issues with people who understand them.

❖ **Explore.** Review your relationship with your parent, and perhaps with others in the family. Write down memories of your parent, focusing on both the good and bad. Describe your relationship and how it changed, or failed to change, through the years. What did you do together? How did you make decisions? Make a list of your parent's traits and the things you agreed and disagreed about. Think about what values or traits of your parent live on in you. Go back and review what you wrote several days later, and add any new thoughts.

was always spent at your father's house. While the change is disorienting, getting together as a family is now a choice, and perhaps a chance to create your own traditions.

With time, old roles may disappear and family alliances shift. A sister who was closer to Dad may create a new, stronger relationship with Mom, which in turn may threaten a brother's intimate relationship with her. Or siblings

*"In the spring after my mother's death, I was planting a tree when I realized that it was my mother's birthday. So I called it Mary's Tree. And I tended to it, and fed it and watered it with care and love.*

*When I'm in the backyard, I look up at this tree, which is quite tall now, and I say 'Hi, Mary.' And it helps."*
— RITA W.

who fought about a parent's care may develop new bonds now that the parent is gone.

This is a time of testing and sampling. Let it happen and participate in it. While it may be uncomfortable at first, your family needs to establish new rituals and relationships.

**A review of other relationships.** In the midst of all this sorting-through, your relationship with your mate may come under review, and problems in the relationship may loom large. Remember that your spouse cannot fill the void that your parent's death has left, or know what you are feeling unless you tell him. As you detach from your parent, you will be better able to see your mate for all he is and all he cannot be.

Your relationship with your own children may also come under scrutiny. You may worry about what kind of a parent you are or have been. Are you repeating your parent's mistakes? Are you a good role model? Are you able to offer your children the positive things your parent gave you? Think about these questions and work on your own shortcomings. You do not have to repeat your

parent's mistakes, and you may be able to emulate her best qualities. Make this a time for growth and enrichment, not despair.

# The Surviving Spouse

Some widows or widowers become extremely depressed and isolated in the months, and even years, following the death of a spouse, especially after the funeral is over and friends and family have resumed their own lives. They may have trouble sleeping and eating normally and may become physically ill. And they often face overwhelming practical hurdles—how to manage finances, cook for one, do household repairs that a mate always took care of, or relate to friends who are still couples. While you need time for your own grief, you also need to support your surviving parent and figure out your new role in her life.

◆ In the immediate aftermath, offer lots of support. Stay in close contact. Call regularly and visit as often as possible. Share your grief and allow her to share hers. As you do this, remember that her relationship with her spouse as well as her role as caregiver was very different than yours—probably far more intense and exhausting. Let her deal with her grief and express her feelings in her own way, without comparison or reproach.

◆ While your parent may not have the energy or the will to go out, social contact is very important now. Encourage her to see friends and include her in family gatherings.

◆ Control your impulse to supply more protection than your parent needs. You may have a lot of caregiving energy on your hands, or you may assume that your mother can't survive on her own. Be careful. She has to adjust, learn about her new life as a single person and regain her confidence and independence. If you take over her affairs or deluge her with advice, it may offend her or cripple her. Love and support her, but let her learn to live her own life.

◆ In general, a surviving parent should not make any major decisions, such as moving, changing jobs or selling a home, immediately after a spouse's death. It's better to get through most of the grieving process (which can take a year or more), let things settle and sort out finances first. In the confusion of mourning, people sometimes make decisions which they later regret.

◆ Encourage your parent to see her doctor regularly and to take care of her physical health. Poor health will make her more susceptible to depression and illness. If she is using antidepressants or sleeping pills, be sure that she understands their side effects and potential dangers.

◆ Mark your calendar with your parent's wedding anniversary, birthday, the anniversary of your parent's death and other special dates, and try to be in touch on these days. They are often painful and lonely times for a surviving spouse.

◆ While she may be feeling too vulnerable to attend a support group at first, your parent may benefit from some one-on-one support. The American Association of Retired Persons (800-424-3410) runs a Widowed Persons Service which links newly widowed people with trained volunteers who offer emotional support as well as practical information (how to handle probate, how to deal with friends who are still couples, etc.). When she is ready, a bereavement or support group for widows can provide guidance, emotional support and friendships. Senior centers, family counseling centers, hospice centers and churches and synagogues often run or know of such groups.

◆ As she starts to heal emotionally, urge your mother to take classes, work, travel and get involved in whatever activities interest her. With time and encouragement, she will find in herself the will to enjoy living again.

◆ You may find that your parent undergoes a surprising personality change now that her spouse is gone. A mother who played second fiddle may prove to be quite capable and even assertive. One who was introverted may become extroverted. Living with your deceased parent may have repressed some of her personality traits and encouraged others. Any perceivable change is likely to be troubling for you—you may prefer the "old Mom"—but try to let your parent find out who she is as a single person, and then let that person thrive.

# Children and Grief

No matter how we may try to shield them, children, even very young children, are profoundly affected by dying and death. They are affected indirectly by your distress, and directly by their own loss. There are no magic words, there is no right way, to address this issue. Give your children room to express and explore their feelings, and then try to respond to their questions as honestly as you can. (See page 237 for more on talking with children when a grandparent is ill.)

**Start the conversation.** Sometimes children don't ask questions because they don't know what questions to ask. They simply know that the household is astir and they are scared by it. Explain briefly what is happening—why Mommy is upset, why the child has been sent repeatedly to a friend's house—and ask if he has questions.

Leave any conversation open for further discussion. A few days later you might ask the child if he has any more questions or if there is anything more he wants to talk about. Be aware that children may ask the same questions over and over. Answer them over and over. Sometimes it takes a few repetitions for the information to sink in.

**Be honest.** Don't say things like "God took him away," "She is asleep and won't ever wake up," or "He went on a long trip and will never come back." Children take things literally. (You may end up with an atheist, insomniac or homebody.) Or if you tell a child that a grandparent is up in the clouds watching over the family, he may worry about practical matters, like where Grandpa is on clear days or whether an all-knowing Grandpa sees every private thing he does.

Explain that Grandpa was old, his body was very sick and it stopped working, so he no longer eats, breathes or talks. Use examples from the child's own experience, like the death of a pet. You might add that the deceased person lives on in everyone's memories, or find an explanation that reflects your religious beliefs.

Be sure to explain that Grandpa is in no pain, that in fact he is out of pain; that death is not a punishment, but a natural thing that happens to everyone eventually; that death is not contagious; and that the child is in no way responsible for the grandparent's death. These are all frequent concerns of children.

**Let them be children.** Although it may be hard for you, allow your children to play and laugh at this time. They are not being disrespectful, they are only being children.

**Let them find their own way to grieve.** Young children sometimes use play to work through their feelings and questions. They may have a doll or stuffed animal that "dies," which they then bury. Or they may lie still, pretending they are dead, as they try to figure out what it means to be dead. They may also express their grief by misbehaving or withdrawing. Everyone deals with hurt and confusion in his or her own way and children need the leeway to grieve in whatever way they can.

Early in adolescence, children learn to be cool, and believe that it is uncool to reveal one's fear or pain.

If your child reacts in this way, don't corner or push him into admitting something he doesn't want to admit. Instead, talk about what you are feeling. Hearing about your emotions may help him deal with, and perhaps even talk about, his.

## BOOKS THAT HELP

A number of books can help a child come to grips with death. (They should be read in addition to, not instead of, open dialogue at home.) Some good ones include:

For preschool children: *The Dead Bird* by Margaret Wise Brown, illustrated by Remy Charlip (Young Scott Books); *The Tenth Good Thing About Barney* by Judith Viorst, illustrated by Erik Blegvad (Atheneum).

For children 5 to 8: *Annie and the Old One* by Miska Miles, illustrated by Peter Par-

nall (Little Brown & Co.); *Nana Upstairs and Nana Downstairs* by Tomie DePaola (Putnam); *My Grandpa Died Today* by Joan Fassler (Human Sciences Press).

For children 8 and up: *A Taste of Blackberries* by Doris B. Smith (Thomas Y. Crowell Co.); *Charlotte's Web* by E.B. White, illustrated by Garth Williams (Harper & Row); *The Birds' Christmas Carol* by Kate Douglas Wiggin (Houghton-Mifflin); *Little Women* by Louisa May Alcott (Grosset & Dunlap).

# APPENDIX

# APPENDIX A
## State Units on Aging and
## Long-Term Care (LTC) Ombudsman

### ALABAMA

**Commission on Aging**
RSA Plaza, Suite 470
770 Washington Ave.
Montgomery, AL
36130
334-242-5743

**LTC Ombudsman**
Same Address
334-242-4446

### ALASKA

**Commission on Aging
Division of
Senior Services**
P.O. Box 110211
Juno, AK 99811
907-465-3250

**LTC Ombudsman**
3601 C St., Suite 260
Anchorage, AK 99503
907-563-6393

### ARIZONA

**Aging and Adult
Administration**
1789 West Jefferson-
950A
Phoenix, AZ 85007
602-542-4446

**LTC Ombudsman**
Same Address/Phone

### ARKANSAS

**Division of Aging and
Adult Services
Arkansas Department
of Human Services**
P.O. Box 1437
Slot 1412
1417 Donaghey Plaza S.
Little Rock, AR 72201

**LTC Ombudsman**
Same Address/Phone

### CALIFORNIA

**Department of Aging**
1600 K St.
Sacramento, CA 95814
916-323-6681

**LTC Ombudsman**
Same Address/Phone

### COLORADO

**Aging and Adult
Services
Department of
Social Services**
110-16th St., Suite 200
Denver, CO 80202
303-620-4147

**LTC Ombudsman**
The Legal Center
455 Sherman St.
Suite 130
Denver, CO 80203
303-722-0300

### CONNECTICUT

**Community Services
Division of
Elderly Services**
25 Sigourney St.
Hartford, CT 06106
203-424-5274

**LTC Ombudsman**
Same Address
203-424-5200; ext. 5221

### DELAWARE

**Department of
Health Services
Division of Aging and
Adults with Physical
Disabilities**
1901 N. DuPont Hgwy.
New Castle, DE 19720
302-577-4791

**LTC Ombudsman**
256 Chapman Road
University Plaza
Suite 200
Newark, DE 19702
302-453-3820

## DISTRICT OF COLUMBIA

**Office on Aging**
441 Fourth St., NW
Suite 900 South
Washington, DC
20001
202-724-5622

**LTC Ombudsman**
601 E St., NW
4th Floor, Building A
Washington, DC
20049
202-434-2188

## FLORIDA

**Department of Elder Affairs**
4040 Esplanade Way
Building B, Suite 152
Tallahassee, FL 32399
904-414-2000

**LTC Ombudsman**
600 South Calhoun St.
Suite 270
Tallahassee, FL 32301
850-488-6190

## GEORGIA

**Division of Aging Services Department of Human Resources**
2 Peachtree St. N.W.
Suite 36-233
Atlanta, GA 30303
888-454-5826

**LTC Ombudsman**
Same Address/Phone

## HAWAII

**Executive Office on Aging**
Office of the Governor
250 South Hotel St.
Suite 107
Honolulu, HI 96813

**LTC Ombudsman**
Same Address
317-232-1750

## IDAHO

**Commission on Aging**
P.O. Box 0007
Boise, ID 83720
208-334-3833

**LTC Ombudsman**
Same Address
208-334-2220

## ILLINOIS

**Department on Aging**
421 East Capitol Ave.
Suite 100
Springfield, IL 62701
217-785-2870
Chicago Office:
312-814-2630

**LTC Ombudsman**
Same Address
217-785-3143

## INDIANA

**Bureau of Aging and In-Home Services**
402 W. Washington St.
P.O. Box 7083
Indianapolis, IN 46207
317-232-1147

**LTC Ombudsman**
Same Address
317-232-1750

## IOWA

**Department of Elder Affairs**
200 10th St., 3rd Fl.
Des Moines, IA 50309

**LTC Ombudsman**
Same Address
515-281-4646

## KANSAS

**Department on Aging**
Docking State Office
Building, Rm. 150 S.
915 S.W. Harrison
Topeka, KS 66612
913-296-4968

**LTC Ombudsman**
610 S.W. 10th St.
2nd floor
Topeka, KS 66612
785-296-3017

## KENTUCKY

**Division of Aging Services Department of Social Services**
275 E. Main St., 5 W
Frankfort, KY 40621
502-564-6930

**LTC Ombudsman**
Same Address/Phone

## LOUISIANA

**Governor's Office of
Elderly Affairs**
4550 N. Blvd., 3rd Fl.
P.O. Box 8037
Baton Rouge, LA
07802

**LTC Ombudsman**
Same Address/Phone

## MAINE

**Bureau of Elder and
Adult Services
Department of
Human Services**
35 Anthony Ave.
State House-Station
#11
Augusta, ME 04333
207-626-5335

**LTC Ombudsman**
1 Weston Court
P.O. Box 126
Augusta, ME 04332

## MARYLAND

**Office on Aging**
State Office Building
Room 1007 301 West
Preston St.
Baltimore, MD 21201
410-225-1102

**LTC Ombudsman**
Same Address
410-767-1074

## MASSACHUSETTS

**Executive Office of
Elder Affairs**
One Ashburton Place
5th Floor
Boston, MA 02108
617-727-7750

**LTC Ombudsman**
Same Address/Phone

## MICHIGAN

**Office of Services to
the Aging**
P.O. Box 30026
Lansing, MI 48909
517-373-8230

**LTC Ombudsman**
Citizens for Better Care
6105 W. St. Joseph
Hgwy. Suite 211
Lansing, MI 48917
516-886-6797

## MINNESOTA

**Board on Aging**
444 Lafayette Road
St. Paul, MN 55155
612-296-2770

**LTC Ombudsman**
121 East 7th Place
Suite 410
St. Paul, MN 55101
651-296-0382

## MISSISSIPPI

**Division of Aging and
Adult Services**
750 N. State St.
Jackson, MS 39202
601-359-4925

**LTC Ombudsman**
Same Address
601-359-4929

## MISSOURI

**Division of Aging
Department of
Social Services**
P.O. box 1337
615 Howerton Ct.
Jefferson City, MO
65102
573-751-3082

**LTC Ombudsman**
Same Address
573-526-0727

## MONTANA

**Office on Aging
Department of
Family Services**
48 North Last Chance
Gulch
P.O. Box 8005
Helena, MT 59604
406-444-5900

**LTC Ombudsman**
P.O. Box 4210
111 Sanders
Helena, MT 59604
406-444-4077

## NEBRASKA

**Department on Aging**
P.O. Box 95044
301 Centennial Mall-
S.
Lincoln, NE 68509
402-471-2306

**LTC Ombudsman**
Same Address/Phone

## NEVADA

**Division for Aging Services**
**Department of Human Resources**
340 North 11th St.
Suite 203
Las Vegas, NV 89101
702-486-3545

**LTC Ombudsman**
Same Address/ Phone

## NEW HAMPSHIRE

**Division of Elderly and Adult Services**
State Office Park South
129 Pleasant St.
Concord, NH 03301
603-271-4680

**LTC Ombudsman**
Same Address
603-271-4680

## NEW JERSEY

**Senior Affairs & LTC Ombudsman**
P.O. Box 807
Trenton, NJ 08625
609-588-3614

## NEW MEXICO

**State Agency on Aging**
La Villa Rivera Bldg.
Ground Floor
228 East Palace Ave.
Santa Fe, NM 87501
505-827-7640

**LTC Ombudsman**
Same Address/Phone

## NEW YORK

**Office for the Aging**
2 Empire State Plaza
Albany, NY 12223
800-342-9871
518-474-5731

**LTC Ombudsman**
Same Address
518-474-7329

## NORTH CAROLINA

**Division of Aging**
CB 29531
693 Palmer Dr.
Raleigh, NC 27626
919-733-3983

**LTC Ombudsman**
Same Address
919-733-8395

## NORTH DAKOTA

**Department of Human Services**
**Aging Services Division**
1929 N. Washington
P.O. Box 7070
Bismarck, ND 58507
701-328-2577

**LTC Ombudsman**
600 S. 2nd St.
Suite 1C
Bismarck, ND 58504
701-328-8910

## OHIO

**Department of Aging**
50 W. Broad St., 9th Fl.
Columbus, OH 43215
614-466-5500

**LTC Ombudsman**
Same Address
614-466-7922
Long-Term Complaint Line: 800-282-1206

## OKLAHOMA

**Aging Services Division**
**Department of Human Resources**
312 N.E. 28 St.
Oklahoma City, OK 73105
405-521-2281

**LTC Ombudsman**
Same Address
405-521-6734

## OREGON

**Senior and Disabled Services Division**
500 Summer St., N.E.
2nd Floor
Salem, Oregon 97310
503-945-5810

**LTC Ombudsman**
3855 Wolverine N.E.
Suite 6
Salem, OR 97310

## PENNSYLVANIA

**Department of Aging
Commonwealth of
Pennsylvania**
400 Market St., 6th Fl.
Harrisburg, PA 17101
717-783-1550

**LTC Ombudsman**
555 Walnut St.
5th Floor
P.O. Box 1089
Harrisburg, PA 17101

## PUERTO RICO

**Governor's Office of
Elderly Affairs**
P.O. Box 50063
Old San Juan Station
San Juan, PR 00902
809-721-5710

**LTC Ombudsman**
Same Address
809-721-1515

## RHODE ISLAND

**Department of
Elderly Affairs**
160 Pine St.
Providence, RI 02903
401-277-2858

**LTC Ombudsman**
422 Post Road
Suite 204
Warwick, RI 02888
401-785-3340

## SOUTH CAROLINA

**Division on Aging**
202 Arbor Lake Drive
Suite 301
Columbia, SC 29223
803-737-7500

**LTC Ombudsman**
1801 Main St.
P.O. Box 8206
Columbia, SC 29202

## SOUTH DAKOTA

**Office of Adult
Services and Aging**
Richard F. Kneip Bldg.
700 Governors Drive
Pierre, SD 57501
605-773-3656

**LTC Ombudsman**
Same Address/Phone

## TENNESSEE

**Commission on Aging**
Andrew Jackson Bldg.
9th Floor
500 Deaderick St.
Nashville, TN 37243
615-741-2056

**LTC Ombudsman**
Same Address/Phone

## TEXAS

**Department on Aging**
P.O. Box 12786
Capitol Station
Austin, TX 78751
512-444-2727

**LTC Ombudsman**
Same Address
512-424-6840

## UTAH

**Division of Aging and
Adult Services**
Box 45500
Salt Lake City, UT
84145
801-538-3910

**LTC Ombudsman**
120 North, 200 West
Room 401
Salt Lake City, UT
84145
801-538-3924

## VERMONT

**Department of Aging
and Disabilities**
Waterbury Complex
103 South Main St.
Waterbury, VT 05671
802-241-2400

**LTC Ombudsman**
VT Legal Aid Inc.
P.O. Box 1367
Burlington, VT 05402
802-863-5620

## VIRGINIA

**Department for the
Aging**
700 East Franklin St.
10th Floor
Richmond, BA 23219
804-225-2271

**LTC Ombudsman**
530 E. Main St.
Suite 428
Richmond, VA 23219
900-552-3402
800-644-2923

WASHINGTON

**Aging and
Adult Services
Administration
Department of Social
and Health Services**
P.O. Box 45600
Olympia, WA 98504
360-493-2500

**LTC Ombudsman**
So. King County
Multi-Service Center
1200 South 336th St.
Federal Way, WA
98093
800-422-1384
253-838-6810

WEST VIRGINIA

**Commission on Aging**
Holly Grove
State Capitol
1900 Kanawha Blvd. E.
Charleston, WV 25305
304-558-3317

**LTC Ombudsman**
Same Address/Phone

WISCONSIN

**Bureau on Aging
Department of Health
and Social Services**
P.O. Box 7851
Madison, WI 53707
608-266-2536

**LTC Ombudsman**
Board on Aging and
Long-Term Care
214 N. Hamilton St.
Madison, WI 53703
608-266-8995

WYOMING

**Department of Health
Division on Aging**
117 Hathaway
Building
Room 139
Cheyenne, WY 82002
800-442-2766
307-777-7986

**LTC Ombudsman**
WY Senior Citizens
2756 Gilchrist St.
P.O. Box 94
Wheatland, WY 82201
307-322-5553

# APPENDIX B

*Yellow Pages of Useful Organizations*

## AFRICAN-AMERICAN SERVICES

**National Caucus and Center on Black Aged**
1424 K St., NW, Suite 500
Washington, DC 20005
202-637-8400

The Center works to improve the quality of life for the African-American and low-income elderly population. While it provides no services directly to the public, it has programs in job opportunities and training, health care, housing options and long-term care.

## ALCOHOL AND DRUG ABUSE

**Alcoholics Anonymous**
P.O. Box 459
Grand Central Station
New York, NY 10163
212-870-3400

The national office in New York can direct you to a local AA chapter, but it may be easier to simply look it up in your local telephone book. AA assists alcoholics become and remain sober through self-help groups.

**Al-Anon Family Groups**
P.O. Box 862
Midtown Station
New York, NY 10018
800-356-9996

These groups help family members and friends of alcoholics to cope. The organization makes referrals to local chapters and will also send out brochures on how alcoholism affects families.

**National Clearinghouse for Alcohol and Drug Information**
P.O. Box 2345
Rockville, MD 20847
800-729-6686

This federal clearinghouse has publications on alcoholism and drug use. The focus of most of the information is prevention, but there are some materials on treatment as well.

**National Council on Alcoholism and Drug Dependence Hopeline**
12 West 21st St.
New York, NY 10010
800-622-2255

The Council has information on alcoholism and referrals to local services.

## ALZHEIMER'S DISEASE

**Alzheimer's Association**
919 N. Michigan Ave.
Suite 1000
Chicago, IL 60611
800-272-3900

Also known as the Alzheimer's Disease and Related Disorders Association, this organization provides information and referrals to local chapters, which in turn refer people to local services and support groups. The information and services are helpful to families dealing with other forms of dementia as well.

**Alzheimer's Disease Education
and Referral Center**
P.O. Box 8250
Silver Spring, MD 20907
800-438-4380
  Directed by the National Institute on Aging, this center has information on all aspects of Alzheimer's Disease.

**National Institute of Neurological
Disorders and Stroke
Information Office**
Building 31, Room 8A16
31 Center Dr., MSC2540
Bethesda, MD 20892
800-352-9424
  Part of the National Institutes of Health, this office has information about stroke and other brain disorders, such as Parkinson's, Alzheimer's and epilepsy and makes referrals to local clinical research centers.

## ARTHRITIS AND OSTEOPOROSIS

**Arthritis Foundation
Information Line**
P.O. Box 19000
Atlanta, GA 30326
800-283-7800
  The Foundation provides information and makes referrals to local chapters that sponsor support groups, events and classes.

**National Arthritis and
Musculoskeletal and Skin Diseases
Information Clearinghouse**
1 AMS Circle
Bethesda, MD 20892
301-495-4484
  This federal clearinghouse has publications covering a host of disorders and diseases that affect bones, joints and skin.

**National Osteoporosis Foundation**
1150 17th St., NW, Suite 500
Washington, DC 20036
800-223-9994
202-223-2226
  This organization sends out reports on the causes, prevention, detection and treatment of osteoporosis.

## CANCER

**American Cancer Society**
1599 Clifton Rd., NE
Atlanta, GA 30329
800-227-2345
404-320-3333
  Staff members can answer questions on a broad range of subjects, such as cancer detection, treatment and the latest research. They also have brochures and can refer callers to local chapters for information about local services.

**Cancer Information Service
National Cancer Institute**
Building 31, Room 10A24
Bethesda, MD 20892
800-422-6237
  The NCI helpline provides information on everything from detection of cancer and treatment to financial help and home care. It gives referrals to local organizations, cancer centers and support groups, and sends NCI brochures.

**National Coalition for
Cancer Survivorship**
1010 Wayne Ave.
Silver Spring, MD 20910
301-650-8868
  This private, nonprofit group offers information on cancer treatments, costs, insurance coverage and employment, and refers people diagnosed with cancer to support groups.

## CAREGIVER SERVICES

**Aging Network Services**
**4400 East West Highway**
**Suite 907**
**Bethesda, MD 20814**
**301-657-4329**
This is a private business which, for a fee, will refer you to a geriatric care manager in your parent's hometown. The manager coordinates services for your parent and serves as a liaison for the family.

**American Association of**
**Retired Persons (AARP)**
**601 E St., NW**
**Washington, DC 20049**
**202-434-2277**
**800-424-3410**
AARP has a number of good brochures on caregiver stress, caring from a distance and a variety of issues facing the elderly and their families. Most of them are free.

**Children of Aging Parents**
**1609 Woodbourne Rd.**
**Suite 302A**
**Levittown, PA 19057**
**215-945-6900**
**800-227-7294**
CAPS provides information on caregiving and referrals to support groups, geriatric care managers and other resources. There is a small charge for brochures and copies of articles from the group's newsletter, which is published six times a year. (An individual membership costs $20 a year.)

**Eldercare Locator**
**800-677-1116**
Run by the National Association of Area Agencies on Aging, this is a good place to start when looking for local services. Its helpline will tell you how to reach the "area agency on aging" that oversees services to the elderly in your parent's hometown.

**National Association of Professional**
**Geriatric Care Managers**
**1604 North Country Club Rd.**
**Tucson, AZ 85716**
**520-881-8008**
Primarily a trade association for care managers, this group will make referrals to geriatric care managers (but only its members).

**National Association of**
**Social Workers**
**750 First St., NE**
**Washington, DC 20002**
**800-638-8799 (ext. 291)**
This is a trade association for social workers, but it can give referrals to local social workers who serve as care managers or therapists.

**National Federation of Interfaith**
**Volunteer Caregivers**
**368 Broadway, Suite 103**
**Kingston, NY 12401**
**914-331-1358**
**800-350-7438**
This private, nonprofit group administers over 400 regional offices that send volunteers into the homes of people who need care, company and supervision. The national headquarters can tell you whether interfaith volunteers are available in your parent's area.

**Well Spouse Foundation**
**P.O. Box 801**
**New York, NY 10023**
**212-644-1241**
The Foundation offers support to people caring for a sick spouse who need a little emotional care themselves. Members are directed to support groups, can be assigned pen pals if desired and receive a newsletter six times a year.

## DEATH AND DYING

**Choice in Dying**
**200 Varick St.**
**New York, NY 10014**
**212-366-5540**
**800-989-9455**

Choice in Dying provides information and advance directives (legal forms that include a living will and durable power of attorney for health care) that are up-to-date and specific to each state. Staff lawyers, nurses and social workers will counsel families.

**Funeral and Memorial**
**Societies of America**
**6900 Lost Lake Rd.**
**Egg Harbor, WI 54209**
**800-765-0107**

The group offers guidance on planning inexpensive and dignified funeral and memorial services.

**Hemlock Society USA**
**P.O. Box 101810**
**Denver, CO 80250**
**800-247-7421**

The Hemlock Society promotes the right to euthanasia—both refusal of life-saving treatment and physician-assisted suicide. It has information and publications as well as telephone counseling and referrals to local chapters and other local organizations.

**National Funeral Directors**
**Association**
**11121 West Oklahoma Ave.**
**Milwaukee, WI 53227**
**414-541-2500**
**800-228-6332**

This association offers guidance in locating a funeral director, and planning memorial services and burials.

**National Right to Life Committee**
**419 Seventh St., NW, Suite 500**
**Washington, DC 20004**
**202-626-8800**

The Committee, a grass-roots organization that opposes abortion and euthanasia, has drafted a "Will to Live" form for each state. The form states a person's wishes to be kept on life support regardless of the medical prognosis. The Committee also helps people seeking treatment that a doctor or hospital refuses to provide.

## DENTISTRY

**National Institute of**
**Dental Research**
**9000 Rockville Pike**
**Bethesda, MD 20892**
**301-496-4261**

Part of the National Institutes of Health, this institute offers general information to the public on dentistry and periodontal care.

## DIABETES

**American Association of**
**Diabetes Educators**
**444 N. Michigan Ave. Ste. 1240**
**Chicago, IL 60611**
**800-338-3633**

This is a professional association for diabetes educators—health workers trained and certified to teach diabetics how to manage the disease. The Association provides referrals to local diabetes educators.

**American Diabetes Association**
**1660 Duke St.**
**Alexandria, VA 22314**
**800-232-3472**

The Association provides information on diabetes, from medical treatment to financial concerns and can direct you to state chapters for referrals to local doctors and support groups.

**National Diabetes Information Clearinghouse**
**1 Information Way**
**Bethesda, MD 20892**
**301-654-3327**
Sponsored by the National Institute of Diabetes and Digestive and Kidney Diseases, the Clearinghouse sends out information on all aspects of diabetes.

## DIGESTIVE DISEASES

**National Digestive Diseases Information Clearinghouse**
**2 Information Way**
**Bethesda, MD 20892**
**301-654-3810**
**800-891-5389**
This information service of the National Institute of Diabetes and Digestive and Kidney Diseases sends out brochures, scientific articles and other data on digestive diseases, from indigestion and gas to ulcers and gallstones.

## DRIVING

**AAA Foundation for Traffic Safety**
**1440 New York Ave., NW**
**Suite 201**
**Washington, DC 20005**
**800-305-7233**
**202-638-5944**
The Foundation has information, pamphlets and videos on driving and safety. One of the items aimed at older drivers is a booklet containing a self-exam to test driving knowledge and skills, and information about a flexibility training program.

**National Safety Council**
**1121 Spring Lake Dr.**
**Itasca, IL 60143**
**800-621-6244**
The Council offers a course for elderly drivers called "Coaching the Mature Driver." Call to find out where it is offered locally.

## EXERCISE

**American Alliance for Health, Physical Education, Recreation and Dance**
**P.O. Box 385**
**Oxon Hill, MD 20750**
**800-321-0789**
The Alliance publishes books on exercise and other physical activity, including books for the elderly and the disabled. There is a charge.

**American Physical Therapy Association**
**1111 North Fairfax St.**
**Alexandria, VA 22314**
**703-684-2782**
A professional association, the APTA has a pamphlet on exercise tips for the elderly. It also makes referrals to state chapters, which have names of local physical therapists. (It is best, however, to get such referrals from a personal physician.)

**Arthritis Foundation**
**P.O. Box 19000**
**Atlanta, GA 30326**
**800-283-7800**
The Foundation has information on exercise and rehabilitation and makes referrals to local chapters, which often offer exercise classes.

**President's Council on Physical Fitness and Sports**
**701 Pennsylvania Ave., NW**
**Room 250**

Washington, DC 20034
202-272-3421

The Council provides information on physical fitness and exercise programs, and also publishes the "Nolan Ryan Fitness Guide" for people over 40. For a copy, write to Nolan Ryan Fitness Guide, P.O. Box 22091, Albany, NY 12201-2091.

## FINANCES

**American Institute of Certified Public Accountants**
**1211 Avenue of the Americas**
**New York, NY 10036**
**212-596-6200**
**800-862-4272**

A professional organization, the Institute has brochures on hiring a CPA, financial planning, estate planning and other related subjects. It also provides referrals from its member list.

**American Society of CLU & CFC (Chartered Life Underwriters and Chartered Financial Consultants)**
**270 South Bryn Mawr Ave.**
**Bryn Mawr, PA 19010**
**800-392-6900**

The Society provides names of members—insurance or financial advisors—in your area. It also has a list of questions to ask when selecting a financial advisor.

**Certified Financial Planner Board of Standards**
**1660 Lincoln St., Suite 3050**
**Denver, CO 80264**
**303-830-7543**

This regulatory board oversees the licensing of certified financial planners and allows you to check on a CFP's current standing or file a complaint.

**Institute of Certified Financial Planners**
**7600 East Eastman Ave., Suite 301**
**Denver, CO 80231**
**800-282-PLAN (7526)**

The Institute, primarily a trade association, offers brochures and books for the general public on selecting a financial planner, retirement planning, financial security in old age and more. It also gives referrals from its list of members.

**International Association for Financial Planning**
**Two Concourse Parkway, Suite 800**
**Atlanta, GA 30328**
**800-945-4237**
**404-395-1605**

This trade association has material on hiring a planner and referrals to local financial planners.

**Internal Revenue Service**

For tax questions or to file a complaint against a tax preparer, call the local IRS office. You can also call the IRS at 800-829-1040 for tax information or 800-829-3676 to order publications and tax forms.

**National Association of Personal Financial Advisors**
**1130 Lake Cook Rd., Suite 105**
**Buffalo Grove, IL 60089**
**800-366-2732**

NAPFA provides referrals to local financial advisors, who charge a fee for drawing up a plan.

**National Association of Securities Dealers**
**9513 Key West Ave.**
**Rockville, MD 20850**
**800-289-9999**

The Association can inform you of any complaints filed against a brokerage firm or individual broker.

**National Center for Home
Equity Conversion
7373 147th St., Suite 115
Apple Valley, MN 55124**

To request an up-to-date list of regional programs that offer reverse mortgages, send a stamped, self-addressed envelope and one dollar. You can also order a detailed consumer guide by calling 800-247-6553 or by sending a check for $24.95 along with your request.

**National Foundation for
Consumer Credit
8611 Second Ave., Suite 100
Silver Spring, MD 20910
800-388-2227**

The Foundation makes referrals to local Consumer Credit Counseling Service offices, which provide free or low-cost counseling on budgeting and debt management.

**Pension Rights Center
918 16th St., NW, Suite 704
Washington, DC 20006
202-296-3776**

The Center provides consumers with information and legal guidance.

**Securities Exchange Commission
450 Fifth St., NW
Washington, DC 20549
202-942-8088**

Anyone giving advice on stocks must be registered with the SEC. Many financial planners register voluntarily. For background information on a planner or advisor, write to the SEC's Public Reference Department (include the advisor's name, address, and company). For information about complaints filed against an advisor, write to the SEC's Freedom of Information Act officer.

**Social Security Administration
800-772-1213**

Call to arrange for direct deposit of social security checks, to notify the agency of a change of address, to check benefits or for general information on social security.

## FOOT CARE

**American Podiatric
Medical Association
9312 Old Georgetown Rd.
Bethesda, MD 20814
800-366-8227**

For pamphlets on foot care and disease, and listings of state associations (some of these provide referrals).

## GENERAL

**American Association of
Retired Persons
601 E St., NW
Washington, DC 20049
202-434-2277
800-424-3410**

AARP is one of the largest and most powerful lobbying and educational organizations in the country. It has free booklets on a wide range of topics such as housing options, home care, caregiver stress, and financial plights. There are money-saving programs for members, such as a travel service and a mail-order pharmacy, and volunteer programs and services. Call to find out about local chapters, membership benefits and publications.

**Consumer Information Center
"Catalogue"
Pueblo, CO 81009
719-948-3334**

This federal agency distributes more than 200 consumer publications from various departments and agencies of the government. Many of the brochures relate to health, nutrition, insurance and aging. To request a catalogue of publications, write to the above address. (Most of the materials are free; some cost less than a dollar.)

**National Association of Area Agencies on Aging (NAAAA)**
**1112 16th St., NW, Suite 100**
**Washington, DC 20036**
This private, nonprofit organization runs an Eldercare Locator (800-677-1116), which directs people to local agencies on aging.

**National Council on the Aging**
**409 Third St., SW**
**Washington, DC 20024**
**202-479-1200**
This private, nonprofit organization initiates programs, trains professionals and advocates on behalf of the elderly. The NCOA has specialized membership units for professionals and volunteers, including the National Institute of Senior Centers, the National Institute of Senior Housing and the National Institute on Financial Issues and Services for Elders. While largely administrative, the NCOA makes referrals to local services and has information and brochures on caregiving and related topics (living arrangements, adult day care, respite care, support groups, social services, legal and financial support, nutrition and health).

**National Council of Senior Citizens**
**1331 F St., NW**
**Washington, DC 20004**
**202-347-8800**
The Council is a membership organization—a much smaller version of AARP—that advocates for the elderly in Washington D.C. and

offers members benefits such as group insurance, low-priced prescription drugs and travel services.

## HEALTH AND MEDICINE

**National Health Information Center**
**P.O. Box 1133**
**Washington, DC 20013**
**800-336-4797**
The Center, sponsored by the Department of Health and Human Services, is a referral service that links people with questions about illness, health or health insurance to the appropriate organizations.

**National Institute on Aging Information Center**
**P.O. Box 8057**
**Gaithersburg, MD 20898**
**800-222-2225**
The NIA, a division of the National Institutes of Health, supports research on aging and health. It produces several free publications, including dozens of "Age Pages" with information on geriatric health issues.

**National Organization for Rare Disorders**
**P.O. Box 8923**
**New Fairfield, CT 06812**
**800-999-6673**
This nonprofit clearinghouse makes referrals to national organizations for rare disorders and provides information about them. The first request is free, but there is a minimal charge for subsequent requests.

**People's Medical Society**
**14 East Minor Street**
**Emmaus, PA 18049**
**610-770-1670**
The Society protects the rights of patients and their families by

monitoring the practices of doctors, nurses, hospital administrators and others in the medical field. Call for information on patients' rights and how to file a complaint.

**United Seniors Health Cooperative**
**1331 H St., NW, Suite 500**
**Washington, DC 20005**
**202-393-6222**
This private, nonprofit organization helps elderly people lead healthy and independent lives. The group puts out a newsletter five times a year and offers a number of publications on insurance and health-related topics.

## HEARING AND SPEECH

**American Academy of**
**Otolaryngology—**
**Head and Neck Surgery**
**1 Prince St.**
**Alexandria, VA 22314**
**703-836-4444**
The Academy, a professional association for otolaryngologists, makes referrals to local doctors and provides general information about head and neck surgery.

**American Hearing**
**Research Foundation**
**55 East Washington St.**
**Chicago, IL 60602**
**312-726-9670**
The Foundation provides information on specific hearing disorders and makes referrals to local otolaryngologists.

**American Speech-Language-**
**Hearing Association**
**10801 Rockville Pike**
**Rockville, MD 20852**
**301-897-8682 (in Maryland)**
**800-638-8255**
A membership organization for audiologists and speech pathologists, the Association provides general information on speech and language disorders, and makes referrals to audiologists and speech pathologists.

**American Tinnitus Association**
**P.O. Box 5**
**Portland, OR 97207**
**503-248-9985**
The Association makes referrals to local support groups, and publishes brochures and a newsletter on tinnitus.

**AT&T Accessible Communication**
**Products Center**
**5 Wood Hollow Rd., Room 1119**
**Parsippany, NJ 07054**
**800-233-1222**
The Center produces a catalogue of equipment for people with impaired hearing and/or speech. (You don't have to be an AT&T customer to order products.)

**Better Hearing Institute**
**Hearing Helpline**
**P.O. Box 1840**
**Washington, DC 20013**
**800-327-9355**
This nonprofit organization publishes educational brochures and pamphlets on various aspects of hearing loss.

**Hearing Aid Helpline**
**20361 Middlebelt Rd.**
**Livonia, MI 48152**
**800-521-5247**
The helpline is run by the International Hearing Society, a professional association for "hearing instrument specialists" (people who fit hearing aids). The Society sends out information on hearing aids and provides referrals to local specialists who are members of the society.

**HEAR NOW**
**9745 East Hampden Ave., Suite 300**
**Denver, CO 80231**
**800-648-4327**
This private, nonprofit group supplies hearing aids and cochlear implants, without charge, to low-income people.

**Modern Talking Picture Service**
**Caption Films/Videos**
**5000 Park St. North**
**St. Petersburg, FL 33709**
**800-237-6213**
The U.S. Department of Education sponsors this program, which loans videos with captioning free of charge to people who have hearing loss.

**National Aphasia Association**
**P.O. Box 1887**
**New York, NY 10156**
**800-922-4622**
The Association promotes public awareness of aphasia, a disorder which interferes with a person's ability to use or comprehend words; and makes referrals to local support groups and representatives who can link you to local services.

**National Association of the Deaf**
**814 Thayer Ave.**
**Silver Spring, MD 20910**
**301-587-1788**
**301-587-1789 (TDD)**
The NAD is a membership organization that advocates for deaf and hard-of-hearing people and their families through its scholarships, teacher certification, youth and volunteer programs, legal services and other projects.

**National Information Center**
**on Deafness**
**Gallaudet University**

**800 Florida Ave., NE**
**Washington, DC 20002**
**202-651-5051**
Gallaudet University has information on every aspect of deafness. Its information services can refer callers to the school's National Center for Law and Deafness, which offers legal information and free legal services to low-income people facing discrimination or civil rights challenges. Callers may also be connected to the Research Institute for statistical information, or to the University Press for catalogues and publications.

**National Institute on Deafness and**
**Other Communication Disorders**
**Information Clearinghouse**
**1 Communication Ave.**
**Bethesda, MD 20892**
**800-241-1044**
Part of the National Institutes of Health, this clearinghouse provides information on disorders related to hearing, balance, smell, taste, speech and language.

**Self-Help for**
**Hard-of-Hearing People**
**7910 Woodmont Ave., Suite 1200**
**Bethesda, MD 20814**
**301-657-2248**
**301-657-2249 (TDD)**
The group distributes information on hearing loss, including tips on coping and help for family members. Its bimonthly journal keeps people abreast of news from regional chapters and support groups.

## HEART DISEASE

**American Heart Association**
**7272 Greenville Ave.**
**Dallas, TX 75231**
**800-242-1793**
The Association provides refer-

rals to local CPR courses and offers information on blood pressure, cholesterol, stroke, heart disease, diet, nutrition, exercise and other topics.

**National Heart, Lung, and Blood Institute Information Center**
**P.O. Box 30105**
**Bethesda, MD 20824**
**301-251-1222**
Part of the National Institutes of Health, this center provides information on ailments of the heart, lungs and blood.

## HISPANIC SERVICES

**National Association for Hispanic Elderly**
**3325 Wilshire Blvd.**
**Los Angeles, CA 90010**
**213-487-1922**
The Association advocates for the Hispanic elderly, especially those on low incomes. It has brochures and other information in Spanish and may be able to give referrals.

## HOME CARE

**National Association for Home Care**
**519 C St., NE**
**Washington, DC 20002**
**202-547-7424**
This professional organization represents a wide range of home-care organizations. On request, it will send out a pamphlet of tips on choosing a home-care agency.

**Visiting Nurse Associations of America**
**3801 East Florida Ave., Suite 900**
**Denver, CO 80210**
**800-426-2547**
The VNAA represents nearly 500 visiting nurse associations across

the country which offer skilled nursing care, therapy, hospice care, counseling, home health aides and homemakers, nutrition counseling, and chore services.

## HOSPICE

**Foundation for Hospice and Home Care**
**320 A St., NE**
**Washington, DC 20002**
**202-547-6586**
The Foundation works to improve public policy on health care, particularly for the elderly. It also certifies home-health care aides. Call for information on home care and hospice, how to choose a home-care and/or hospice agency, and for referrals to local organizations that offer home-care and hospice services.

**Hospice Association of America**
**519 C St., NE**
**Washington, DC 20002**
**202-546-4759**
Part of the National Association of Home Care, this trade association makes referrals to local hospices and has information—brochures, videos, books—on hospice care.

**Hospice Helpline**
**National Hospice Organization**
**1901 N. Moore St., Suite 901**
**Arlington, VA 22209**
**800-658-8898**
The National Hospice Organization represents hospices across the country. Through its Helpline, it provides information about hospice care and makes referrals to local hospices.

## HOUSING

**American Association of Homes
and Services for the Aging
901 E St., NW, Suite 500
Washington, DC 20004
202-783-2242**

The Association has consumer brochures on various housing options, nursing homes and community services. It also publishes the *Consumers' Directory of Continuing Care Retirement Communities* (available for $24.95, or through many public libraries), which lists and describes more than 550 retirement communities. The Association sponsors the Continuing Care Accreditation Commission (202-508-9413), which has a list of approved continuing care retirement communities that meet certain standards with regard to finances, medical care, resident life and management.

**Assisted Living Facilities
Association of America
9411 Lee Highway
Plaza Suite J
Fairfax, VA 22031
703-691-8100**

This professional association puts out a couple of helpful brochures—one defines assisted living and another discusses what to look for when choosing an assisted-living home.

**National Shared Housing
Resource Center
321 East 25th St.
Baltimore, MD 21218
410-235-4454**

The Center provides information about shared housing and makes referrals to local organizations that help bring together roommates.

## HUNTINGTON'S DISEASE

**Huntington's Disease Society
of America (HDSA)
140 West 22nd St., 6th Floor
New York, NY 10011
212-242-1968
800-345-4372**

This society publishes information about all aspects of Huntington's disease, and offers medical referrals (to genetic counseling clinics, nursing homes, neurologists, etc.) and to local chapters that can link individuals to local support groups and services.

## INCONTINENCE AND URINARY TRACT DISORDERS

**American Foundation for
Urologic Disease
300 West Pratt St., Suite 401
Baltimore, MD 21201
800-242-2383**

The Foundation educates patients by providing information on urinary tract infections, incontinence, diseases and disorders of the prostate and bladder and other urinary tract and rectal disorders.

**Help for Incontinent People (HIP)
P.O. Box 544
Union, SC 29379
800-252-3337**

This nonprofit organization has brochures, books, videos and audio-cassette tapes giving detailed information about incontinence. It also sends out a catalogue of special products that are available and a national listing of doctors who specialize in incontinence.

**International Foundation for
Bowel Dysfunction
P.O. Box 17864
Milwaukee, WI 53217
414-241-9479**

The Foundation has brochures, articles and other information on irritable bowel syndrome, constipation, diarrhea, fecal incontinence and other disorders of the bowels.

**National Kidney and Urologic Diseases Information Clearinghouse**
**3 Information Way**
**Bethesda, MD 20892**
**301-654-4415**
Sponsored by the National Institute of Diabetes and Digestive and Kidney Diseases, the Clearinghouse provides up-to-date information on incontinence, as well as other disorders and diseases of the kidneys, prostate and urinary tract.

**Simon Foundation for Continence**
**P.O. Box 815**
**Wilmette, IL 60091**
**800-237-4666**
A consumer education organization, the Foundation puts out books, videos, tapes, newsletters and reprints of articles on urinary incontinence.

## INSURANCE

**Center for Medicare Advocacy**
**P.O. Box 350**
**Willimantic, CT 06226**
**203-456-7790**
**800-262-4414**
This center offers free legal help to Connecticut residents struggling with the Medicare bureaucracy. It also provides general advice to people from other states and makes referrals to similar organizations in other states.

**Medicare Hotline**
**800-638-6833**
**800-492-6603 in Maryland**
The Hotline answers questions about Medicare, Medigap and state insurance departments. It also reports on Medicare fraud and other illegal practices.

**National Association of Claims Assistance Professionals**
**5329 South Main St.**
**Downers Grove, IL 60515**
**800-660-0665**
This organization represents medical claims agents—people hired to file health insurance claims forms and appeals. While set up to help professionals, the Association also provides a brochure for consumers describing the field and makes referrals (only to agents who can provide three letters of recommendation).

**National Consumers League**
**1701 K St., NW**
**Washington, DC 20006**
**202-835-3323**
This nonprofit organization educates the public about a variety of issues, from food and drug safety to financial services. The League has brochures on Medicare, Medicaid and other insurance issues.

**National Insurance Consumer Helpline**
**1025 Connecticut Ave., NW**
**Suite 1200**
**Washington, DC 20036**
**800-942-4242**
This industry-sponsored hotline answers questions concerning home and life insurance, as well as government insurance programs.

**United Seniors Health Cooperative**
**1331 H St., NW, Suite 500**
**Washington, DC 20005**
**202-393-6222**
This private, nonprofit organization teaches elderly people how to lead healthy and independent lives. The group has a number of publica-

tions on insurance and health and publishes a newsletter.

## LEGAL ADVICE

**American Bar Association**
**750 North Lake Shore Drive**
**Chicago, IL 60611**
**312-988-5000**
**800-964-4253**

The ABA primarily serves lawyers, but it has some brochures for the public. It makes referrals to local bar associations which have more specific information and often make referrals.

**Commission on Legal Problems**
**of the Elderly**
**American Bar Association**
**1800 M St., NW, South Lobby**
**Washington, DC 20036**
**202-662-8690**

A resource for lawyers, this ABA commission has technical books and brochures available to the public and makes referrals to local agencies and legal aid societies.

**Legal Counsel for the Elderly**
**American Association of**
**Retired Persons**
**601 E St., NW**
**Washington, DC 20049**
**800-424-3410**

This organization, with hotlines in Arizona, Florida, Maine, Michigan, New Mexico, Northern California, Ohio, Pennsylvania and Texas, offers free legal advice on general matters, and referrals to low-cost legal help on more specific issues. For the local hotline number, call AARP's central office.

**National Academy of Elder**
**Law Attorneys**
**1604 North Country Club Road**
**Tucson, AZ 85716**
**602-881-4005**

For a fee, this organization will send you a list of its members.

## LIVING WITH DISABILITIES

**Access Foundation**
**1109 Linden St.**
**Valley Stream, NY 11580**
**516-568-2715**

This information clearinghouse, on the Internet, helps elderly, disabled, and handicapped people and their families to find local services, equipment, referrals and answers. The fee is about $5 per search; a $45 membership fee per year covers unlimited searches.

**Adaptive Environments Center**
**374 Congress St., Suite 301**
**Boston, MA 02210**
**617-695-1225**

The Center is a private, nonprofit organization that trains professionals in making buildings accessible to people with disabilities. Its booklet, "A Consumer's Guide to Home Adaptation," describes possible modifications to each area of a home and has information on buying special equipment (cost, $12).

**American Association of**
**Retired Persons**
**601 E St., NW**
**Washington, DC 20049**
**800-424-3410**

AARP puts out a free booklet called "The Do-Able, Renewable Home," that describes how to make a home more accessible for people with disabilities. A second booklet, "A Perfect Fit," offers technical design information for contractors.

**"Center for Universal Design"**
**North Carolina State University**
**P.O. Box 8613**
**Raleigh, NC 27695**
**800-647-6777**
The Center, which conducts research into accessible housing, makes available brochures and other publications on accessible housing and home modification.

**National Rehabilitation**
**Information Center**
**and ABLEDATA**
**8455 Colesville Rd., Suite 935**
**Silver Spring, MD 20910**
**800-346-2742**
**800-227-0216**
**(Internet address:**
**naric@capaccess.org)**
These federally-funded resources share a database of information on disabilities and rehabilitation, including ways to make a home more accessible, and lists of equipment and products. They can also make referrals to rehabilitation centers and organizations serving the disabled. The cost of a search depends upon the amount of information needed.

**Paralyzed Veterans of America**
**801 18th St. NW**
**Washington, DC 20006**
**800-424-8200**
This private, nonprofit advocacy group provides information on getting benefits, living with a disability, modifying a home and other topics. It also makes referrals to local services.

## LUNG DISEASE

**American Lung Association**
**G.P.O. Box 596**
**New York, NY 10016**
**800-586-4872 (LUNG USA)**
The Association will refer you to a local office that can offer information about lung diseases such as asthma, emphysema, tuberculosis and cancer. It makes referrals for medical care, support groups, smoking cessation programs and other local services.

**National Heart, Lung, and**
**Blood Institute**
**Information Center**
**P.O. Box 30105**
**Bethesda, MD 20824**
**301-251-1222**
As part of the National Institutes of Health, this center provides information about ailments of the heart, lungs and blood.

## MENTAL HEALTH AND SUPPORT GROUPS

**American Association for Marriage**
**and Family Therapy**
**1100 17th St., NW, 10th Floor**
**Washington, DC 20036**
**800-374-2638**
AAMFT makes referrals to local therapists who specialize in problems facing families of the elderly.

**American Psychiatric Association**
**1400 K St., NW**
**Washington, DC 20005**
**202-682-6220**
The Association has a catalogue of brochures and publications available to the public.

**American Psychological Association**
**750 First St., NE**
**Washington, DC. 20002**
**800-374-2721**
This organization provides information and makes referrals to state associations, for help in finding local clinical psychologists.

**American Self-Help Clearinghouse**
**25 Pocono Rd.**
**St. Clares-Riverside Medical Center**
**Denville, NJ 07834**
**201-625-7101**
The Clearinghouse provides referrals to self-help groups (or support groups) in New Jersey and can link you to similar organizations in more than a dozen other states.

**National Alliance for the**
**Mentally Ill**
**2102 Wilson Blvd., Suite 302**
**Arlington, VA 22201**
**800-950-6264**
NAMI provides information on mental illness, and gives individuals and families referrals to local support groups and services.

**National Association of**
**Social Workers**
**750 First St., NE**
**Washington, DC 20002**
**202-408-8600**
The Association makes referrals to local care managers, therapists and social workers in other specialties.

**National Foundation for**
**Depressive Illness**
**P.O. Box 2257**
**New York, NY 10116**
**800-248-4381**
This foundation makes referrals to local doctors who specialize in treating depression, and makes available a number of publications on depression.

**National Institute of Mental Health**
**Public Inquires Office**
**Room 7C-O2**
**5600 Fishers Lane**
**Rockville, MD 20857**
**301-443-4513**
**FAX: 301-443-4513**
NIMH is a research institute which has a list of publications for the general public. Its Depression Awareness, Recognition and Treatment (DART) program (800-421-4211) provides information on depression and makes referrals to local organizations.

**National Mental Health Association**
**1021 Prince St.**
**Alexandria, VA 22314**
**800-969-6642**
The Association provides information on mental health issues and makes referrals to local organizations.

**National Self-Help Clearinghouse**
**25 West 43rd St., Room 620**
**New York, NY 10036**
**212-354-8525**
The Clearinghouse directs people to national or regional organizations that can connect you to a local support group. If no local groups exist, the National Clearinghouse can help you start a group.

## NATIVE AMERICAN SERVICES

**National Association of Area**
**Agencies on Aging**
**1112 16th St., NW, Suite 100**
**Washington, DC 20036**
The Association serves area agencies on aging and represents 190 Native American organizations that serve elderly members of federally recognized tribes. To contact a local Native American organization, call

the NAAAA's Eldercare Locator at 800-677-1116.

## NURSING HOMES

**National Citizens' Coalition for Nursing Home Reform**
**1424 16th St., NW, Suite 202**
**Washington, DC 20036**
**202-332-2275**

This coalition of advocacy organizations, ombudsman programs and individuals works to improve nursing home care. It offers guidance in selecting a nursing home and in filing complaints. It can also explain laws regulating nursing homes and provides referrals to local ombudsman programs.

**Nursing Home Information Service**
**National Council of Senior Citizens**
**1331 F St., NW**
**Washington, DC 20004**
**202-347-8800 ext. 340/341**

The Council is a nonprofit membership organization that has limited information about long-term care nursing homes, life-care communities, adult day-care centers and home health-care agencies.

## NUTRITION AND MEAL SERVICES

**National Association of Meal Programs**
**101 North Alfred St., Suite 202**
**Alexandria, VA 22314**
**703-548-5558**

A membership organization for providers, the Association will make referrals to local community dining and meals-on-wheels programs.

**National Meals on Wheels Foundation**
**2675 44th St., SW, Suite 305**

**Grand Rapids, MI 49509**
**800-999-6262**

The Foundation receives private donations and makes grants to meal programs. Through its toll-free number it makes referrals to local meal-delivery programs and congregate or group dining programs.

**Nutrition Hotline**
**American Dietetic Association**
**216 West Jackson Blvd., Suite 800**
**Chicago, IL 60606**
**800-366-1655**

Call the Hotline for up-to-date information on nutrition, to speak with a registered dietitian or for a referral to a local dietitian.

## OCCUPATIONAL THERAPY

**American Occupational Therapy Association**
**P.O. Box 31220**
**4720 Montgomery Dr.**
**Bethesda, MD 20824**
**301-652-2682**

This professional association has consumer brochures on topics such as making a home safe, recovery, Alzheimer's disease and living with disabilities. Call or write for a catalogue of publications.

## PARKINSON'S DISEASE

**American Parkinson's Disease Association**
**60 Bay St., Room 401**
**Staten Island, NY 10301**
**800-223-2732**

The Association sends out general information on Parkinson's disease and links people to local APDA centers.

National Institute of Neurological
Disorders and Stroke
Information Office
Building 31, Room 8A06
31 Center Dr., MSC2540
Bethesda, MD 20892
800-352-9424
Part of the National Institutes of
Health, this office provides information about stroke and other brain
disorders, such as Parkinson's,
Alzheimer's and epilepsy. It reports
on the latest scientific research and
makes referrals to local clinical research centers.

National Parkinson's Foundation
1501 N.W. 9th Ave.
Miami, FL 33136
800-327-4545
This foundation reports on all
aspects of Parkinson's disease and
makes referrals to local services and
medical experts specializing in the
disease.

Parkinson's Disease Foundation
710 West 168th St.
New York, NY 10032
212-923-4700 in New York
800-457-6676
This organization sponsors
research and professional education,
educates the public about Parkinson's disease, and makes referrals to
specialists.

## SKIN

American Academy of Dermatology
P.O. Box 681069
Schaumburg, IL 60168
708-330-0230
The Academy sends out infor-
mation on specific skin diseases.
Requests must be accompanied by a
stamped, self-addressed envelope.
(No phone calls please.)

National Arthritis and
Musculoskeletal and Skin Diseases
Information Clearinghouse
1 AMS Circle
Bethesda, MD 20892
301-495-4484
This federal clearinghouse provides publications on many disorders
and diseases affecting the skin.

## SLEEP

National Sleep Foundation
1367 Connecticut Ave., NW
Suite 200
Washington, DC 20036
This foundation sends brochures
on sleep disorders and makes referrals to local sleep clinics. (They ask
that you write, rather than call, for
information.)

## STROKE

American Heart Association
7272 Greenville Ave.
Dallas, TX 75231
800-242-1793
Call for referrals to local chapters which have information on
stroke and support groups.

American Physical Therapy
Association
111 North Fairfax St.
Alexandria, VA 22314
703-684-2782
APTA has a bibliography on
stroke and makes referrals to rehabilitation centers.

American Speech-Language-
Hearing Association
10801 Rockville Pike
Rockville, MD 20852
301-897-8682
800-638-8255
The Association has information

and makes referrals to pathologists and organizations.

**Family Caregiver Alliance**
**425 Bush St., Suite 500**
**San Francisco, CA 94108**
**415-434-3388**
The project is part of a California information clearinghouse for people caring for someone with stroke or other cognitive impairment. It offers some guidance and referrals to those outside the state.

**National Aphasia Association**
**P.O. Box 1887**
**Murray Hill Station**
**New York, NY 10156**
**800-922-4622**
The Association has information on aphasia and makes referrals.

**National Institute of Neurological Disorders and Stroke**
**Information Office**
**Building 31, Room 8A16**
**31 Center Dr., MSC2540**
**Bethesda, MD 20892**
**800-352-9424**
The Institute provides information on stroke and other brain disorders, such as Parkinson's, Alzheimer's, and epilepsy and makes referrals to local clinical research centers.

**National Stroke Association**
**8480 East Orchard Rd., Suite 1000**
**Englewood, CO 80111**
**800-787-6537**
The Association offers information on stroke and makes referrals to medical experts, support groups, rehabilitation centers and other services.

## VETERANS

**Department of Veterans Affairs**
**810 Vermont Ave., NW**
**Washington, DC 20420**
**800-827-1000**
Veterans can call this office for general information about benefits and eligibility and for referrals to regional offices and VA medical centers.

## VISION

**American Council of the Blind**
**1155 15th St., NW, Suite 720**
**Washington, DC 20005**
**800-424-8666**
This council advocates for the blind and makes referrals to state affiliates and other organizations that provide information, services and equipment to the blind.

**American Foundation for the Blind**
**11 Penn Plaza**
**New York, NY 10001**
**800-232-5463**
The Foundation provides referrals to rehabilitation centers, state agencies, low-vision clinics and other services, and has information on the emotional and practical aspects of coping with vision impairment and loss.

**Association of Late-Deafened Adults**
**P.O. Box 930075**
**Rochester, NY 14692-7375**
**708-445-0860 (TDD or fax only)**
This membership organization publishes a newsletter and sponsors an annual convention.

**Association for Macular Diseases**
**210 East 64th St.**
**New York, NY 10021**
**212-605-3719**

The association is run by volunteers who provide emotional support, information and referrals.

**Better Vision Institute**
**1800 North Kent St., Suite 904**
**Rosslyn, VA 22209**
**800-424-8422**
This nonprofit group works to increase public awareness about vision care. It has some information on eye disease and aging.

**Blinded Veterans Association**
**477 H St., NW**
**Washington, DC 20001**
**202-371-8880**
The Association helps veterans get VA benefits, rehabilitation and other services.

**Glaucoma Research Foundation**
**490 Post St., Suite 830**
**San Francisco, CA 94102**
**415-986-3162**
**800-826-6693**
The Foundation runs a self-help hotline called the Glaucoma Support Network, that hooks patients and family members up with others who have faced a similar situation and can offer support. It puts out a free guide, "Understanding and Living with Glaucoma," and a newsletter and provides referrals to local glaucoma specialists.

**The Lighthouse National Center**
**for Vision and Aging**
**111 East 59th St.**
**New York, NY 10022**
**212-821-9200**
**800-334-5497**
Contact the Lighthouse for information on every aspect of vision loss and eye disease, as well as for referrals to state agencies, local services, support group and low-vision centers.

**National Association for the**
**Visually Handicapped**
**22 West 21st St.**
**New York, NY 10010**
**212-889-3141**
This association provides information on vision, eye diseases, low-vision aids and the emotional aspects of vision loss. It offers referrals to low-vision specialists and clinics, and it has a lending library of large-print books and a catalogue of visual aids that can be ordered by mail.

**National Eye Care Project**
**American Academy of**
**Ophthalmology**
**P.O. Box 7424**
**San Francisco, CA 94120**
**800-222-3937**
The Project provides information on eye diseases and makes referrals to ophthalmologists who offer low-cost eye care to people over 65.

**National Eye Institute**
**Information Office**
**31 Center Dr., MSC2510**
**Building 31, Rm. 6A32**
**Bethesda, MD 20892**
**301-496-5248**
The Institute, which supports research projects, has fact sheets on eye disease and information on the latest research and treatments.

**National Federation of the Blind**
**1800 Johnson St.**
**Baltimore, MD 21230**
**410-659-9314**
The Federation runs a number of programs for the blind, provides information on blindness (including medical, social, emotional, legal and financial issues) and makes referrals to services and support groups.

**National Library Service for the
Blind and Physically Handicapped
Library of Congress
1291 Taylor St., NW
Washington, D.C. 20542
800-424-8567**
The Library lends out books on tape, on disk, and in Braille (as well as equipment for playing tapes and disks). All of this is free.

**Prevent Blindness America
500 East Remington Rd.
Schaumburg, IL 60173
800-331-2020**
Through its toll-free line, known as the National Center for Sight, the organization provides information on eye diseases and referrals to local support groups.

## VOLUNTEERING, WORKING AND LEARNING

**Elderhostel
P.O. Box 1959
Wakefield, MA 01880
617-426-7788**
Through Elderhostel, universities, colleges, museums, theaters, and national parks offer low-cost, short-term courses for people 60 and over.

**National Senior
Service Hotline
ACTION
1201 New York Ave.
Washington, DC 20525
800-424-8867**
ACTION runs federal volunteer programs, including the Foster Grandparent Program, the Senior Companion Program and the Retired Senior Volunteer Program.

## WOMEN'S SERVICES

**Older Women's League
666 11th St., NW, Suite 700
Washington, DC 20001
800-825-3695**
OWL is a grass-roots organization advocating for economic and social equity of midlife and older women. It offers fact sheets on issues such as pensions, women's health and caregiving, and provides some referrals. (It prefers that requests be made in writing, accompanied by a self-addressed, stamped envelope.)

# APPENDIX C

## *A Patient's Bill of Rights**

1. The patient has the right to considerate and respectful care.

2. The patient has the right to and is encouraged to obtain from physicians and other direct caregivers relevant, current, and understandable information concerning diagnosis, treatment, and prognosis.

Except in emergencies when the patient lacks decision-making capacity and the need for treatment is urgent, the patient is entitled to the opportunity to discuss and request information related to the specific procedures and/or treatments, the risks involved, the possible length of recuperation, and the medically reasonable alternatives and their accompanying risks and benefits.

Patients have the right to know the identity of physicians, nurses, and others involved in their care, as well as when those involved are students, residents, or other trainees. The patient also has the right to know the immediate and long-term financial implications of treatment choices, insofar as they are known.

3. The patient has the right to make decisions about the plan of care prior to and during the course of treatment and to refuse a recommended treatment or plan of care to the extent permitted by law and hospital policy and to be informed of the medical consequences of this action. In case of such refusal, the patient is entitled to other appropriate care and services that the hospital provides or transfer to another hospital. The hospital should notify patients of any policy that might affect patient choice within the institution.

4. The patient has the right to have an advance directive (such as a living will, health care proxy, or durable power of attorney

---

*These rights can be exercised on the patient's behalf by a designated surrogate or proxy decision maker if the patient lacks decision-making capacity, is legally incompetent, or is a minor.*

for health care) concerning treatment or designating a surrogate decision maker with the expectation that the hospital will honor the intent of that directive to the extent permitted by law and hospital policy.

Health care institutions must advise patients of their rights under state law and hospital policy to make informed medical choices, ask if the patient has an advance directive, and include that information in patient records. The patient has the right to timely information about hospital policy that may limit its ability to implement fully a legally valid advance directive.

5.  The patient has the right to every consideration of privacy. Case discussion, consultation, examination, and treatment should be conducted so as to protect each patient's privacy.

6.  The patient has the right to expect that all communications and records pertaining to his/her care will be treated as confidential by the hospital, except in cases such as suspected abuse and public health hazards when reporting is permitted or required by law. The patient has the right to expect that the hospital will emphasize the confidentiality of this information when it releases it to any other parties entitled to review information in these records.

7.  The patient has the right to review the records pertaining to his/her medical care and to have the information explained or interpreted as necessary, except when restricted by law.

8.  The patient has the right to expect that, within its capacity and policies, a hospital will make reasonable response to the request of a patient for appropriate and medically indicated care and services. The hospital must provide evaluation, service, and/or referral as indicated by the urgency of the case. When medically appropriate and legally permissible, or when a patient has so requested, a patient may be transferred to another facility. The institution to which the patient is to be transferred must first have accepted the patient for transfer. The patient must also have the benefit of complete information and explanation concerning the need for, risks, benefits, and alternatives to such a transfer.

9.  The patient has the right to ask and be informed of the existence of business relationships among the hospital, educational

institutions, other health care providers, or payers that may influ-
ence the patient's treatment and care.

10. The patient has the right to consent to or decline to participate in proposed research studies or human experimentation
affecting care and treatment or requiring direct patient involvement, and to have those studies fully explained prior to consent. A
patient who declines to participate in research or experimentation
is entitled to the most effective care that the hospital can otherwise provide.

11. The patient has the right to expect reasonable continuity of
care when appropriate and to be informed by physicians and other
caregivers of available and realistic patient care options when hospital care is no longer appropriate.

12. The patient has the right to be informed of hospital policies
and practices that relate to patient care, treatment, and responsibilities. The patient has the right to be informed of available resources
for resolving disputes, grievances, and conflicts, such as ethics
committees, patient representatives, or other mechanisms available
in the institution. The patient has the right to be informed of the
hospital's charges for services and available payment methods.

# APPENDIX D
## The ABC's of Diet

As your parent ages, it is more important than ever that she maintain a healthful diet. Since age and a more sedentary lifestyle lead to a slower metabolism, older people typically burn about one-third fewer calories than younger people. And because they are less hungry, older people eat less food. (They eat less for a variety of other reasons as well, all discussed in Chapter Eight.) However, they still need as many vitamins, minerals and nutrients as they ever did. In fact, they may need them more than ever. They just have to get them from less food. So the bottom line is, every bite counts.

But what is a good diet? If you follow the daily news, you'll never be able to sort out what your parent or anyone else should be eating. Dietary recommendations and scientific findings change faster than a weather vane in a tornado.

If your parent ignores the latest findings and sticks with a few basic principles (and any special medical orders), she will be eating just fine. The general guidelines for an elderly person, stated most simply, are: low-fat, low-caffeine, low-alcohol, high-fiber, high-fluid, high-fruit and high-vegetable. Beyond that, the key words are *variation* and *moderation*. That is, don't let your parent fall into a rut even if it's a healthful rut. A good diet should include lots of different vegetables, fruits, rice, grains, nuts, etc. And it shouldn't go to extremes. An occasional doughnut is fine; a pound of broccoli a day is not necessary.

Here are the nuts and bolts, or nuts and grains, if you will, of a good diet:

## Vitamins

Vitamins help all the systems of the body run efficiently, but all bodies do not need vitamins equally. Recent studies of the elderly have found that they have different dietary needs than their younger counterparts, in part because of changes in weight, activity and the body's ability to absorb vitamins. While the research is still scant, scientists now know that older people are often lacking in a number of essential vitamins, particularly in folate and vitamins B-6, B-12, D and E.

Vitamins come in two types, fat-soluble and water-soluble. Fat-soluble ones (A,D, E and K) are stored in fat, where they can be retrieved for use at a later time, so

| Vitamin | Daily RDA* (for adults over 50) | Foods that Provide It |
|---------|------------------------------|----------------------|
| **Vitamin A/ Beta carotene** Foods that are rich in beta carotene, an antioxidant the body converts into vitamin A, are thought to lower the risk of cancer and heart disease. | 5 to 6 milligrams of beta carotene (800 to 1,000 retinol equivalents of vitamin A) | Liver, cheese, egg yolks, fortified milk, cantaloupe and apricots (Beta carotene is in carrots, squash, sweet potatoes, broccoli and other dark green vegetables.) |
| **Vitamin B-6** B-6 strengthens the immune system. | 1.6 to 2 milligrams | Whole-grain breads and cereals, beans, nuts, chicken, avocado, liver, legumes, potatoes, ba- nanas, spinach, fish |
| **Vitamin B-12** Older people often have atrophic gastritis, which hinders absorption of B-12 and can cause confusion. | 2 micrograms | Liver, kidney, beef, eggs, cheese, milk and shellfish (Older people who have trouble absorbing B-12 may have to take supple- ments of the vitamin.) |
| **Folate, or folic acid** A deficiency causes de- pression and fatigue, and may increase the risk of stroke, heart disease and some cancers. | 180 to 200 micrograms | Dried peas and beans, whole grains, liver, kid- neys, nuts, wheat germ and dark green, leafy vegetables |
| **Vitamin C** Vitamin C may lower the risk of heart disease and cancer, but too much can block absorption of B-12. | 60 milligrams | Citrus fruits, strawberries, tomatoes, cantaloupe, potatoes, broccoli, brussels sprouts, cabbage and other dark green vegeta- bles |
| **Vitamin D** Vitamin D helps the body to absorb calcium, which strengthen bones. | 400 to 800 I.U. (international units) | Fortified milk, egg yolks, liver and oily fish (such as salmon, sardines, herring and tuna). |
| **Vitamin E** Vitamin E may lower the risk of cataracts and help prevent heart disease. Deficiency can lead to anemia. | 8 to 10 I.U. | Vegetable oils, dark green, leafy vegetables, wheat germ and nuts |

*Recommended Dietary Allowances, from the National Academy of Sciences.

people don't need them daily; they can eat them on Monday and use them up on Wednesday. Water-soluble ones (C and the B vitamins) can't be stored in the body so should be consumed daily.

# Minerals

Of the 13 minerals that humans need, your parent should be most concerned about two: calcium, because it wards off osteoporosis, and sodium, which raises blood pressure and should be limited if your parent has high blood pressure (hypertension).

CALCIUM. If you are female and doing a little aging yourself, you might join your parent in some high-calcium meal planning. Calcium makes bones strong, which is particularly important for women, whose bones tend to atrophy after menopause. The recommended dose of calcium is 800 to 1,000 milligrams a day; however some experts recommend that women should take up to 1,500 milligrams a day after menopause, especially if they are not taking estrogen supplements. The fact is, most women get only about 400 milligrams of calcium a day. If getting enough calcium through diet is a problem, your parent should consider taking calcium supplements. (Be sure your mother also gets ample vitamin D, which enables the body to absorb calcium.)

The best source of calcium is low-fat or nonfat dairy products, but the mineral is also in dark green, leafy vegetables, such as broccoli, collards, mustard greens and kale; and in tofu, salmon and sardines (with the bones), oysters, dried beans and peas and citrus fruits. Some brands of orange juice and bread are now fortified with calcium.

| Food | Serving Size | Milligrams of Calcium |
|---|---|---|
| Plain yogurt | 1 cup | 400 |
| Sardines (with bones) | 3 ounces | 370 |
| Collards | 1 cup | 360 |
| Milk | 1 cup | 300 |
| Hard cheese | 1 ounce | 150-200 |
| Cottage cheese | 1 cup | 140 |
| Broccoli, raw | 1 cup | 130 |

SODIUM. Sodium helps to regulate the body's water level and keeps the heart in rhythm and the nerves conducting. It is present in almost all foods, but the major contributor is table salt. There are inordinate levels of sodium in most prepared meals and processed foods, deli cheese, cured meats, pickles and snack foods. Most Americans eat far more sodium than they need, which leads to high blood pressure, heart disease, stroke, kidney damage and fluid retention.

However, in some cases, a person can have too little sodium. For instance vomiting, diarrhea, heavy sweating and diuretic drugs all reduce the body's level of sodium. Because of these problems and because elderly bodies are less able to regulate the balance of sodium and water, ask your parent's doctor about his individual sodium needs or limits.

IRON. Too little iron shouldn't be a problem unless your parent has an ulcer, hemorrhoid or some other condition that causes bleeding, or is taking large doses of antacids, which hinder the body's absorption of iron. Your parent may also be at some risk of iron deficiency if she is what dietitians refer to as a tea-and-toaster—an elderly lady who sits around sipping tea and nibbling on toast. The bread may be fortified with iron, but ingredients in the tea combine with the iron to form another substance that is excreted by the body, and in the process iron is lost.

Too much iron can contribute to heart attacks in some cases, so your parent shouldn't take extra doses of iron except under her doctor's orders.

ZINC. People with diabetes or cirrhosis of the liver, or those who take diuretics can become zinc-deficient. This mineral is important for healing wounds, and it plays a role in appetite and taste. Zinc is found in fish and other seafood.

MAGNESIUM. Magnesium is

---

## A NOTE ABOUT VITAMIN AND MINERAL SUPPLEMENTS

The experts are still hemming, hawing and disagreeing about the virtues and dangers of dietary supplements. Certainly, the best way to get nutrients is through a healthful diet. A good diet (especially five servings of fruits and vegetables a day) provides lots of things that a body needs beyond vitamins and minerals.

However, most people fail miserably when it comes to eating well, and the elderly often have health problems that make it impossible for them to get all the nutrients they need through diet alone.

A general rule of thumb: For a relatively healthy older person a multivitamin can't hurt, and may help. However, supplements should not exceed twice the recommended dietary allowances since megadoses of vitamins can be dangerous. When in doubt, get a doctor's or dietitian's okay.

important for normal nerve impulses and muscle contractions. Alcoholics are at risk of magnesium deficiency. Low levels of magnesium can cause tremors, seizures and muscular pain. The mineral is found in whole grains, dried peas and beans, nuts, seafood and milk.

# Protein

While most people get plenty of protein, the elderly often have lower levels of protein in their bodies than their more youthful counterparts because they don't make as much of it as they used to.

Proteins are lengthy molecular strings of tiny amino acids. They make up many hormones, form cell walls and serve as the major structural basis of many body tissues—skin, hair, muscles and tendons. To repair or grow new cell walls, the body needs ample protein.

Most of the 20 amino acids that the body needs to make proteins are manufactured internally, but at least nine of them—the "essential amino acids"—must come from outside sources. The most complete sources of protein are meat, chicken, fish, dairy and eggs. But rice, peanuts, kidney beans, peas and tofu are all rich in protein.

# Carbohydrates

Carbohydrates are the sugars and starches that fuel the body, not just for running around the track but for processing and operating even when you are just lying on the couch. Carbohydrates come from cereals, fruits, potatoes, rice, pasta, bread, corn and dried beans and peas. Sugar and white flour also have lots of carbohydrates, but cakes and cookies should be consumed with moderation as they are full of fat and lack any real nutritional value.

# Fluids

Drinking water seems almost like a waste of time—no calories, no vitamins, no energy. But the human body is about 70 percent water and it's important to keep it that way. Fluids keep the volume of blood high, they keep the digestive track running smoothly, and they help kidneys work effectively. A lack of fluids can lead to dehydration, constipation, confusion and dry skin, mouth and eyes.

You will have to push your parent to drink enough fluids. Elderly people often forgo fluids because going to the bathroom can be a tiresome trip. If your parent is incontinent, he may become obsessed with avoiding liquids. But drying the body out is not the way to treat incontinence and usually just makes it worse.

Water is so cheap, so available and, with a few ice cubes or a squeeze of lemon, so good. A bit of juice mixed with seltzer makes a wonderful treat. Your parent should always have a glass of something close at hand. If she sucks on hard candies all day because her mouth is dry or it has a bad taste, get her to sip on a glass of minty water instead. (If you're worried about the purity of tap water, call the EPA's Safe Drinking Water Hotline 800-426-4791.) Limit caffeine, which acts as a diuretic (expelling liquids from the body) and also buzzes the central nervous system, speeding up the heart rate and making a person jittery. Also, be cautious about herbal teas, especially odd, uncommon brews. Most are fine, but some are medicinal and may not mix well with the drugs your parent takes.

# Fiber

Anyone who's heard of constipation has heard of fiber. Fiber keeps things moving, through the body and out. It is the indigestible part of plants. Fiber is found in roughage—fruits, vegetables and grains. Bran, which is the outer coating of whole wheat, corn and oats, is high in fiber, with wheat bran having the highest fiber content.

In the intestines, fiber acts like a sponge, soaking up liquids (but your parent has to drink those fluids so there is something to soak up!) and making the bowels softer and, thus, easier to pass. Fiber is helpful in preventing and treating constipation, diverticular disease and irritable bowel syndrome. It also helps lower blood cholesterol and stabilizes blood sugar levels. Most adults should have about 20 to 35 grams of fiber each day in their diets.

But wait. Your parent should not suddenly start pouring bran on

| High-fiber Foods | Amount | Grams of Fiber |
|---|---|---|
| Dried apricots | 100 grams | 24 |
| All-Bran or 100% Bran cereal | 1 cup | 23 |
| Prunes | 100 grams | 16 |
| Green peas, cooked | ½ cup | 7.7 |
| Grape-Nuts cereal | ⅓ cup | 5 |
| Corn | ⅔ cup | 4.2 |
| Lentils (cooked) | ½ cup | 4 |
| Carrots (raw) | 1 medium | 3.7 |
| Potatoes, cooked | ⅔ cup | 3.1 |
| Apple | 1 small | 3.1 |
| Grapefruit | ½ | 2.6 |
| Strawberries | ½ cup | 2.1 |
| Broccoli, cooked | ¾ cup | 1.6 |
| Grapes | 16 | 0.4 |
| Rice, white, cooked | 1 cup | 0.4 |

his food or gobbling up fiber pills to reach his daily requirement or to treat a case of constipation. A sudden and unusually large dose will tie his stomach in knots and give him gas. Instead, he should start slowly, adding a little more to his diet each day, and drinking plenty of water to help the fiber do its job. Your parent should also try several sources of fiber, such as vegetables, fruits, whole-grain bread, cereal and pasta, rather than gulping down a bowl of high-fiber cereal every morning and calling it quits. High-fiber cereals are helpful, but if overused they can interfere with the absorption of important trace minerals.

Look at the label on various foods to find out exactly how much fiber they contain. (Convenience foods, which are popular among the elderly, are practically fiber-free.)

# Fat and Cholesterol

Fat, that almost four-letter word, is actually a necessary part of every diet. It is used by the body to supply energy and maintain cell structure, and it provides important vitamins. It also makes food more appealing, and helps it slide down the throat more easily, which is particularly important for elderly people who have trouble swallowing.

Unfortunately, because it tastes so good, most people get more than enough fat without trying, and could stand to eat less of the stuff. Too much fat increases the risk of some cancers, heart disease and diabetes. While the risk is greatest for younger people, elderly people, especially those suffering from high cholesterol levels or obesity, should be concerned as well.

Fat, which is made primarily of something known as fatty acids, is saturated or unsaturated depending upon the number of hydrogen atoms attached to the fat molecules. Saturated means just that; there is no more room on the molecule. Unsaturated fats have some room for more hydrogen, and polyunsaturated fats have plenty of room.

Saturated fats come primarily from animal fat, but are also found in the oils of tropical plants, such as coconuts and palms. Mono-unsaturated fats come from peanuts and olives for the most part—peanut oil, peanut butter, olive oil —some of which are thought to be benign, or even good, for the heart, as they lower blood cholesterol levels. Polyunsaturated fats come from vegetable oils—safflower, corn, sunflower, soybean, canola oils—and fish oils. The easiest rule, which applies in most cases, is that if something is solid at room temperature (butter, lard, animal fat and milk products) it should be consumed sparingly.

The infamous fatty substance, cholesterol, is also an essential dietary element, but too much is a bad thing. At high levels, it can clog up arteries and cause heart disease or stroke.

Cholesterol is made in the liver from saturated fats, or absorbed directly from foods such as dairy products, meat and eggs. (A prod-

## DIETARY ADVICE

If you are worried about your parent's eating habits and the doctor isn't much help, your parent, or you, may want to consult a nutritionist. Anyone can claim to be a nutritionist, so be sure to look for a "registered dietitian," a certification that means the person has, at the very least, received a bachelor's degree in nutrition or a related field, passed an exam in nutrition and an internship. To find a registered dietitian or to get more information on nutrition, call the state dietetic association, look through the Yellow Pages, ask at the hospital or doctor's office or call the American Dietetic Association's Nutrition Hotline (800-366-1655). The Hotline has recorded messages about several current nutritional issues and registered dietitians on staff who can answer questions or refer you to a dietitian in your parent's hometown.

uct can have "no cholesterol," but still can be loaded with saturated fats and, therefore, raise cholesterol levels in the body.) Cholesterol roams the body wrapped in a package called a lipoprotein. High-density lipoproteins (HDLs) are "good" in that they actually transport cholesterol out of the body and reduce the risk of heart disease. Low-density lipoproteins (LDLs), or very low-density lipoproteins (VLDLs), are "bad" because they tend to be slovenly and sit around on cell walls, narrowing the passageways.

While it's always good to keep to a low-fat diet and exercise, there is evidence that people over 70 shouldn't become suddenly concerned about cholesterol. Those over 70 who have not suffered any heart problems probably either have low cholesterol or are genetically protected in some way from the effects of high cholesterol. If your parent has been working at keeping his cholesterol down with diet, exercise and medication, he shouldn't stop

his efforts, as they may be what is keeping him alive. But if he has no symptoms of heart disease and is told that he has a high cholesterol level, he probably doesn't need to start aggressive efforts to lower it now. In fact, for some elderly people, the benefit of protein from eggs, cheese and other high-cholesterol foods outweighs any adverse effects of high cholesterol.

# The Five Food Groups

Despite lots of new information about food and diet, the four basic food groups still hold merit for people of any age. They are shown on the facing page, with a fifth group tacked on, and a few minor variations to reflect recent nutritional data. (Note that a "serving" is not whatever amount you dump on a plate; in fact, it is a pretty small portion of food.)

# THE FIVE FOOD GROUPS

| Food Group | Sample Servings | Notes |
|---|---|---|
| Bread, pasta, rice, grains (Six to eleven servings a day) | 1 slice bread ½ to ¾ cup pasta ½ to ¾ cup rice 1 ounce dry cereal ½ to ¾ cup cooked cereal | Lean towards whole-grain bread, brown rice, grains. Limit doughnuts, croissants, sugary cereal and other desserts masquerading as breakfasts. Try something new, like couscous, polenta, bulgur and other grains. |
| Fruits and vegetables (Five or more servings a day) | ½ cup chopped vegetables or fruits ½ medium grapefruit ½ medium melon 1 orange | Fresh is best. Frozen is fine, but canned foods are often high in sodium and sugar. Do not overcook or soak vegetables and do not chop them in advance. Include at least one serving of dark green vegetables and one of citrus fruits. |
| Dairy (Two servings a day) | 8 ounces (1 cup) milk 2 cups cottage cheese 1¼ ounce hard cheese 1 cup plain yogurt | Use nonfat or low-fat products. Don't fulfill dairy requirements with ice cream or cheesecake. People with lactose intolerance can try Lactaid (artificial lactose enzyme) or Dairy Ease instead of milk. |
| Beans, nuts, fish, poultry, eggs and meat (Two servings a day) | 1 to 1½ cups cooked dried beans or peas 4 tablespoons peanut butter 2 to 3 ounces of fish, poultry or lean meat 1 to 2 eggs | Choose beans and peas and stick to lean meats. Limit bacon, bologna, ribs and other fatty meats. Use tuna canned in water, not oil. Remove the skin from poultry. And watch the PB&Js. Peanut butter is loaded with calories. |
| Fluids: water, juice, seltzer, broth (Eight servings a day) | 8 ounces (1 glass) | Fluids are included as a fifth food group because they are so important. Limit caffeinated drinks, which act as diuretics. |

# APPENDIX E

## *Catalogues: Where to Find What*

There is no end to the gadgets and gizmos you can order from catalogues or find in medical supply stores to make eating, dressing, reading, walking and just living a little easier for your parent. From loud telephones to special fishing gear for stiff fingers, if your parent needs it, someone sells it. Some of the merchandise is very helpful, some is silly and some of it you can duplicate with a little ingenuity. Request catalogues from several companies and flip through the pages for ideas.

PRODUCTS FOR
DAILY LIVING

**Access to Recreation**
(Recreational and
household aids)
800-634-4351

**adaptAbility**
800-243-9232

**Bruce Medical Supply**
800-225-8446

**Enrichments**
800-323-5547

**LS&S Group**
(Low-vision aids)
800-468-4789

**Independent
Living Aids**
800-537-2118

**Sears Home
Health Care**
800-326-1750

**Smith & Nephew**
(Specializing in
rehabilitation products)
800-558-8633

**The Lighthouse**
(Low-vision products)
800-346-9579

EASY-TO-WEAR
CLOTHING

**Wardrobe Wagon**
800-992-2737

**Fashion Ease, M&M
Health Care Apparel**
800-221-8929

**JC Penney Easy
Dressing Fashions**
800-222-6161

**American Health
Care Apparel**
800-252-0584

**Mature Wisdom**
(Household gadgets
and clothing)
800-691-9222

**Avenues Unlimited**
(For people using
wheelchairs)
800-848-2837

**Wishing Well**
818-840-6919

**Buck & Buck**
800-458-0600

ELECTRIC
SCOOTERS

**Electric Mobility**
800-662-4548

**Lark of America**
800-446-4522

If you don't find what you need in these catalogues, call the National Rehabilitation Information Center (800-346-2742) or the Access Foundation (516-568-2715); both have extensive information on products for people with disabilities. These organizations can tell you what equipment is available, where to buy it and how you might borrow or rent equipment at a discount.

# APPENDIX F

## Choosing a Nursing Home
## • A Resident's Bill of Rights

When touring nursing homes (or assisted-living homes or other homes for the elderly), look for a place where your parent will be safe and comfortable, keeping in mind her particular needs and preferences (especially if she cannot join you on the tour). What's most important in a residence? Proximity to you and other family? Religious affiliations? Quality medical care? You might want to make a list of things to look for and questions to ask. Here are some questions and issues to consider:

### AT FIRST GLANCE

❖ Is the residence conveniently located for anyone who might visit your parent regularly? If your parent is still able to get around, is it near shops or restaurants? Is it near public transportation?

❖ Are the buildings, grounds and interiors clean, well-kept and maintained? Do the premises smell fresh, airy and odor-free? Or do they smell of chemicals meant to conceal odors? (At least a few rooms will smell of urine because some patients are apt to be incontinent, but the odor should be minimal and limited to only a few rooms.)

❖ Is the residence well-lit, attractive and cheery? Does it feel comfortable and homey?

❖ Is the building safe and accessible? Are there clearly-marked fire exits, smoke alarms, fire doors, fire alarms and ample security? Are there grab bars by the toilets and beds and handrails along the hallways? Are pathways kept clear of clutter? Is it designed for wheelchairs, with ramps, wide hallways and elevators? Are toilets wheelchair-accessible? Are residents required to climb stairs?

❖ Is the building kept at a comfortable temperature?

❖ How is the noise level? For example, is a television constantly blaring in the only public room? Are disruptive or noisy residents allowed to dominate public spaces?

❖ What are the grounds like? Is there a garden or nearby park? Are there benches and paths? Is there a solarium? Do residents have ready access to these areas?

### THE RESIDENTS

❖ How are residents dressed? Are their clothes clean and appropriate for the weather or temperature? Are they wearing scanty clothing in public places, or left in soiled or wet clothing?

❖ What is the level of functioning—physical and mental—of the residents? Will your parent find people at his general level of functioning?

❖ Do residents say they are happy here? What do they like best about this residence and what troubles them? Do they like the staff?

❖ Are residents encouraged to be independent, to care for themselves and make decisions for themselves as much as possible?

❖ Is there a written plan of care for each resident? How is the plan determined, how often is it reassessed and how closely is it followed?

❖ Is the schedule flexible? For instance, can your parent stay up and watch television until 1 A.M. and have a snack at midnight, if that is his habit?

❖ Do residents and families have a voice in how the home is managed? Is there a resident and/or family council? When was the last time it recommended a change that was adopted?

## THE STAFF

❖ Does the staff seem to treat the residents with respect, kindness and affection? Is the same care given to all alike?

❖ Is the staff friendly, accommodating and courteous when you visit? Are they open and direct in answering your questions?

❖ Does the staff seem harried and overworked? Are patients neglected and chores left undone, or does the staff-to-patient ratio seem adequate? (A good ratio is 1 to 8 during the day, although that ratio might be 1–15 at night.) There should be at least one registered nurse on every shift.

❖ Do staff members seem content and do they receive support from colleagues and supervisors? (The morale of the workers will make a big difference in the quality of care your parent receives.)

❖ Does the staff have experience in dealing with people who have the same disabilities as your parent?

❖ How are family members regarded by the staff—with respect or as a nuisance? Ask other family members who are visiting or talk with a member of the family council, if there is one.

❖ Does the staff encourage phone calls, so you can routinely inquire about your parent's well-being?

## MEDICAL CARE

❖ What are the arrangements for medical care, dentistry, psychiatric services, foot care, eye care and other health-related needs? Do residents receive regular checkups by a doctor or nurse? Can they continue to use their personal doctors, if they so choose? (By law, they can.)

❖ Is a physician on call at all times for emergencies?

❖ Is there a hospital within a reasonable distance?

❖ What percentage of patients are restrained—physically with straps or chemically with sedative drugs—at any given time? (See page 225 for more on use of restraint.)

❖ What percentage are incontinent and how is incontinence handled? Are patients put on a regime to improve continence? (If a large number of patients are incontinent—half or more—it may be because the staff uses diapers and catheters in place of good toileting habits.)

❖ Do you notice any patients with sores, wounds or other problems that may not have received medical attention?

## ROOMS

❖ Are bedrooms private or shared? Are bathrooms private or shared?

❖ How are rooms assigned and roommates matched? Do residents have any choice? If roommates don't get along, can they change?

❖ Are the rooms pleasant? Is there enough space? Are there windows and views?

❖ Are the rooms furnished nicely? Is there a comfortable bed, a bureau and closet for personal belongings, a lamp and sitting chair? Is personal furniture allowed?

❖ Do the rooms reflect their individual inhabitants? Are residents encouraged to decorate their rooms with their own touches and fill them with personal mementos? Or do they look sterile and institutional?

❖ Is there privacy? Are there curtains around the beds in shared rooms?

❖ Is there a locked place to store valuables?

❖ Are there emergency call buttons that can be easily reached from both the bed and toilet?

❖ In general, are visits encouraged and visitors made to feel welcome? What are the rules regarding visiting hours and visitors? Can visitors come for meals? Are young children allowed? Can residents have private time in their rooms with mates or spouses? Are there private places where you can be alone with your parent?

❖ What are the rules regarding smoking?

❖ What accommodations are there for televisions and telephones?

## MEALS

❖ Are meals nutritious and well-balanced? Is the food fresh and relatively appetizing? Is it served at an appropriate temperature? Is there variety and choice in the daily menus? Is the menu that is posted adhered to?

❖ Is there a registered dietitian on staff, or one who consults with the cook regularly?

❖ Can the kitchen accommodate special diets (kosher, low-salt, fat-free, soft foods)?

❖ Is the kitchen clean?

❖ Are the hours for meals flexible? Is food available between meals?

❖ Can residents keep food of their own? Where?

❖ Will the staff help residents who have trouble eating on their own?

❖ Do patients confined to beds have help or company at meals?

❖ Is the dining room attractive, neat and intimate? How is seating decided? Can residents choose their own dining companions?

## ACTIVITIES

❖ What are residents doing when you visit? Are they bored, staring at a television set? Or are they engaged in projects and activities?

❖ Is there a monthly activity calendar and does it look interesting? Are there frequent movies, lectures, classes, outings, games and meetings that your parent might enjoy, given his abilities? If there is an activity during your visit, how many people are involved and why aren't more taking part in it?

❖ Are there exercise classes, physical trainers or physical therapists?

❖ Is there a library? Lounge? Card room? Exercise room?

❖ Is the nursing home involved with the community? For example, are there school groups that visit on holidays? Cultural activities from the community? Adopt-a-grandparent program? Are volunteer visitors encouraged?

❖ What are the rules on leaving the grounds? Are residents encouraged to spend time outdoors? Are there planned outings? How are residents monitored if they leave the building?

❖ What sort of transportation is available to residents?

❖ What provisions are there for religious worship? Are there services in-house? Can residents go to churches or synagogues in the community? Is transportation provided? Do clergy visit frequently?

❖ Can residents do paid or volunteer work?

❖ Do residents who are confined to their rooms because of illness or disability receive any kind of physical and social stimulation?

## COSTS

❖ Is this nursing home certified to participate in Medicare or Medicaid? If only a certain number of beds are covered by Medicaid, what will happen if your parent goes on Medicaid while he is living in the facility and no such beds are available?

❖ What are the entry fees, monthly fees and additional costs? Find out exactly what is included and what is extra, such as laundry, haircuts, special meals, outings, physical therapy, dental visits, lab work, medical equipment and prescription drugs.

❖ How long will your parent's bed be reserved in the event that he needs to be hospitalized or is temporarily absent for some other reason? What happens if he exceeds that limit? (This is particularly important if your parent is on Medicaid, as the facility's time limit may be quite short or it may not hold a bed at all. If your parent loses his place, the residence must give him the first Medicaid bed available, but you need to be persistent to make sure that he gets it.)

❖ What has the increase in monthly fees been over the past three years? What sort of increases are expected in the coming years?

❖ Can contracts be terminated? Under what conditions? What is the refund policy?

❖ How stable is this residence financially? (Ask to see the most recent annual report and/or financial records. You may also want to ask the state's long-term care ombudsman about the financial stability of a particular nursing home). What happens to your parent if the home becomes part of another facility or goes out of business?

❖ Do residents maintain control over their personal finances?

# A Resident's Bill of Rights

To participate in Medicare or Medicaid, nursing homes must meet standards outlined in the Nursing Home Reform Law (the Omnibus Budget Reconciliation Act, 1987). Among the law's provisions:

**Residents Have a Right to:**

❖ be treated with dignity and respect

❖ exercise their rights, file complaints or voice grievances without fear of discrimination, restraint, interference, coercion or reprisal, and to expect prompt efforts for the resolution of grievances

❖ equal access to care and services without discrimination

❖ privacy concerning their personal and medical care, telephone calls, visits, letters and meetings with family and resident groups

❖ inspect and purchase photocopies of their records

❖ confidentiality regarding their medical and personal records

❖ full information about their health, and the right to participate in decisions regarding their care and treatment

❖ refuse treatment and refuse to participate in experimental research

❖ information concerning Medicare and Medicaid benefits and how to apply

❖ information regarding all facility services and charges

❖ information regarding advocacy groups and ombudsman programs

❖ manage their own financial affairs; they are not required to deposit personal funds with the facility

❖ choose a personal physician

❖ self-administer drugs unless determined unsafe by an interdisciplinary team

❖ perform or refuse to perform services for the facility; payment for any work done must be at or above prevailing rates

❖ advance notice of any change in room or roommate

❖ share a room with a resident spouse

❖ choose their own activities, schedules and health care and any other aspect affecting their lives within the facility

❖ organize or participate in resident councils or other groups

❖ be free from verbal, sexual, physical or mental abuse, corporal punishment and involuntary seclusion.

## The Nursing Home Must:

❖ not require a third-party guarantee of payment or accept any gifts as a condition of admission or continued stay

❖ not require residents to waive their right to receive or apply for Medicare or Medicaid benefits

❖ provide a copy of the latest inspection report and any written plans to correct violations

❖ provide residents with individualized financial reports quarterly and upon request

❖ protect resident funds with a security bond

❖ notify residents when their balance comes within $200 of the Medicaid eligibility limit

❖ not charge Medicaid residents for items or services covered by Medicaid, including routine personal hygiene items and services

❖ not use physical restraints or psychoactive drugs for discipline or convenience; restraints must not be used without a doctor's written orders to treat medical symptoms or to ensure the safety of the resident and others

❖ provide access to any relevant agency of the state or any entity providing health, social, legal or other services

❖ use identical policies regarding transfer, discharge and services for all residents

❖ not discharge or transfer a resident unless his needs cannot be met, safety is endangered, services are no longer required or payment has not been made

❖ notify a resident of reason(s) for transfer or discharge and provide sufficient preparation to ensure a safe transfer or discharge

❖ provide written notice of state and facility bed-hold policies before and at the time of a transfer

❖ follow a written policy for readmittance if the bed-hold period is exceeded

❖ thoroughly investigate all alleged violations and report the results

❖ provide a private space for residents' group meetings, and then listen to and act upon requests of the group

❖ provide social services to maintain each resident's highest level of well-being

❖ provide a safe, clean, comfortable, home-like environment

❖ allow residents to use personal belongings to the extent possible

❖ provide housekeeping and maintenance services; clean bath and bed linens; private closet space; adequate and comfortable lighting and sound levels; comfortable and safe temperature levels.

# APPENDIX G

## *The Aftermath: Funerals and Burials*

After a parent has died, in the midst of your grief or even before you have had a chance to grieve, there is work to be done—people to be called, services to be planned, obituaries to be written. While these tasks may seem overwhelming, they also can be therapeutic.

Funeral and memorial services are valuable rituals, allowing you and others to accept the reality of your parent's death, bring closure and move forward in the grieving process. Planning the service, picking out the music, choosing readings and deciding who will speak give you a chance to think about your parent and to honor her life. The service allows you to openly mourn her death and share your grief with others who also want to remember and pay their respects. A funeral or memorial service allows you to see, in the midst of your emotional disarray, that life still has some order and to experience the comfort that rituals and customs can bring.

Do what feels right to you, but do take an active part in planning this last farewell.

# Finding a Funeral Director

For most people, the first step in planning a funeral is to talk to a funeral director, who will guide you through the rest of the process. (You may prefer to contact a memorial society, which helps people arrange simple, low-cost funerals. See box on page 435.)

Find a funeral director who has a good reputation and make sure the funeral home is in a convenient location, particularly important if you are going to hold a service or reception there. Ask friends or family who have held funerals in the area for recommendations. Once you have a few names, contact some funeral homes and compare prices.

If you are planning this funeral from a distance, you can call the National Funeral Directors Association (414-541-2500) for a listing of funeral homes in the area. You might also ask reputable funeral directors in your area for a recommendation, as they often know funeral directors in other places.

You should also contact a member of the clergy or whoever will officiate at the services to plan the program. If the minister, priest or rabbi did not know your parent, talk to him about your parent so he can personalize the service, readings and remarks. If you do not have anyone in mind, the funeral director should be able to recommend someone.

# A FUNERAL CHECKLIST

❏ Make a list of people who should be notified. Split it up and have others make some of the calls.

❏ Choose a funeral director.

❏ Once you have decided the place and time for the service, write an obituary and send it to local newspapers and other appropriate publications (alumni or company magazines, newspapers in other places he has lived).

❏ Decide whether the body will be cremated or embalmed.

❏ If the body or ashes are to be buried, find out if your parent owns a plot or if there is a family plot. If not, visit local cemeteries. Find out the rules of the cemetery. (Do you need a grave liner? Can you hold a service on the weekend or evening?)

❏ Pick out a casket or urn.

❏ Decide whether you want a viewing, grave-side service, funeral and/or memorial service.

❏ Decide the date of the services. Pick a day when all immediate family members can be present, leaving ample time to make the necessary preparations.

❏ Choose the place for services—a church, synagogue or other religious building, the funeral home, a private home or a rented hall or club—and make sure it is available.

❏ Decide whom you would like to officiate and then meet with them to plan what will be included in the services—prayers, songs, readings, and speakers.

❏ Select music. Will there be instruments, an organ, a choir, a soloist? Do you need to pass out songbooks, hymnals or sheet music? Talk to the music director or organist at the

# The Obituary

Obituaries needn't be poetic, just jot down the facts. (Most newspapers will rewrite what you send them anyway.) The funeral director can help you. An obituary should include the full legal name of your parent, his date of birth, schooling, career (where he worked, in what positions and during what years), memberships in organizations, military service, awards received, hobbies and full names of siblings, children, spouse and other survivors. (You can simply send a resume and list of the names of relatives.) You should include the time and place of a funeral or memorial service, and note the fund or charity where people can send donations in lieu of flowers. You may want to send a photo as well. (Some newspapers charge a fee to print death church and to relatives who might know your parent's favorite hymns.

❏ Decide what kind of flowers, candles, guest books or other extras you would like and where you will buy them. (Do you want photos or other mementos of your parent on display at the service?)

❏ Ask people to serve as pallbearers and/or ushers at the service.

❏ If there is to be a graveside service, decide whether the casket or urn will be lowered into the grave or placed in the columbarium while people are present and, if so, who will perform the honors.

❏ Ask a neighbor who will not be attending the services, or the police if you live in a small community, to keep an eye on your parent's home during the services, for any suspicious activity.

❏ Decide whether there will be

a gathering after the service. (If so, where and when? Will everyone be invited or just a select few? Will a meal be served or just coffee?)

❏ If you want a program for the funeral, you need to write it and get it printed. (Sometimes funeral directors keep a few sample programs on hand that you can look at for ideas. They should also be able to recommend printers.) Be sure to order a few extra copies for friends and family who will be unable to attend the service.

❏ Think about where visitors will stay and how they will get from the airport or train station to the services. You are not responsible for this, but it's helpful, if you can, to make recommendations.

❏ If you have chosen an earth burial, then at some point you need to select a grave marker or headstone. (This can be done later, however.)

notices, which include information about the services, and a few charge to print obituaries.)

Local papers and school alumni magazines may print longer and more personal obituaries, in which case you need to provide more detailed information about your parent's past, his personality, gifts and traits. You might include anecdotal stories, especially ones that occurred in that town or at that school.

# Handling the Body

If your parent had specific wishes about how his body is handled, they should be honored. If not, what would make you and others in the family feel most comfortable?

If your parent's wishes and yours conflict, think about the

## ACCEPT ALL HELP

If, during this time, people ask if they can do anything to help—and many people will—by all means say yes. Ask them to baby-sit, run errands, prepare a meal, call to tell people the time and place of the service or pick up out-of-town guests.

If they are close friends of your parent, you might ask them to write down their memories of him, especially if they start reminiscing over the phone to you. You may be too raw and too busy to absorb such stories, but you will want to hear them later. Save all notes and recorded memories for yourself and other members of the family.

strength of your parent's convictions—was he simply trying to be organized and helpful or did he have personal or religious feelings about this?—and weigh that against your own needs. While you should try to respect his choices, the funeral and other final rituals are truly meant for those left behind. Some of the options you will need to consider include:

AUTOPSY. An autopsy is an examination of the body performed by a coroner, medical examiner or physician, usually when a death is regarded as suspicious or unnatural. However, a doctor might suggest an autopsy if such an examination would be useful for medical research or teaching purposes. You must give your permission before such an exam is performed.

Ask the doctor exactly what the procedure would entail in your parent's case. Sometimes physicians want to examine a large portion of the body, which may mean severe disfigurement, and sometimes they simply want to look at one particular organ or bit of tissue. The decision depends solely on your own beliefs and feelings. If you think your parent would want to give this one last contribution to medicine, or if you want to, and you don't mind any disfigurement that might occur, then this is a noble gesture. But if the idea makes you squeamish, don't be pushed into it.

ORGAN DONATION. Older organs are not accepted for donation, although eye banks will usually take healthy corneas from someone under the age of seventy. Some medical schools will accept older bodies for medical research and education. If your parent expressed an interest in donation, you can call local medical schools or call the National Anatomical Service (800-727-0700).

INTERMENT. Interment is the traditional form of burial underground in which the body is placed in a casket and buried in the ground, usually in a cemetery.

ENTOMBMENT. The casket is put in a mausoleum, a structure usually made of marble, stone or concrete, with rows of crypts or, in some cases, individual rooms for caskets.

**CREMATION.** The body is placed in a box and then in a special crematory furnace, where over several hours, intense heat reduces it to a few pounds of bone fragments and ashes. The ashes, or "cremains," are then returned to the family in a box of cardboard, metal or plastic, or placed in an urn or other container (known as an inurnment).

The ashes are buried in the earth, put in a niche at a cemetery or church columbarium, kept by family or friends or scattered in some meaningful place. (It is illegal to sprinkle ashes in some places, so check with local health officials first.)

Cremation simply speeds up the natural process of decay (all bodies, even those buried in expensive caskets, decay), and it is generally less expensive than an earth burial. You can still have all the rites of a funeral—a viewing before the cremation, a memorial service and burial in a cemetery with a gravestone. Most religions now allow cremation, although the Greek and Jewish orthodox faiths oppose it.

**EMBALMING.** People began embalming bodies in this country during the Civil War, when the bodies of soldiers had to be shipped long distances. The custom has continued, but is not necessary in most cases. Embalming is sometimes required when a body is going to be transported a long distance, when there is to be a viewing, or when the dead person carried certain communicable diseases. It does not prevent the body from decaying, it only delays the process.

During an embalming, the body is washed and disinfected. Blood and other body fluids are drained out and chemicals—perfumed formaldehyde, glycerin, alcohol and water—are injected into the arteries to make the tissue gel and to prevent the growth of bacteria. The undertaker then prepares the body for the viewing by dressing it and, in some cases, applying make-up. He or she can repair any damaged areas, rebuild sunken skin and replace missing hair.

# The Cemetery

Most communities have a municipal cemetery as well as several cemeteries owned by religious or private organizations. Veterans have the added option of being buried at a national cemetery. (See box, page 434.)

Your parent may have made plans for his burial (if he has not told you, look through his important papers and safe-deposit box to see if he has already reserved a cemetery plot). If not, choose a cemetery that appeals to you. Though you may not have the energy or heart for it, you should compare prices as well.

Within a cemetery, you can buy a single grave plot or a family plot. Some cemeteries also sell space in a mausoleum, an above-ground building that has crypts for caskets, or a columbarium, which has stacks of niches for urns of ashes. Find out if the cemetery has any restrictions on markers, monuments or plantings.

Some cemeteries, for example, are set up like gardens and allow only flat markers and no headstones.

A growing number of cemeteries now offer a full range of services, with a funeral home on the premises and, in some cases, a crematorium, flower shop and grave-stone supplier.

## Services

The service should be whatever, whenever, and wherever you want it to be. People usually schedule the service within a week or two of the death because they need it then, emotionally. But you can wait several weeks or even months if you want to. Or you can have a cremation or burial service soon after the death, and then hold a memorial service months later when you have the energy to make arrangements,

and when friends and family can all be present.

Once you know when to hold the service, you have to decide what it will be. A funeral or memorial usually follows the tradition of your parent's religion. But you can personalize even a formal service by giving it whatever touch you feel is appropriate. You can hold communion, have speakers, read poems, prayers or letters, or play music that has special meaning. You might hold a memorial walk or have an open, unstructured service that allows people in the congregation to stand and share memories and thoughts about your parent. You can even tell jokes or funny stories. This service can and should be whatever you want it to be. It is, after all, for you and others who are mourning this death and honoring this life.

As you decide what the mood and the message will be, think about

## CHILDREN AND FUNERALS

While children are often excluded from funerals, wakes and memorial services, they often want to be included in the ritual and they stand to learn from it. Describe what the event will be like and let them decide for themselves if they want to attend. Most children, even as young as four or five, can make such decisions for themselves. If the service is going to be quite long—too long for a child to sit still or remain quiet—bring a supply of toys and snacks, or include her for only part of the service and arrange for a sitter to be nearby.

In the weeks after the funeral, give your child a chance to talk about your parent. You might give her a photo or help her make a scrapbook about her grandmother's life (as soon as you can handle such a project). Don't be surprised if your child has nightmares. They are normal and they will end.

## A PRIVATE REMEMBRANCE

If you can't go to the funeral, hold your own service where you live. Invite a few close friends to come over and share in a memorial. Put out photos, flowers and candles. Ask a member of the clergy to come. Have a reception. Or have your own private memorial so you can say good-bye.

what you want out of this service and what you want others to feel as they walk away. Do you want a joyous gathering that celebrates and remembers your parent's life or a solemn, religious service that attempts to help people come to terms with death?

A service can last for ten minutes or more than an hour. In the Jewish tradition of *shivah*, the family stays at home for seven days after the funeral service to receive guests. Funeral ceremonies and receptions are usually held at a funeral home, graveside, a private home, a hall, a church or a synagogue, but they can be held at any favorite spot—on the beach, in a park, near a summer cottage.

**VIEWING.** The casket is usually present at a funeral—opened or closed—and not present at a memorial service. Either type of service may be preceded by a viewing or wake.

An open casket, which allows people to view the body, provides an opportunity to accept the reality of death, to see, quite literally, that this person is gone, and to say good-bye. It may be helpful for family and close friends who were not present at the time of death and who feel that they missed something important, but it is certainly not for everyone. Do what is right for your family; don't be swayed by what others say.

# The Cost

Money may seem like a crass subject at a time like this, but it is not. You can spend an exhorbitant amount of money now, at this time of great stress and little time to think. Do not let anyone make you feel that the amount you spend has any bearing on how much you cared for your parent. The service—what is said and who is present—is far more important than the size and price of a casket or the number of floral arrangements. Make this a remembrance that is right for you, but don't be pressured into spending more than you want to or can afford.

If you have the strength for it, compare prices and negotiate. There is absolutely nothing wrong with getting the best price possible. In fact, if your parent was at all frugal, he would want you to shop around. Do it in that spirit.

Funeral homes are required, under the Funeral Rule of the Federal Trade Commission, to quote prices over the phone. Or you can have them sent to you, which gives you more time to study them. Cemeteries are not bound by the same rules, but most will quote prices to you as well.

Be sure to get all costs from each home so you are comparing apples and apples. Find out what costs are not included in the price and what the total bill will come to? Once you have received a price, ask if that is the best price the funeral home can offer or if there is any way of reducing it. (For instance, you could ask whether picking up the death certificates from Town Hall and bringing the ashes from the crematorium to the cemetery will save on expenses.)

Once you have calculated the total cost, you may find that you need to trim back a little—buy a simpler casket, hold the reception at a private home instead of at a hall or make the coffee and sandwiches yourself. Funerals can be terribly expensive, but there are many ways to cut costs.

The following list will give you some idea of the services offered and the average price of those services. The prices listed here are from a survey conducted by the National Funeral Directors Association in 1995. They are only averages; actual costs will depend upon the cost of living in the area, the specific services you require and the rates of an individual funeral home. For example, the average funeral director's fee was $1,148 in New England, while it was $840 in the Mountain states. The average cost of a 20-gauge steel casket was more than $1,295 in the Pacific states, while it was $853 in the

mid-Atlantic states. Here are some general guidelines to follow.

**FUNERAL DIRECTOR'S SERVICES.** These are fixed, basic charges that are not optional if you use a funeral director. They cover overhead, paperwork, meetings with the funeral director and the cost of supervising and arranging the ceremony.

Average price: $952

**CARE OF THE BODY.** Although the funeral director may suggest it, embalming is not required or necessary in most cases. By federal law, a funeral home must seek permission before embalming a body and, unless it is required under state law, you do not have to pay for the service if you did not authorize it.

Dressing the body and putting it in the casket is usually, but not always, included in the price of embalming, but find out exactly what is covered. You may be charged extra for fixing hair, putting on makeup and restoring a body that is damaged by autopsy or disease.

Average price:
Embalming: $322
Other body preparations: $117

**TRANSPORTATION.** The transportation price quoted to you may cover only the price of getting the body to the funeral home; most funeral homes charge an additional fee for transporting the body to the church, grave site or crematorium, and for other transportation, such as picking up the death certificate or burial permit. You will also have to pay extra for services such as a hearse, a limousine for the family, a flower car or a motorcycle escort for the funeral procession.

If you need to transport the body from one funeral home to another, the cost of the funeral can soar. Funeral homes charge, on average, $1,060 to send a body to another funeral home, and then you can be charged another $890 or so by the funeral home that is receiving the body. You can skip these expenses by making arrangements directly with an airline, cremating the body and sending the ashes or carrying them with you on the plane.

Average price:
Transporting the body to the funeral home: $118
Other transportation costs: $ 74
Local hearse: $145
Local limousine: $117

**SERVICES.** You can hold services in a private home, church, synagogue or hall, or you may be able to hold them at the funeral home. Be sure that any price quoted includes everything, because funeral homes may suddenly add charges for overhead expenses, the use of lounges, parking lots, offices, dressing rooms, tents and chairs.

Average price:
Visitation/viewing : $258
Funeral: $306
Memorial service: $322
Graveside service: $300

**MISCELLANEOUS ITEMS.** The funeral director will usually require a cash advance to pay for copies of the death certificate, death notices and obituaries. You may also choose to order acknowledgment cards through the funeral home. These usually cost about $20 for one hundred.

**RECEPTIONS, FLOWERS, ETC.** You can spend as much or as little as you want to on flowers, guest books, music, food, alcohol and rented halls. You may also be expected to pay (usually by way of a donation) for the use of the church or synagogue and for the services of the clergy.

**CASKETS.** Walking through rows of caskets is unsettling. If you have a good idea of what you want and how much you want to spend, it ex-

## FILING COMPLAINTS

Funeral directors are regulated by state licensing boards and by the Funeral Rule of the Federal Trade Commission. If you have questions, have trouble with a funeral home or feel that you have been misled or cheated in any way, you should contact the state examining or licensing board and/or write the FTC at:

Federal Trade Commission
Division of Marketing Practices
Funeral Rule Staff
6th St. & Pennsylvania Ave, NW
Washington, DC 20580

pedites the process. If it's too unpleasant a task, do it quickly, over
the phone, or ask a friend or relative to do it for you. At the very
least, have someone accompany you.

Caskets come in wood, metal,
fiberglass or plastic. The wooden
ones may be hardwood, softwood
or plywood; they may be solid wood
or veneer. The metals include stain-
less or rolled steel, or copper bronzes
of varying thicknesses. They may be
lined with cloth, twill, crepe, velour
or velvet (although you can use your
favorite cloth, quilt or comforter).
Some have mattresses in them, and
you can opt for a spring contrap-
tion that raises and lowers the body
for viewing.

You will also have to decide if
you want the casket to be sealed,
which is usually done with a rubber gasket, to prevent water and
rust from entering it. As with embalming, sealing a casket does not
prevent the body from decaying.
Some unscrupulous funeral directors will talk about preserving the
body in order to sell more expensive caskets, but their claims simply are not true.

Prices vary widely. At the lower end, a simple pine box sells for
under $200 in most places. This is
commonly used for cremation, but
is perfectly fine for earth burials as
well. At the upper end, a copper casket, with sealers and a velvet interior, can sell for more than $3,500.

It's up to you. Buy only what
you want. Your love for your parent
is not measured by the amount of
silver, satin or velvet you sink into
the ground. If you want a simple,
inexpensive casket, ask for it. Some-

times they are not on display or they
are hidden in a corner, covered with
dust. Don't let that deter you. Get
what you want.

And don't be afraid or embarrassed to negotiate over the price of
caskets. Most funeral homes jack up
their prices substantially, but faced
with the prospect of losing a customer, they will usually come down.
Negotiating may be more than you
can handle now, but if you want to
or want someone else to do it for
you, you should know that people
do it all the time and that it is perfectly acceptable, even in a time of
mourning.

You can also have a casket made
or buy it elsewhere, which is often
cheaper than buying it from the funeral director. Under the latest version of the Funeral Rule, funeral

## A SIMPLE CASKET

If you are cremating the
body, holding an immediate
burial or donating the body
to science, you don't need a
casket at all. A simple box
made of heavy cardboard,
particle board or pine is the
most you need. Any funeral
director who suggests otherwise is violating the federal
Funeral Rule.

If you want a fancy casket
for a viewing, but not for a
burial, you can usually rent a
casket with a removable liner
for about a third of the retail
price.

directors cannot charge any "non-declinable fees" beyond the funeral director's fee which means they cannot charge for "casket handling" if you buy a casket elsewhere.

**VAULTS AND LINERS.** In addition to a casket, some cemeteries require that you buy a grave liner or vault to prevent the ground from sinking as the casket deteriorates. You can buy these from the funeral director, the cemetery or a third party.

A liner is a simple concrete box that costs several hundred dollars. Sealing or lining the concrete with asphalt adds several hundred dollars to the price. A vault of ungalvanized steel costs almost twice as much as concrete, and a vault of galvanized steel triples the price.

The funeral director may advise you to choose a steel vault in order to preserve the body. Again, nothing prevents the body from decomposing. Also, if the funeral director tells you that the cemetery requires the heavier vault, check for yourself.

Average price:
Concrete box: $495
Galvanized steel vault: $1,310

**CREMATION.** A cremation should be relatively inexpensive—under $300. You will not need a casket or embalming, unless you have a viewing. Funeral homes may charge you $100 to $200 for a simple box (although you can buy one elsewhere or make one yourself usually for less than $50). If you think you are being charged too much and you have the energy, call the crematorium directly to ask about their prices.

The ashes will be returned to you in a cardboard box unless you select an urn, which can cost anywhere from $100 to $1,000.

**IMMEDIATE BURIAL AND DIRECT CREMATION.** Many funeral homes offer package deals that are simple and inexpensive. The body is buried in the ground or cremated immediately after death, and there is no viewing or embalming. You can then hold a memorial service, with all the fixings you choose, at a later date.

## HOME FUNERAL

**S**ome people find it therapeutic and meaningful, not to mention a lot less expensive, to plan the funeral, build the casket, and bury the body themselves. This do-it-yourself style of dealing with death is an age-old tradition, just as natural, difficult and rewarding as allowing someone to die at home.

Most states allow you to arrange the funeral and burial or cremation without a funeral director, as long as you comply with public health codes. Home burials are described in the book, *Caring for Your Own Dead*, by Lisa Carlson, published by Upper Access Book Publishers (800-356-9315).

Prices include the funeral director's fees, transportation of the body, care of the body and a simple container or casket. They usually do not include the cost of any cash advance items, such as medical examiner's fees or death certificates. Funeral homes offer wide variations on these themes, so be sure you understand exactly what is included in the plan you select.

Average price:
Immediate burial,
with container: $1,383
Direct cremation,
with container: $1,155

CEMETERIES. The price of cemetery plots and services depends largely upon the cost of land and labor in the area. Visit several and be sure that you will get the plot or crypt shown to you. (And don't be talked into a family plot, a common selling tactic, if you don't want one.)

In addition to the cost of a plot or space in a mausoleum, you may be charged a few hundred dollars for "perpetual care." This money is usually put in a permanent trust to pay for the upkeep of the grounds. Some cemeteries also charge for opening and closing the grave (anywhere from $200 to $2,000) and for installing the gravestone or marker ($200 and up), so be sure you find out all the costs involved.

You will have to pay for any gravestone, bench or marker you choose. And you may have to buy a vault or liner. You can pay extra to have the grave decorated on holidays, or to have a slot for a vase installed by the grave. You may also be charged extra for burials on weekends or during the evening.

---

## BENEFITS FOR VETERANS

**M**ost military veterans are eligible for a free burial (including opening and closing of the grave, care of the grounds, headstone and grave marker) in a national cemetery, and in some cases the spouse of a veteran may also be buried in a national cemetery.

If your parent is buried elsewhere, the Department of Veterans Affairs will reimburse families of qualified veterans about $300 for funeral and burial expenses; $150 for a plot or inurnment; and, in some cases, a small amount for the cost of transporting the body from a nursing home or VA hospital. The VA will also provide a grave marker, cover some of the cost of a gravestone, and send a large American flag to drape over the casket. A funeral director or the regional VA office should be able to help you apply for these benefits.

(Be leery of any private cemeteries offering free burials to veterans. They often charge other fees that cancel out any savings.)

# Taking Care of Business

If you weren't taking care of your parent's business before he died, you can only hope that he was well-organized, because there is a lot of paperwork to be done now. Most of it doesn't have to be done immediately. Take time to grieve, then attend to these tasks when your head and heart are a little more stable.

◆ *Contact relevant parties*, such as your parent's lawyer, financial planner or accountant. If your parent didn't have a lawyer, you may need to hire one now.

◆ *Locate the will* by checking the safe-deposit box, files and desk drawers and/or call your parent's lawyer. If there is no will and no lawyer, then the estate will be doled out according to state laws.

◆ *Check with the probate clerk's office* in your parent's town to get a list of deadlines. If your parent has property in more than one state, be sure to check with the probate clerk's office in each state.

◆ *Contact your parent's bank* to close accounts, and to find out if there is a safe-deposit box. These boxes are closed at the time of death in some states, but you can usually check the box for a will and list the contents for tax purposes.

◆ *Get five to ten copies of the death certificate* from the funeral director or health department. You will need these when reporting your parent's death to insurance companies, the social security office, the IRS, veterans affairs, etc.

## FUNERAL AND MEMORIAL SOCIETIES

The high cost of dying, even back in 1939, so outraged a group of Seattle residents that they organized a society to help people plan simple, dignified and affordable funerals. Today, the Funeral and Memorial Societies of America represents 147 societies in some 40 states and has more than 500,000 members. The societies are nonprofit and are run by volunteers elected by the members.

Most of these societies have contracts with funeral directors who offer low-cost funerals or discounts to society members, while some simply supply members with price lists of local funeral homes and examples of package prices. All of the groups provide information on arranging a low-cost funeral. A membership costs between $10 and $30.

To find out about local memorial societies or to get information about planning an affordable funeral, contact the association at 800-765-0107.

◆ *Find your parent's marriage certificate* if your parent's spouse is alive and will be applying for benefits. The town clerk in the town where your parents were married should be able to provide copies if you can't find them in your parent's files. You may also need birth certificates for any dependent children, which are available from the town clerk's office in the town where the children were born.

◆ *Notify insurance companies* (life, health, mortgage, accident, auto, credit card, employer policies). File all claims, switch any policies over to a spouse's name, and/or change the names of beneficiaries. Do this early so beneficiaries can receive their money as soon as possible. (Some health insurance policies provided by an employer can be continued in a spouse's or in childrens' names.)

◆ *Contact the social security and veterans affairs offices.* You may receive a death benefit to cover funeral costs and other benefits to help a surviving spouse. Call the Social Security Administration at 800-772-1213 for information, and if your parent served in the military, contact the local veterans affairs office. (To apply for funeral benefits, you will need to find his military papers. If you can't find them, write to the Department of Defense's National Personnel Record Center at 9700 Page Blvd., St. Louis, MO 63132.)

◆ *Contact former employers.* Your parent may be owed pension benefits, salary, or pay for unused vacation or sick leave.

◆ *Make a list of all assets.* You will need to gather titles and deeds to any property, automobiles, boats; ownerships or partnerships in businesses; stocks, bonds, savings and checking accounts; profit-sharing plans, pension plans and retirement accounts. You'll need to change the name on any titles and deeds if property is transferred to a surviving parent or child.

◆ *List all debts* from mortgages, unpaid bills, charge accounts, etc. Cancel all credit cards and pay the balance out of the estate.

◆ *Find a copy of your parent's most recent income tax return.* If your parent was required to file a tax return (see page 270), you will have to file one for the year in which he died. You can get an extension, if necessary. Call the local IRS office for information. Federal taxes are also due on estates worth more than $600,000. Get form 706 from the IRS for federal taxes, which are due within nine months of the death. There are usually state estate and inheritance taxes as well.

◆ *Revise the will of a surviving spouse.* The will of a surviving spouse may have to be changed if it lists your deceased parent as a beneficiary. Likewise with any insurance policies. She will also need to adjust anything held under joint names, such as bank accounts, property, credit cards, etc.

# INDEX

# INDEX

# D

# G

# O

Obesity, 147
Obituaries, 424-25
Occupational therapy, 93, 140, 181, 249
  resources for, 399
Only children, 230
Oral cancer, 84
Oral hygiene, 84-86, 146
Organ donation, 426
Organization, 9-12
  community services and, 172
  from distance, 11-12
Osteoarthritis, 88, 92
Osteoporosis, 88-91
  combatting, 89-91
  resources for, 93, 384
  symptoms of, 88, 89
Overflow incontinence, 95
Overmedication, 70-75, 302
  symptoms of, 57
Over-the-counter medications, 72
Ownership, 289-91, 293
  joint, with right of survivorship, 289-90
  sole, 289

# P

Pain, dying and, 346, 349, 350, 352, 359
Pain medication, 286, 361
  for dying parent, 349, 350, 352
  inadequate, 127-28
"Panic buttons," 139
Parent-child relationship, 14-26
  adapting to new roles in, 15-19
  emotional minefields and, 32-36
  expectations about, 21-22, 26
  intervention and, 16-19
  living together, 194-98
  managing day-to-day in, 24-26

parent's death and, 367-68, 369, 370
  remembering earlier days and, 15
  removing blame from, 24
  resolving old struggles in, 19-24
  unrealistic hopes and, 21-22, 28
Parkinson's disease, 300
  resources for, 399-400
Patient advocates, 123
Patient's Bill of Rights, 404-6
Peer review organizations (PROs), 123
Pensions, 9, 436
  resources for, 389
People's Medical Society, 124
Periodic leg movements, 67-68
Persistent vegetative state, 358-59
Pet-facilitated therapy (PFT), 164
Pharmacies, 169
Physical exams:
  for aging parent, 44-46, 47
  for caregiver, 39
Physical therapy, 93, 140, 181, 249
Physician-assisted suicide, 359
Pill boxes, 74
Placebo effect, 52
Planning ahead, 1-13
  dementia and, 309
  denial and, 5-7
  discussing future with parent and, 2-7
  financing long-term care and, 246
  housing and, 207
  information gathering and, 6, 7-9
  intransigent parent and, 7
  need for, 1-2
  organization in, 9-12
Pneumococcal vaccines, 46
Police, 334
Polyunsaturated fats, 413
Power of attorney, 280-83
  see also Durable power of attorney
Presbyopia, 58
Pressure-sensitive alarms, 334
Preventive care, 46, 249

Saturated fats, 413, 414
Schedules, 9-10
Scooters, electric, 416
Seat belts, 153
Second opinions, 54, 117, 356
Security alarm systems, 139
Sedatives, 125-26, 210, 218, 225
Senior apartments, 200-1, 203-4
Senior centers, 163, 168, 176, 170
Senior Companion Program, 172
Setting limits, 28-31
Sexual behavior, inappropriate, in
    dementia, 337
Shared housing, 200-1, 202-3, 204
Shingles (herpes zoster), 81
Shoes, 84, 143
Shower, chairs for, 145
    see also Bathing
Siblings, 229-35
    accepting and enlisting help from,
        29
    dividing estate between, 295-97
    dividing up duties with, 235
    family meetings with, 231, 232-35
    family spokesperson role and, 54,
        234-35
    financial issues and, 244, 246
    primary caregiver role and, 231-32
    problems with, 232
Skin cancer, 82
Skin problems, 57, 79-83
    bedsores, 82-83, 126, 348
    fungal infections, 81
    itchiness and dryness, 79-81
    reactions to medications, 81-82
    resources for, 400
    shingles (herpes zoster), 81
Sleep, 110-11, 155
    caregiver's need for, 39
    dementia and, 326-27
    tips for good night of, 68-69
Sleep apnea, 68
Sleep disorders, 57, 66-70
    in parent, your sleep disrupted by,
        69-70

resources for, 68, 400
restless leg syndrome and periodic
    leg movements, 67-68
Sleeping pills, 66-67, 68, 70, 368
Small estate administration, 295
Smoke detectors, 137
Smoking, 78
    bone mass and, 89, 90
    dementia and, 315
    sleep disorders and, 69
Snacks, 151, 152, 326
Snoring, 68
Soap, 79-80
    dispensers for, 142, 144
Social isolation, of caregiver, 37, 320
Social life, 110-11, 164
    of caregiver, 36-37, 40
    including parent in, 40, 320
    of parent, 163
    of surviving spouse, 371-72
Social security, 8, 247, 389, 436
    gathering information about, 9
    tax on, 271
Social workers, 19
    in-home care and, 170, 181
    resources for, 183, 385, 398
Sodium, 410
Sole ownership, 289
Sound-activated lights, 143
Space heaters, 137
Spastic colon, 101
Specified Low-Income Medicare
    Beneficiary Program (SLMB),
    251
Speech therapy, 181, 249
    resources for, 391-92
Spinal taps, 306
Spiritual needs, 41-42, 133, 161
Sports, 163
Spouse of aging parent:
    intervention and, 17
    Medicaid eligibility and, 262
    resources for, 115, 385
    when spouse is ill, 115
Spouse of caregiver, 235-37

# Y

# We Welcome Your Views

*How to Care for Aging Parents* tries to address the wide range of concerns and questions that caregivers face, in as much detail as possible. But there is always room for improvement. Please let us know your thoughts on the book—advice that was helpful, questions that weren't addressed, facts we might have missed—so that we can make adjustments and include your views in any future editions. We look forward to hearing from you.

Write to:

> *How to Care for Aging Parents*
> c/o Workman Publishing Company
> 708 Broadway
> New York, New York 10003-9555

To contact the author, order books, or find helpful internet addresses, visit our website: http://www.careforagingparents.com.